ESSENTIALS OF

Pharmacokinetics and Pharmacodynamics

SECOND EDITION

ESSENTIALS OF

Pharmacokinetics and Pharmacodynamics

SECOND EDITION

Thomas N. Tozer

Malcolm Rowland

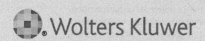

Wolters Kluwer

Philadelphia • Baltimore • New York • London
Buenos Aires • Hong Kong • Sydney • Tokyo

Acquisitions Editor: Shannon Magee
Product Development Editor: Stephanie Roulias
Marketing Manager: Lisa Zoks
Production Project Manager: Bridgett Dougherty
Design Coordinator: Stephen Druding
Manufacturing Coordinator: Margie Orzech
Prepress Vendor: S4Carlisle Publishing Services

2nd edition

9 8 7 6 5 4

Printed in The United States of America

Library of Congress Cataloging-in-Publication Data

Tozer, Thomas N., author.
[Introduction to pharmacokinetics and pharmacodynamics]
Essentials of pharmacokinetics and pharmacodynamics / Thomas N. Tozer,
Malcolm Rowland. –
Second edition.
p. ; cm.
Preceded by Introduction to pharmacokinetics and pharmacodynamics : the quantitative
basis of drug therapy /
Thomas N. Tozer, Malcolm Rowland. c2006.
Includes index.
ISBN 978-1-4511-9442-5
I. Rowland, Malcolm, author. II. Title.
[DNLM: 1. Pharmacokinetics. 2. Dose-Response Relationship, Drug. 3. Drug
Therapy–methods. 4. Pharmaceutical
Preparations–administration & dosage. QV 38]
RM301.5
615'.7–dc23

2015021592

LWW.com

To Margaret and Dawn—
ever patient, ever understanding

ABOUT THE AUTHORS

THOMAS N. TOZER

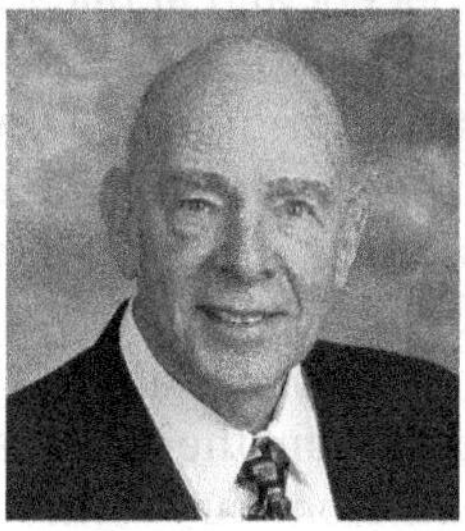

Dr. Tozer, Professor Emeritus of Biopharmaceutical Sciences and Pharmaceutical Chemistry, School of Pharmacy, University of California, San Francisco, California, received his BS, PharmD, and PhD degrees from the University of California, San Francisco. After a 2-year postdoctoral fellowship in the laboratory of Dr. B. B. Brodie, National Institutes of Health, Bethesda, Maryland, he joined the Faculty of the School of Pharmacy in San Francisco in 1965. Since obtaining emeritus status, he has taught courses and workshops in pharmacokinetics/pharmacodynamics and clinical pharmacokinetics at several institutions in the United States and Europe. For 10 years he was an Adjunct Professor of Pharmacology at the University of California, San Diego, where he taught biopharmaceutics and clinical pharmacokinetics at the Skaggs School of Pharmacy and Pharmaceutical Sciences.

Dr. Tozer, together with Dr. Malcolm Rowland, University of Manchester, authored the textbook, *Clinical Pharmacokinetics and Pharmacodynamics: Concepts and Applications.* He has published more than 155 scientific papers and book chapters on a variety of research topics with emphasis on the development and application of kinetic concepts in drug therapy. Dr. Tozer's research before retirement was focused in four areas: colon-specific drug delivery; toxicokinetics; kinetics of potential contrast agents for magnetic resonance imaging; and nonlinear pharmacokinetics. Other research included determination of drug disposition in disease states, particularly end-stage renal disease. Emphasis here was placed on evaluating and predicting when and how drug administration to renal disease patients should be altered.

Dr. Tozer was a corecipient of the 2000 Meritorious Manuscript Award, American Association of Pharmaceutical Scientists, and was a Visiting Professor (1996–1999) at the University of Manchester, Manchester, England. He is a Fellow of the American Association of Pharmaceutical Scientists and has served as a consultant to the Food and Drug Administration and to many pharmaceutical companies.

MALCOLM ROWLAND

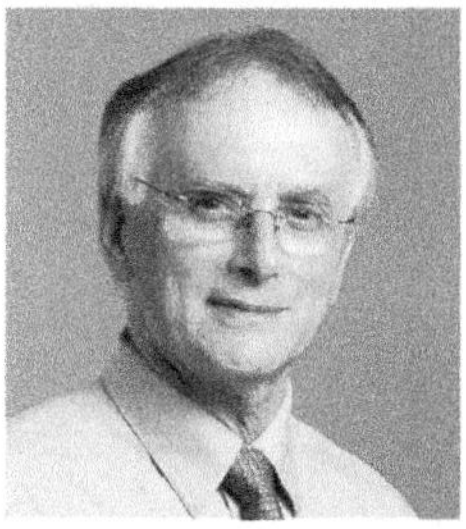

Malcolm Rowland is Professor Emeritus and former Dean (1998–2001), Manchester School of Pharmacy, University of Manchester, and Adjunct Professor, Department of Bioengineering and Therapeutic Sciences, Schools of Pharmacy and Medicine, University of California, San Francisco. He served as a Vice-President, International Pharmaceutical Federation (FIP, 2001–2009), the organization that represents and serves pharmacy and pharmaceutical sciences around the globe, and was President, European Federation of Pharmaceutical

Sciences (1996–2000). He received his Pharmacy degree and PhD from the University of London, and was on the faculty at the School of Pharmacy, University of California, San Francisco (1967–1975), before taking up a professorship at Manchester (1975–2004).

Dr. Rowland, together with Dr. Thomas Tozer, has authored the textbook *Clinical Pharmacokinetics and Pharmacodynamics: Concepts and Applications.* He has authored more than 300 scientific articles and chapters. His research interest is primarily in physiologically based pharmacokinetics and its application to drug development and clinical use. In particular, he has pioneered the concept and application of clearance, and developed approaches to the prediction of pharmacokinetics of drugs from a combination of physicochemical properties and in vitro information. He served as an editor of *Journal of Pharmacokinetics and Pharmacodynamics* (1973–2007), the premiere speciality journal dedicated to the subject, and has established workshops for teaching both basic and advanced level pharmacokinetics. He is an advisor to the pharmaceutical industry and sits on various scientific advisory boards.

Dr. Rowland has been awarded honorary doctorate degrees from the University of Poitiers (France), Uppsala (Sweden), and Athens (Greece), and Honorary Membership of the Royal College of Physicians (London). He received various awards including the 2012 Sheiner-Beal Award in Pharmacometrics, American Society of Clinical Pharmacology and Therapeutics; the 2011 Host Madsen Award, FIP; and the 2007 American College of Clinical Pharmacology (ACCP) Distinguished Investigator Award. He has been made a fellow of various professional organizations including the Academy of Medical Sciences, ACCP (Hon), the Royal Pharmaceutical Society of Great Britain, and the British Pharmacological Society.

PREFACE

This is the second edition of this textbook, which lays down the foundations of how exposure of drug within the body and response following drug administration are quantified and integrated, and how this vital information provides a rational approach to the establishment, optimization, and individualization of dosage regimens in patients. The title of the first edition began "*Introduction to...*," but so many readers of the first edition expressed the view that this textbook contained the very essence of the quantitative basis of drug therapy that we decided to change the title to *Essentials of Pharmacokinetics and Pharmacodynamics: The Quantitative Basis of Drug Therapy.* The book is intended for students and practitioners of pharmacy and medicine, as well as other health professionals, who need to understand the basic principles upon which quantitative decisions in drug therapy are based. It will also be a valuable resource and primer for those in the pharmaceutical and biotech industries involved in drug development, especially those from other backgrounds who have been given responsibility for the clinical development and evaluation of new drugs and those involved in the registration and regulation of drugs.

We are perhaps best known for our larger textbook *Clinical Pharmacokinetics and Pharmacodynamics: Concepts and Applications*, now in its fourth edition. This widely read, more in-depth, textbook serves a more advanced readership. In a sense, this smaller *Essentials* textbook aims to meet the needs of another wide audience, those who apply the principles in clinical practice or who work on the clinical side of drug development, who are in need not only of a more simplified textbook but, in particular, one that links drug exposure within the body to drug response—that is, to the pharmacodynamics of drugs. It provides the key quantitative tools and principles of drug therapy without recourse to an extensive use of mathematics, although some use of mathematics is essential when dealing with the quantitative aspects of drug therapy. Furthermore, many examples of currently prescribed drugs are included in the book to emphasize its utility to contemporary practice.

The book begins with the basic principles underlying pharmacokinetics and pharmacodynamics, and finishes with the application of these principles to the establishment, maintenance, and optimization of dosage regimens for the individual patient. Relative to the first edition, the second has many more Study Problems, including many in the multiple choice format used in licensing examinations. There are also practice questions that allow the reader to calculate and appreciate the quantitative aspects of pharmacokinetics and pharmacodynamics. As some readers may have less familiarity with some of the medical terms needed to convey the therapeutic setting in which pharmacokinetic and pharmacodynamic data are acquired and applied, an appendix of medical terms and words used in the text has been included. Chapters 5 and 6 of the first edition have been expanded to four chapters on: Quantifying Events Following An Intravenous Bolus, Physiologic and Physicochemical Determinants of Drug Disposition, Quantifying Events Following An Extravascular Dose, and Physiologic and Physicochemical Determinants of Drug Absorption. The second edition also has a greater emphasis on protein drugs and has been reorganized and updated from the first. With its emphasis on the integration of basic concepts, as well as concern for clarity of content in each chapter, great attention has been devoted to ensuring that the material content builds on knowledge from prior chapters as one progresses through the book.

Key elements in the organization of each chapter include Objectives at the beginning and a Summary and a Key Term Review toward the end. The Key Relationships of each chapter and Study Problems are provided at the end of each chapter. Detailed answers to the problems are provided in Appendix F. Definitions of Symbols and Medical Terms and Words used throughout the book are located in Appendices A and B. Appendices C, D, and E are intended as supplemental material for the interested reader. They also contain a few practice problems with answers to them in Appendix F. Further details on the organization of the book are given at the end of Chapter 1. Intentionally, coverage of the many concepts is not comprehensive; the book is meant to provide selected examples that illustrate the principles presented and to encourage the reader to give further thought to the concepts.

As an introductory text, this book should be particularly helpful to those teaching pharmacy and medical students within a separate course or within a pharmacology course or elective course in clinical pharmacology. In general, the textbook should be useful in all courses designed to train health professionals in the fundamental principles underlying the establishment of dosage regimens and individualization of drug administration to optimize drug therapy. We recognize that, in addition, some readers will treat this as a self-study textbook. Indeed, it has been written and organized to facilitate this mode of learning.

We wish to acknowledge all the students and colleagues, both in academia and the industry—too numerous to name individually—whose interactions over the years have provided the very "food for thought" for many parts of this book. Without their input, this book would not have been possible. Finally, and most importantly, our special thanks to our wives, Margaret and Dawn, for putting up with the many hours and temporary separations needed for us to work together to write this book.

THOMAS N. TOZER
South San Francisco, California

MALCOLM ROWLAND
London, England

CONTENTS

CHAPTER 1

Opening Comments

THE CLINICAL SETTING

When asked, most patients can readily proffer the names of the drugs they are taking, or, if they do not know the names, they know the general reason they are taking them, such as for a heart problem, a backache, high blood pressure, or recurrent depression. They also know how often the medicine should be taken and whether it should be taken before, with, or after eating, although how well they adhere to the prescription label is another matter. However, when it comes to the question of dose, most patients are at best unsure or even have no idea of the strength of their medicine or the amount they are taking. This is because most patients, and many clinicians, think qualitatively rather than quantitatively, but dose is of paramount importance. To paraphrase Paracelsus, who lived some 500 years ago, "all drugs are poisons, it is just a matter of dose." A dose of 25 mg of aspirin does little to alleviate a headache; a dose closer to 300–600 mg is needed, with few ill effects. However, 10 g taken all at once can be fatal, especially in young children.

What determines the therapeutic dose of a drug and its manner and frequency of administration, as well as the events experienced over time by patients on taking the recommended dosage regimens, constitutes the body of this introductory book. It aims to demonstrate that there are principles common to all drugs, and that equipped with these principles, not only can many of the otherwise confusing events following drug administration be rationalized, but also the very basis of dosage regimens can be understood by addressing the key questions about a specific drug: How much? How often? For how long? That is, the principles form the quantitative basis of drug therapy. The intended result is the better and safer use of drugs for the treatment or amelioration of diseases or conditions suffered by patients. Keep in mind, for example, that still today some 7% of patients admitted into hospital are there because of adverse reactions, some life threatening, due to the inappropriate use of drugs, much of which is avoidable. Many additional patients receive suboptimal dosage or have adverse reactions, but not severe enough to require hospitalization.

It is possible, and it was common practice in the past, to establish the dosage regimen of a drug through trial and error by adjusting such factors as the dose and interval between doses and observing the effects produced, as depicted in Fig. 1-1 (next page). A reasonable regimen might eventually be established, but not without some patients experiencing excessive toxicity and others ineffective therapy. Certainly, this was

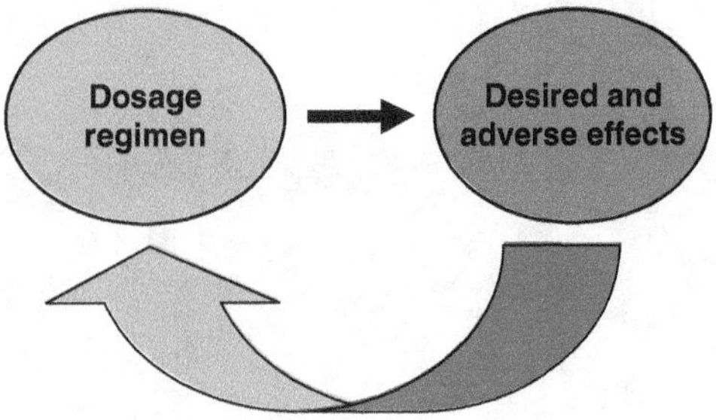

FIGURE 1-1 An empirical approach to the design of a dosage regimen. The effects, both desired and adverse, are monitored after the administration of a dosage regimen of a drug, and used to further refine and optimize the regimen through feedback (*curved arrow*).

the procedure to establish that digoxin needed to be given at doses between 0.1 and 0.25 mg only once a day for the treatment of congestive cardiac failure. On the other hand, morphine sulfate needed to be administered at doses between 10 and 50 mg up to six times a day to adequately relieve the chronic severe pain experienced by patients suffering from terminal cancer. However, this empirical approach not only fails to explain the reason for this difference in the regimens of digoxin and morphine, but also contributes little, if anything, toward establishing effective dosage regimens of other drugs. That is, our basic understanding as to how drugs behave and act within the body has not been increased.

Components of the Dose–Response Relationship

Progress in understanding the relationship between drug administration and response has only been forthcoming by realizing that concentrations at active sites—not doses—drive responses, and that to achieve and maintain a response, it is necessary to ensure the generation of the appropriate exposure profile of drug within the body. This in turn requires an understanding of the factors controlling this exposure profile. These ideas are summarized in Fig. 1-2, where now the relationship between drug administration and response produced, which we will refer to as **"dose–response,"** is divided into two components, **pharmacokinetics** and **pharmacodynamics** (with the root of both terms derived from the Greek *pharmacon*, meaning a drug, or, interestingly, also a poison). The pharmacokinetic component covers the relationship between the dosage regimen, which comprises such adjustable factors as dose, dosage form, frequency, and route of administration, and the concentration or exposure achieved in the body *with time*. The pharmacodynamic phase covers the relationship between drug exposure within the body and both the desired and adverse effects produced *with time*. In simple terms, pharmacokinetics

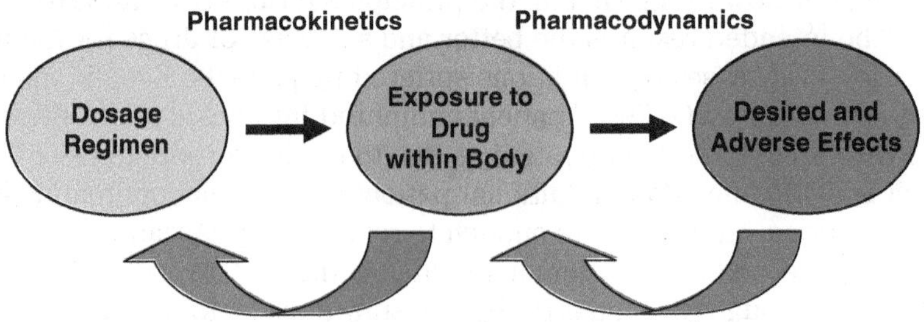

FIGURE 1-2 A rational approach to the design of a dosage regimen. The pharmacokinetics and the pharmacodynamics of the drug are first defined. Then, responses to the drug, together with pharmacokinetic information, are used as a feedback (*curved arrows*) to modify the dosage regimen to achieve optimal therapy.

may be viewed as the time-course of the body's handling of a drug, and pharmacodynamics as the body's response to drug exposure there.

Several other basic ideas have helped to place drug administration on a more rational footing. The first (partially alluded to above) is that the intensity or likelihood of an effect increases with increasing exposure to the drug, but only to some limiting, or maximum, value above which the response can go no higher. Second, drugs act on different components within the body, so that the maximum measured clinical effect produced by one drug may be very different from that of another. For example, both aspirin and morphine relieve pain. Whereas aspirin may relieve mild pain, it cannot relieve the severe pain experienced by patients with severe trauma or cancer even when given in massive doses. Here, morphine, or another opioid analgesic, is the drug of choice. The third (which follows in part from the second idea) is the realization that drugs produce a multiplicity of effects, some desired and some undesired, that when combined with the first idea, has the following implication. Too low an exposure within the body results in an inadequate desired response, whereas too high an exposure increases the likelihood and intensity of adverse effects. Expressed differently, there exists an optimal range of exposures between these extremes, the **therapeutic window,** shown schematically in Fig. 1-3. For some drugs, the therapeutic window is narrow, and therefore the margin of safety is small. For others, the window is relatively wide.

Armed with these simple ideas, one can now explain the reason for the differences in the dosing frequency among morphine, digoxin, and adalimumab. All three drugs have a relatively narrow therapeutic window. However, morphine is eliminated very rapidly from the body, and must be given frequently, up to 6 times a day, to maintain an adequate concentration to ensure relief of pain without excessive adverse effects, such as respiratory depression. Digoxin is more stable within the body, and so with

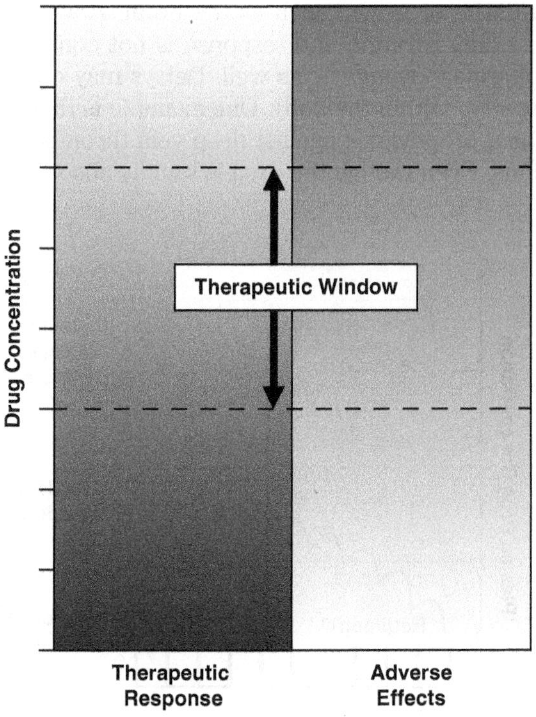

FIGURE 1-3 At higher concentrations or higher rates of administration on chronic dosing, the probability of achieving a therapeutic response increases (*shaded from black* [no response] *to white*), but so does the probability of adverse effects (*shaded from white* [no adverse effect] *to burnt orange* [severe adverse effects]). A window of opportunity, called the "therapeutic window," exists, however, in which the therapeutic response can be attained without an undue incidence of adverse effects.

little lost each day, a once-daily regimen suffices to treat atrial fibrillation and other heart diseases. For adalimumab, a subcutaneous dose given once every 2 weeks to treat rheumatoid arthritis patients is adequate because less than one-half of a dose is eliminated from the body within this time period. Unlike morphine and digoxin, adalimumab, a protein drug, is given subcutaneously because it is not absorbed when given orally.

These principles also helped to explain an enigma at the time concerning the pattern of effects seen with the synthetic antimalarial drug, quinacrine, developed during World War II. Given daily, quinacrine was either ineffective acutely against malaria, or eventually produced unacceptable toxicity when a dosing rate sufficiently high to be effective acutely was maintained. Only after its pharmacokinetics had been defined were these findings explained and the drug used successfully. Quinacrine is eliminated even more slowly than digoxin, with very little lost each day, such that it accumulates extensively with repeated daily administration of the same dose, as depicted schematically in Fig. 1-4. At low daily doses, the initial concentrations are too low to be effective, but eventually, the plasma concentration rises to within the therapeutic window. Increasing the daily dose shortens the time for the concentration to be within the therapeutic window, but, with the concentration still rising, eventually it becomes too high, and unacceptable toxicity ensues. Yet what was needed was rapid achievement, and subsequent maintenance, of adequate antimalarial concentrations without undue adverse effects. The answer developed was to give large doses over the first few days to rapidly achieve therapeutic concentrations, followed by smaller daily doses to maintain the concentration within the therapeutic window.

The lesson to be learned from the case of quinacrine, and indeed most drugs, is that only through an understanding of the temporal events that occur after the drug's administration can meaningful decisions be made regarding its optimal use.

Delays in drug response may also occur due to slow distribution to the target site, which is often in a cell within a tissue or organ, such as the brain. However, the issue of time delays between drug administration and response is not confined to pharmacokinetics, but extends to pharmacodynamics, as well. Delays may occur because of the nature of the affected system within the body. One example is that of the oral anticoagulant warfarin, used as a prophylaxis against deep vein thrombosis and other thromboembolic complications. Even though the drug is rapidly absorbed,

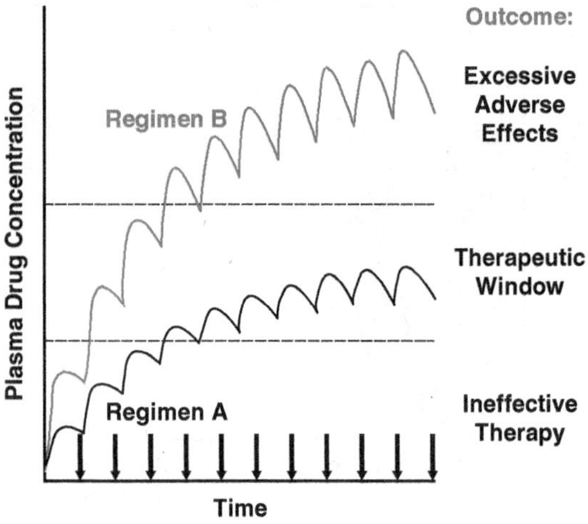

FIGURE 1-4 When a drug is given repetitively in a fixed dose and at a fixed time interval (*arrows*), it accumulates within the body until a plateau is reached. With regimen A, therapeutic success is achieved, although not initially. With regimen B, the therapeutic objective is achieved more quickly, but the drug concentration is ultimately too high, resulting in excessive adverse effects.

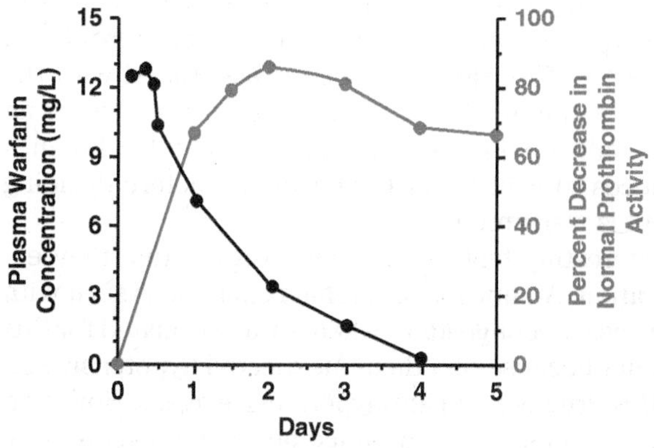

FIGURE 1-5 The sluggish response in the plasma prothrombin complex activity (*colored line*), which determines the degree of coagulability of blood, is clearly evident after administration of the oral anticoagulant, warfarin. Although the absorption of this drug into the body is rapid with a peak concentration seen within the first few hours, for the first 2 days after giving a single oral 1.5 mg/kg dose of sodium warfarin, response (defined as the percent decrease in the normal complex activity) steadily increases, reaching a peak after 2 days. Thereafter, the response declines slowly as absorbed drug is eliminated from the body. The data points are the averages of five male volunteers. (From Nagashima R, O'Reilly RA, Levy G. Kinetics of pharmacologic effects in man: the anticoagulant action of warfarin. *Clin Pharmacol Ther* 1969;10:22–35.)

yielding high early concentrations throughout the body, as seen in Fig. 1-5, the peak effect, as manifested by prolongation of the clotting time, occurs approximately 2 days after a single dose of warfarin. Clearly, it is important to take this lag in response into account when deciding how much to adjust the dose to achieve and maintain a given therapeutic response. Failing to do so and attempting to adjust the dosage based on the response seen after 1 day, before the full effect develops, increases the danger of subsequently overdosing the patient. This can have serious consequences, such as internal hemorrhage, with this low margin-of-safety drug.

Another problem with drugs of a low margin of safety is that individualization of dosage is essential because of interindividual differences in both the pharmacokinetic behavior and pharmacodynamic response to the drug. For warfarin, this is accomplished by titrating the dosage in an individual to obtain a desired in vitro clotting measure, which serves as a surrogate to its clinical response.

Another example of a pharmacodynamic delay is seen with the statin drugs, as shown in Fig. 1-6 with atorvastatin. This class of drugs is used to lower blood cholesterol as a prophylaxis against cardiovascular complications such as atherosclerosis,

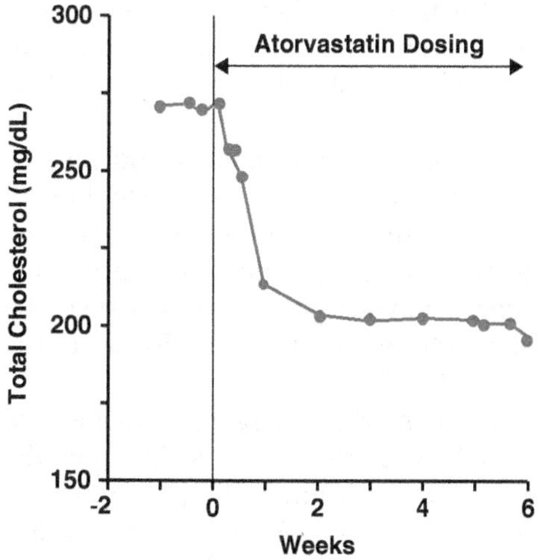

FIGURE 1-6 Plot of total cholesterol against time after oral administration of 5 mg atorvastatin once daily for 6 weeks. Atorvastatin is a selective, competitive inhibitor of HMG-CoA reductase, the rate-limiting enzyme that converts 3-hydroxy-3-methylglutaryl-coenzyme A to mevalonate, a precursor of sterols, including cholesterol. Note that despite the relatively short half-life of atorvastatin (14 hours, not shown), it takes almost 2 weeks to see the full effect of inhibition of cholesterol synthesis. (Redrawn from Stern RH, Yang BB, Hounslow NJ, et al. Pharmacodynamics and pharmacokinetic-pharmacodynamic relationship of atorvastatin, an HMG-CoA reductase inhibitor. *J Clin Pharmacol* 2000;40:616–623.)

signaling the likely occurrence of myocardial infarction and stroke. Despite this statin being rapidly eliminated from the body, the full lowering of blood cholesterol takes from 2 to 3 weeks after chronic dosing. This slow response is associated with the slow turnover of the cholesterol pool within the body. Dose adjustment to ensure an adequate lowering of cholesterol in individual patients is common, and the findings shown in Fig. 1-6 imply that one needs to wait for at least 1 month before deciding whether any further dose adjustment is warranted.

As mentioned previously, an interesting feature of many drugs is that they exhibit different effects with concentration. An unusual but telling example is seen with clonidine. Originally developed as a nasal decongestant, when it was evaluated for this indication, some subjects became faint because of a then-unexpected hypotensive effect. Today, the therapeutic use of this drug is as an antihypertensive agent. However, further investigation showed that it was possible to produce not only a hypotensive effect but also hypertension, depending on the concentration. Clonidine acts on two classes of receptors, one causing a lowering of blood pressure and the other causing an elevation in blood pressure. At low concentrations within the body, and those achieved with therapeutic doses, the lowering effect on blood pressure predominates. However, at high concentrations, as might be achieved during an overdose, the hypertensive effect predominates, although this effect subsides and the hypotensive effect again predominates as the concentration within the body falls. For other drugs, such as warfarin, the mechanism of action is the same for producing desired and adverse effects. Warfarin's almost singular action is anticoagulation. Yet, this effect is defined as therapeutic when warfarin's concentration is such that it minimizes the risk of embolism and it is defined as adverse at higher concentrations, where the risk of internal hemorrhage is high, that is, where the anticoagulation effect becomes excessive. The lesson is clear. Understanding the specific concentration–response relationship of a drug helps in its management and optimal use.

Variability in Drug Response

If we were all alike, there would be only one dose strength and regimen of a drug needed for the entire patient population. But we are not alike; we often exhibit great interindividual variability in response to drugs. This is generally not so important for drugs with wide therapeutic windows, because patients can tolerate a wide range of exposures for similar degrees of benefit, particularly when the dose ensures that the beneficial effect is experienced by essentially all patients. In this case, a single dose of drug, the "one-dose-for-all" idea, suffices. Still, even then, some patients may not respond to therapy because they lack the receptor on which the drug acts or their receptor is different.

The problem of variability in both pharmacokinetics and pharmacodynamics becomes particularly acute for drugs with a medium-to-low therapeutic window, of which there are many. Examples include the immunosuppressive agent cyclosporine, used to prevent organ rejection after transplantation, and the antiepileptic drug phenytoin (Fig. 1-7), in addition to morphine, digoxin, and warfarin. For these drugs, the solution is the availability of an array of dose strengths, with titration of dosage to the patient's individual requirements.

The variability in the concentration of phenytoin is primarily pharmacokinetic in origin. Pharmacodynamics is also a cause of variability in response, as shown by the minimum alveolar concentration (deep in the lungs) of desflurane (Suprane), a general inhalation anesthetic, required to give the same depth of anesthesia in various age

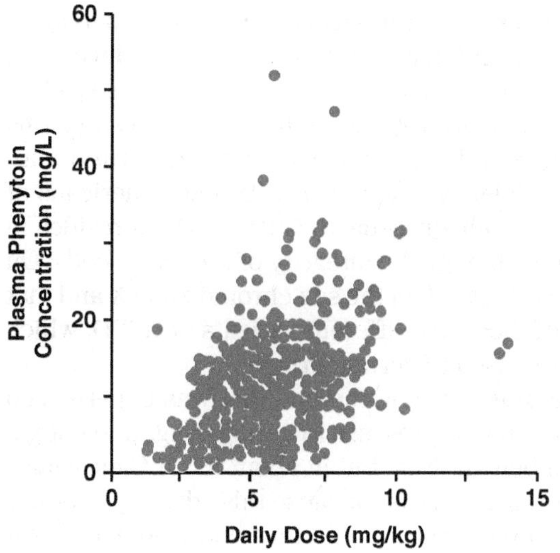

FIGURE 1-7 Although the average plasma concentration of phenytoin on chronic dosing tends to increase with the dosing rate, there is very large variation in the individual values for a given daily dose, even when normalized on a body weight basis. (Redrawn from Lund L. Effects of phenytoin in patients with epilepsy in relation to its concentration in plasma. In: Davies DS, Prichard BNC, eds. *Biological Effects of Drugs in Relation to Their Plasma Concentration.* London and Basingstoke: Macmillan, 1973.)

groups (Fig. 1-8). The sensitivity to the drug is much greater in the elderly patient than in any other age group. The alveolar concentration has been used to measure systemic exposure to the drug in much the same way as a breath test has been used to assess blood levels of alcohol, another volatile substance.

The causes of variability in dose response are manifold. One important and pervasive cause is genetics. It has been known for many years that, when evaluated, identical twins exhibit only minute differences in the pharmacokinetics and response to drugs, even when they live apart and in different social environments, compared with the often experienced wide differences in response between nonidentical twins. The importance of genetics is also known from familial studies and studies in different ethnic groups. One example, again arising during World War II, which occurred when

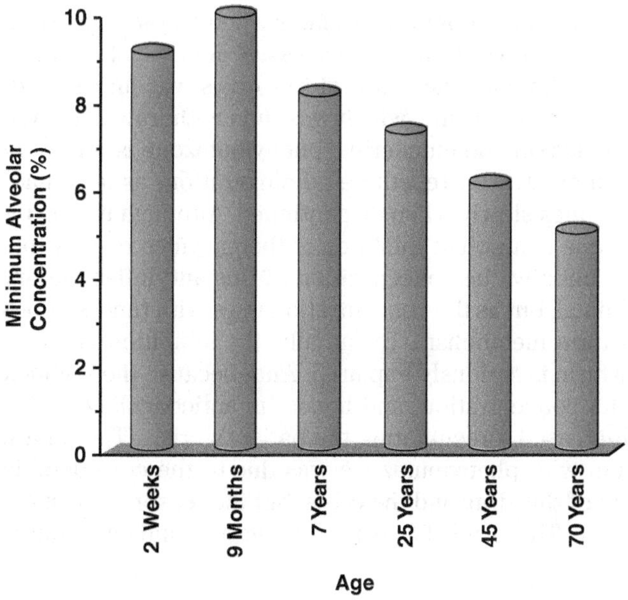

FIGURE 1-8 The minimum alveolar concentration (%, v/v) of desflurane required for general anesthesia varies with age. Elderly patients are clearly more sensitive to the anesthetic effect of the drug. (From table of data in *Physician's Desk Reference.* 60th Ed. Montvale, NJ: Medical Economics Co.; 2006:832.)

the fighting spread to tropical regions where malaria was rife, was the observation that approximately 10% of African American soldiers, but few Caucasians, developed acute hemolytic anemia, due to the abnormal and acute breakdown of red cells, when given a typical dose of the antimalarial drug primaquine. Subsequent investigations showed that this sensitivity to primaquine and some other chemically related antimalarial drugs was due to an inherited deficiency among many African Americans of an important enzyme, glucose 6-phosphate dehydrogenase (G6PD), which resides in red blood cells and is a component responsible for the integrity of the blood cells. On further checking, it was found that G6PD is located on the sex chromosome X and that more than 400 million people carry one of the many different variants of G6PD, which places them at risk for hemolysis when exposed to certain drugs.

Another example of the importance of genetics is the one that was experienced with the drug debrisoquine, a now defunct blood pressure lowering drug. In most patients, this proved to be an effective and benign drug, but in about 8% of Caucasians, even a modest dose caused a major hypotensive crisis. Because this adverse response was then unpredictable, in that there was no means of predicting who would manifest this severe adverse effect, the drug was withdrawn. With progress in deciphering the human genome or, more accurately, human genomes, we are beginning to understand the molecular basis of genetic differences. In the case of the debrisoquine-induced crisis, the cause was eventually traced to the presence within this minority Caucasian group of defective variants of a cytochrome-metabolizing enzyme located within the liver, which is almost exclusively responsible for metabolism of debrisoquine and many other drugs. Normally, debrisoquine is rapidly eliminated from the body, but an inability to readily remove this drug results in the usual doses of debrisoquine producing excessively high concentrations within the body and thus excessive effect. Today, increasingly, genomic information is helping to improve and individualize drug therapy.

In the 1970s, an elderly male patient suffered a bout of inflammatory pain, for which he was prescribed the effective anti-inflammatory drug phenylbutazone at the typical regimen of 100 mg three times daily. He was also susceptible to the development of deep vein thrombosis, for which he was prophylactically receiving warfarin. Everything was under satisfactory control until about a week later when a crisis occurred, caused by the sudden loss of control on warfarin with excessive anticoagulation and the danger of internal hemorrhage. Initially, the cause of this crisis was unclear, but eventually it was traced back to phenylbutazone, which was then withdrawn, and the crisis subsided, but slowly. Like digoxin and quinacrine, phenylbutazone is relatively stable within the body and accumulates on repetitive administration, as schematically depicted in Fig. 1-4, and declines slowly when discontinued. Although it was not known at the time, phenylbutazone is a potent inhibitor of the enzymes responsible for the metabolism of warfarin. Initially, the concentration of this anti-inflammatory drug is low, and inhibition is minimal, but as the concentration rises with time, so does the degree of inhibition of warfarin metabolism. Eventually, the inhibition is so severe that the elimination of warfarin is seriously impaired. And, because the regimen of warfarin was not changed, its concentration, and hence its anticoagulant effect, progressively and insidiously increased, precipitating the patient's crisis. The failure to initially associate the problem with phenylbutazone was due to the considerable time delay between the initiation of this drug and the crisis, but the reason, as just explained, is really all too plain to see. The issue of time is all-pervasive, and one ignores this component at one's peril.

Today, we are well aware of the problem of drug–drug interactions, which are a major source of variability in drug response in clinical practice. Phenylbutazone, despite its being an effective anti-inflammatory agent, was subsequently withdrawn from the market, in part because of its potent inhibition of some of the drug-metabolizing enzymes, but mainly because it caused severe and sometimes fatal blood dyscrasias.

Adherence to Regimen

If only patients adhered to the prescribed dosage regimen of their medicines, we would at least have some idea whether a failure to respond or an excessive response can be attributed to the drug itself. However, the problem of nonadherence, or what was previously called noncompliance, is, to some extent, part and parcel of human behavior. Many patients are compulsive in taking their medicines as instructed, but many others are less reliable, missing doses or times of dosing or even stopping the drug before the full course of treatment is complete, referred to as a lack of persistence of treatment. This is clearly evident in Fig. 1-9, which shows that in a cohort of patients prescribed once daily antihypertensive medication, approximately 50% had discontinued therapy 1 year after starting treatment, even though reducing blood pressure to within the normal adult range is known to decrease the likelihood of premature morbidity and mortality. Reasons for discontinuance are manifold, for example, because patients feel better or because they experience some adverse effect that they had not anticipated and believe it to be worse than the condition for which they are being treated. The

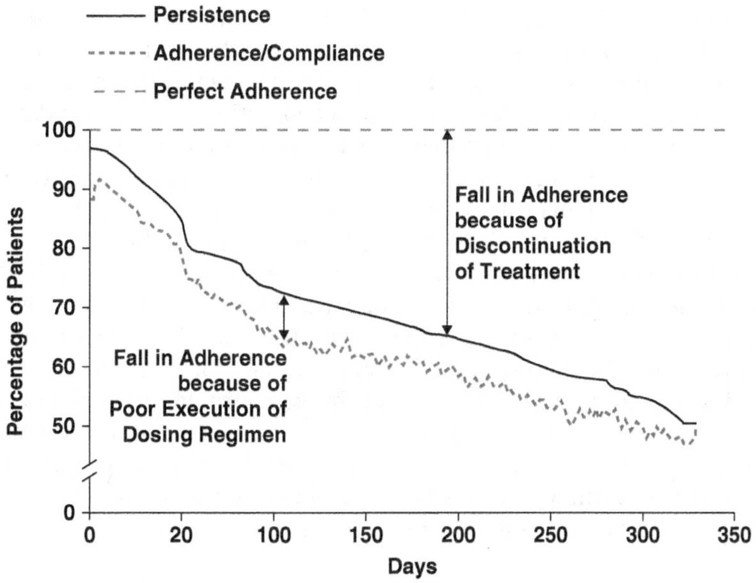

FIGURE 1-9 Nonadherence to prescribed medication is a major source of variability in drug therapy. Shown is the gradual but persistent decrease in adherence in the percentage of 4783 patients prescribed a variety of once-a-day antihypertensive therapies due to discontinuation of treatment, such that by the end of the first year only 50% of the patients prescribed the treatment for an indefinite duration continue to take the prescribed medication. The initial 3% drop in adherence is due to some patients never even starting the medication. The data were obtained using an electronic monitoring device that detects and logs each time the container with the medication is opened. (Taken from Vrijens B, Vincze G, Kistanto P, et al. Adherence to prescribed antihypertensive drug treatments: longitudinal study of electronically compiled dosing histories. *Brit Med J* 2008;18:1-6.)

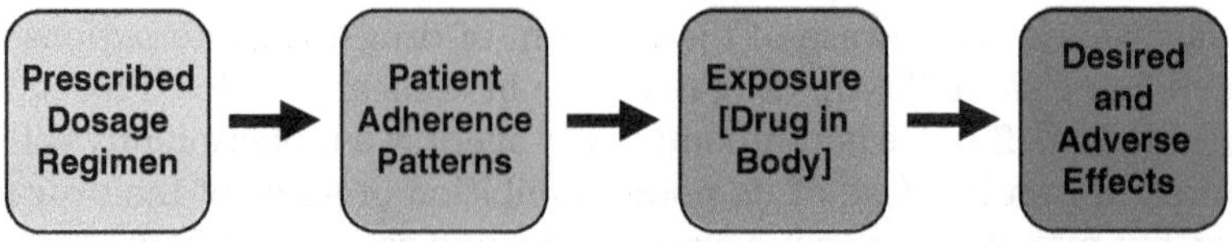

FIGURE 1-10 To adequately relate prescribed dosage regimens of drugs to response outcomes in patients in the real world of clinical practice, it is necessary to insert the adherence pattern of drug usage between the prescribed regimen and systemic exposure in the body. A low response may be a result of the patient not responding to a usual exposure or to a low exposure due either to a pharmacokinetic problem, e.g., low absorption or rapid elimination, or an adherence issue.

result is that we need to broaden the scheme depicted in Fig. 1-2 to include the issue of adherence, as shown in Fig. 1-10, if we wish to relate drug response to prescribed regimens in the real world. In the past, reliance was placed on what the patient said about adherence to the prescribed dosage. However, it has become clear, based on more objective evidence using electronic monitoring devices that record each time the patient opens the bottle to take a tablet, that many patients are untruthful or forgetful about their adherence pattern. For some drugs, a certain degree of nonadherence is tolerable without major therapeutic consequences; for others, close adherence to the prescribed regimen is vital to the success of therapy. This is particularly true in the case of drugs used in the treatment of many infections, such as those due to the human immunodeficiency virus (HIV, the cause of AIDS) and to tuberculosis. Failing to ensure an adequate exposure to the medication at all times can lead to the emergence of resistant strains, with fatal consequences, including those to whom the infection spreads. But fully adhering to a regimen to achieve this goal is often very demanding on a patient, particularly one suffering from AIDS, who is often receiving a combination of many drugs taken several times a day and sometimes at different times of the day. Some argue that we would not be in the situation we are in today—that is, the emergence of resistant microorganisms (such as methicillin-resistant staphylococcus aureus [MRSA], which has caused so many deaths in hospitals, where this organism is increasingly prevalent)—if we had ensured full adherence to the regimens of the existing armament of antibiotics for the full duration of treatment.

To make a point, many of the above examples are extreme. Usually, the therapeutic situation is less stark or of lesser concern. One reason is that drugs are metabolized by several enzymes, so that genetic variation, or inhibition, of any one of them has only a partial effect on overall elimination. Also, for many drugs, the therapeutic window is wide, so that a wide variation in exposure among patients or within the same patient does not manifest in any appreciable variation in drug response. Still, there are many exceptions, so it is important to deal with each drug on a case-specific basis. Nonetheless, the principles briefly enumerated here and stressed throughout this book hold and help to rationalize and optimize drug therapy.

THE INDUSTRIAL PERSPECTIVE

Awareness of the benefits of understanding pharmacokinetics and concentration–response relationships has led in recent years to the extensive application of such information by the pharmaceutical industry to drug design, selection, and development. For example, a potent compound found to be poorly and unreliably absorbed and intended for oral administration may be shelved in favor of a somewhat less potent but more extensively and reliably absorbed one. Also, many of the basic processes

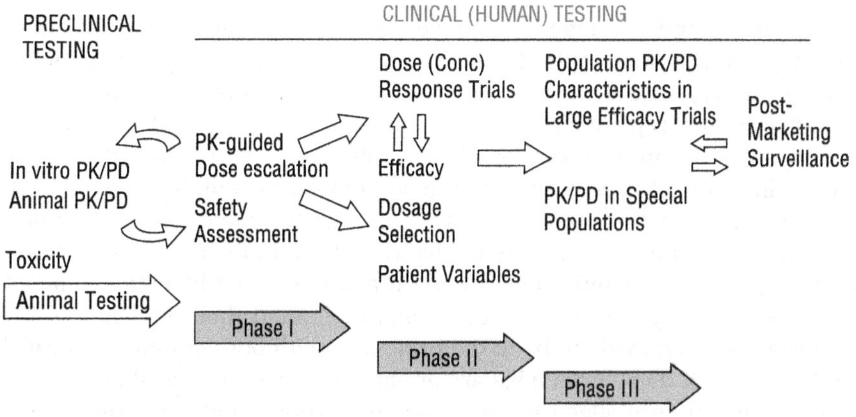

FIGURE 1-11 The development and subsequent marketing of a drug. The preclinical data help to identify promising compounds and to suggest useful doses for testing in humans. Phases I, II, and III of human assessment generally correspond to the first administration to humans, early evaluation in selected patients, and the larger trials, respectively. PK and PD data gathered during all phases of drug development help to efficiently define appropriate dosage regimens. Postmarketing surveillance, particularly for safety, helps to refine the PK/PD information. PK, pharmacokinetic; PD, pharmacodynamic.

controlling both pharmacokinetics and response are similar across mammalian species, such that data in animals can be extrapolated to predict quantitatively the likely behavior in humans. In vitro systems using human or human-expressed materials are increasingly being used to further aid in the prediction. This quantitative framework improves the chances of selecting not only the most promising compounds but also the correct range of safe doses to first test in humans. Incorporation of both pharmacokinetic and pharmacodynamic elements in these early phase I studies, usually in healthy subjects, together with assessment of any acute side effects produced, help to define candidate dosage forms and regimens for evaluation in phase II studies, conducted in a small number of patients to test whether the drug will be effective for the intended indication, commonly known as the "proof of concept" stage. These learning studies are also aimed at defining the most likely safe and efficacious dosage regimens for use in subsequent larger confirmatory phase III clinical trials, often involving many thousands of patients. Ultimately, some compounds prove to be of sufficient therapeutic benefit and safety to be approved for a particular clinical indication by drug-regulatory authorities. Even then, the drug undergoes almost continual postmarketing surveillance to further refine its pharmacotherapeutic profile. This sequence of events in drug development and evaluation, often referred to as a learn–confirm paradigm, is depicted schematically in Fig. 1-11. Lessons learned at each stage often help to improve the overall process of drug development.

ORGANIZATION OF THE BOOK

The problems and issues encountered in ensuring optimal drug therapy (discussed above) are expanded on in the balance of the book. The book is arranged so that each chapter builds on preceding chapters. It is divided into four sections. Section I: Basic Considerations, examines the basic concepts involved in relating exposure in the body to drug administration and response to exposure. Section II: Exposure and Response After a Single Dose, deals with the physiologic and anatomic features governing the pharmacokinetic and pharmacodynamic events after administration of a single dose of drug. Section III: Therapeutic Regimens, covers the principles used to achieve and maintain drug response with time. Constant rate of input by intravenous infusion or specific devices and repeated fixed-dose regimens are emphasized. Finally, Section IV: Individualization, examines sources of variability and how to adjust drug administration in the individual to accommodate the omnipresent variability.

This introductory book unashamedly deals with the quantitative principles underlying drug therapy and how events evolve over time following drug administration. With an emphasis on quantitation, a certain amount of mathematics is inevitable if one is to be able to grasp the concepts and understand their application. However, every effort has been made to back the principles with both graphic illustrations and examples in which these principles are applied to drugs in clinical practice. In addition, appendices are provided for those wishing to know more about the basis of some of the material contained in the body of the book. In common with many aspects of mathematics, symbols are used as a form of shorthand notation to denote common terms for ease of reading and presentation. Each of these symbols is defined the first time it is used, and, in addition, a list of all symbols, with their definitions, and units, where appropriate, are provided in *Appendix A*.

Throughout the book, a number of medical words or terms are used that may not be familiar to some readers. To this end, we have added an appendix, *Appendix B*, to define these words or terms.

A word on generic and brand names of drugs is warranted. During its patent life, a drug is registered worldwide not only by its nonproprietary or generic name, but also under the innovator company's brand name, which may vary from country to country (although today global branding is common). In practice, a drug is marketed as a formulation, such as a tablet or capsule, aimed at ensuring not only the optimal quality and performance of the drug but also its acceptability to patients, and it is this product (or series of products containing the active compound) that carries the brand name. Once the patent has expired, however, other companies may produce versions that are sufficiently similar so that they may be considered interchangeable with the original product. In such cases, the products are known as generic products. Throughout this book, the policy has been to use the generic name as the default when describing a drug product. However, it is recognized that during its patent life, the product is usually referred to by its brand name, which is familiar to both clinician and patient. For example, the brand name of the chemical sildenafil is Viagra; few people, when asked, would know the generic name of this widely used drug. Accordingly, for drugs still under patent, we have provided the brand name at its first mention in the book.

To aid in the learning of the material, at the beginning of each of the 13 subsequent chapters is a list of objectives, which you should regard as points that you might reasonably be expected to address after you have read and studied the concepts of the chapter, and completed the *Study Problems*. At the end of each chapter is a summary, a list of key words and phrases, which were emboldened within the text where these are first introduced, and a list of key relationships. They are intended to aid in identifying the major points, terms, and relationships of the chapter. Study problems follow the *Key Relationships* at the end of each chapter to help you learn the basic concepts and to test your understanding of the material. The problems are of two kinds: multiple-choice, like that used in some licensing examinations, and numerical problems both to aid in learning the basic concepts of the chapter and to build on concepts learned in previous chapters.

Finally, there are several appendices to the book. *Appendix A: Definition of Symbols* and *Appendix B: Medical Words and Terms*, were previously mentioned. Expansions on selected technical points of subsequent chapters are given in *Appendices C–E*. Detailed answers to the Study Problems are in *Appendix F*. To aid the learning process, we strongly encourage you, the reader, to attempt all Study Problems before checking the answers.

So, with these opening thoughts and comments, let us proceed to *Section I: Basic Considerations*.

SECTION I

Basic Considerations

CHAPTER 2

Input–Exposure Relationships

OBJECTIVES

The reader will be able to:

- Explain why plasma drug concentrations are most frequently used to assess drug in the body.
- Define the following terms: bioavailability, compartment, disposition, distribution, enterohepatic cycle, excretion, extravascular administration, first-pass loss, intravascular administration, local administration, metabolism, parenteral administration, pharmacokinetics, regional administration, systemic absorption, systemic exposure.
- Discuss the limitations to the interpretation of pharmacokinetic data imposed by assays that fail to distinguish between compounds administered (e.g., *R*- and *S*-isomers) or between drug and metabolite.
- Show the general contribution of mass balance concepts to drug absorption and disposition.

Pharmacokinetics and pharmacodynamics play many key roles in the development and use of medicinal agents. This section defines basic terms and examines input–exposure and exposure–response relationships. This chapter defines systemic exposure and describes basic models and methods for evaluating systemic drug absorption and disposition.

Before beginning the subject of exposure, a distinction must be made between drugs that act locally and those that act systemically. Locally acting drugs are administered at the local site where they are needed. Examples of products for **local administration** of drugs are eye drops, inhalation products (for pulmonary diseases), nasal sprays, intravaginal creams, and topical preparations for treating skin diseases. This chapter, and indeed much of the book, emphasizes those drugs and situations in which delivery to the site of action by the blood circulation is required. In general terms, we say such drugs act **systemically**.

SYSTEMIC EXPOSURE

The response produced by a systemically acting drug is related in one way or another to the amount entering the body and its duration there. Although responses can be observed, often noninvasively and with ease (such as monitoring blood pressure), measuring the sojourn of drug within the body that caused the change in blood pressure in the first place is difficult. Still, to understand the relationship between the administration of drugs and the responses produced, we need to be able to follow the events affecting the movement of drug to and from the site of action. Here, our options are very limited. It is rare when we can measure drug directly at the site of action, such as the brain or heart. Rather, we turn to more accessible sites to assess exposure to the drug on the assumption that drug at this site reflects exposure at the active site.

Sites of Measurement

Various sites of exposure assessment are used, including plasma, serum, whole blood, urine, milk, and saliva. The first three of these fluids (plasma, serum, and blood) are obtained by invasive techniques. The differences among drug concentrations in these three fluids are listed in Table 2-1. Urine, milk, and saliva are obtained noninvasively.

The two fluids most commonly sampled are plasma and urine. Drug within blood generally equilibrates rapidly with drug in blood cells and on plasma proteins. Accordingly, plasma or serum, as well as whole blood, can be used to reflect the systemic time course of drug. In practice, plasma is often preferred over whole blood for several reasons: it is considered a cleaner fluid to handle and store; it is viewed as a closer reflector than whole blood of the unbound plasma water concentration (see below); and blood constituents can cause interference in some assays. Although plasma and serum yield essentially equivalent drug concentrations, plasma is considered easier to prepare because blood must be allowed to clot to obtain serum. During this process, hemolysis can occur, producing a concentration that is neither that of plasma nor that of blood, or causing an interference in the assay.

TABLE 2-1 | Differences Among Plasma, Serum, and Whole Blood Drug Concentrations

Fluid	Comment
Plasma	Whole blood is centrifuged after adding an anticoagulant, such as heparin or citric acid. The supernate, plasma, contains plasma proteins that often bind drugs. The plasma drug concentration includes drug-bound and unbound to plasma proteins.
Serum	Whole blood is centrifuged after the blood has been clotted. Cells and material forming the clot, including fibrinogen and its clotted form, fibrin, are removed. Binding of drugs to fibrinogen and fibrin is insignificant. Although the protein composition of serum is slightly different from that of plasma, the drug concentrations in serum and plasma are virtually identical, unless hemolysis of the blood cells containing drug has occurred during isolation of the serum.
Whole blood	Whole blood contains red blood cells, white blood cells, platelets, and various plasma proteins. An anticoagulant is commonly added and drug is extracted into an organic phase often after denaturing the plasma proteins. The blood drug concentration represents an average over the total sample. Concentrations in the various cell fractions and in plasma may be very different.

Unbound Drug Concentration

The total plasma (or serum) drug concentration includes both unbound and protein-bound drug. However, it is only unbound drug that passes across cell membranes to reach sites of storage, elimination, or activity; protein-bound drug and the binding protein are generally too large to do so. Because the ratio of unbound to total drug, **fraction unbound**, in plasma usually does not change, it makes little difference whether total or unbound drug is measured. However, in conditions in which binding is altered, such as the presence of another drug that displaces the drug of interest from its binding protein, renal disease, hepatic disease, surgery, and severe burns, the unbound concentration is generally a better correlate of drug at the active site than the total concentration.

Exposure–Time Profile

The systemic exposure–time profile is a function of the rate and extent of drug input, distribution, and elimination. Fig. 2-1 shows the salient features of the systemic exposure–time profile after a patient has ingested a single oral dose. The highest measured concentration is called the **maximum concentration, C_{max},** or **maximum systemic exposure**. The time of its occurrence is called the **time of maximum concentration, t_{max},** or **time of maximum exposure**. Both depend on how quickly the drug enters into and is eliminated from the body, and the frequency of sampling. The area under the concentration–time curve over all time, abbreviated as **AUC**, is a measure of the **total systemic exposure** to the drug. The concentration profile before the peak is a function of how quickly the drug enters the systemic circulation. The area under the curve up to t_{max} is a measure of **early exposure** to the drug.

The measured peak concentration (peak systemic exposure) of the example in Fig. 2-1 is 96 µg/L, and the peak time is 3.0 hours. To get the AUC, the concentration must be integrated with respect to time. A common way to accomplish this is by approximating the areas between measurements as trapezoids and summing up the areas of the successive trapezoids (see Appendix D for further details).

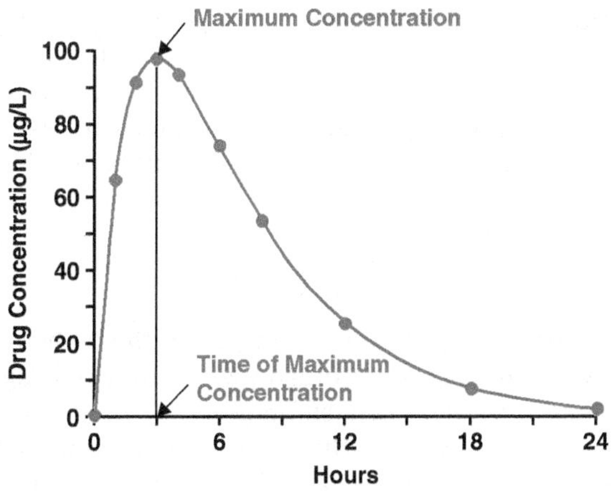

FIGURE 2-1 Drug concentration–time curve after a single extravascular dose showing the maximum systemic exposure (C_{max}) and the time of its occurrence (t_{max}). The area under the curve (AUC) represents total systemic exposure to drug; the area up to t_{max} is a measure of early exposure to the drug. The concentration could represent drug in whole blood, plasma, or serum.

PERIOD OF OBSERVATION

A basic kinetic principle is to make observations within the time frame of the events of interest. An atomic physicist measures atomic events that occur within microseconds or nanoseconds. A geologist, on the other hand, may be studying plate tectonics, which occur on the scale of hundreds of thousands to millions of years. To appreciate the events, both of these individuals must make their observations consistent with the time frame of the kinetic events.

The same principles apply to drugs. Sometimes, drugs have a very short sojourn within the body. After an intravenous bolus dose of such drugs, most of the dose may leave the body within minutes to hours. Other drugs remain in the body for days, weeks, or months. The period of measurement of systemic exposure must then be tailored to the kinetics of the specific drug of interest.

ANATOMIC AND PHYSIOLOGIC CONSIDERATIONS

Measurement of a drug in the body is usually limited to plasma, and occasionally to blood. Nonetheless, the information obtained at these sites has proved to be very useful. Such usefulness can be explained by anatomic and physiologic features that affect a drug's passage through the body after its administration.

Blood is the most logical site for measurement of drug in the body. Blood receives drug from the site of administration and carries it to all the organs, including those in which the drug acts and those in which it is eliminated. This movement of drug is depicted schematically in Fig. 2-2.

Sites of Administration

There are several sites at which drugs are commonly administered. These sites may be classified as either intravascular or extravascular. **Intravascular** administration refers to the placement of a drug directly into the blood—either intravenously or intra-arterially.

Extravascular modes of administration include the intradermal (into the skin), intramuscular, oral, pulmonary (inhalation), subcutaneous (into fat under skin), rectal, and sublingual (under the tongue) routes. After extravascular administration, an additional step, namely, absorption, is required for the drug to reach the systemic site of measurement relative to that required after intravascular administration.

Another term often used is **parenteral administration**. This refers to administration *apart from* the *intestines*. Today, the term is generally restricted to those routes of administration in which drug is injected through a needle, and includes intramuscular, intravascular, and subcutaneous routes. Thus, although the use of skin patches or nasal sprays (for systemic delivery) are strictly forms of parenteral administration, this term is not used for them.

Events After Entering Systemically

Once entered systemically, a drug is distributed to the various organs of the body by the blood. Distribution is influenced by organ blood flow, organ size, binding of drug within blood and in tissues, and movement across tissue membranes.

The two principal organs of elimination, the liver and the kidneys, are shown separately in Fig. 2-2. The kidneys are the primary organs for excretion of the chemically

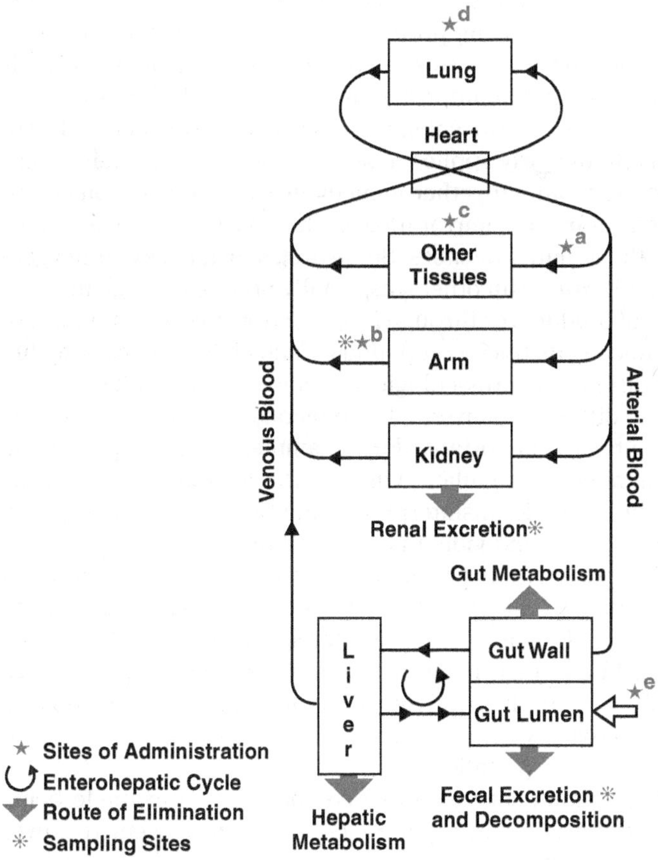

FIGURE 2-2 Once absorbed from any of the many sites of administration, drug is conveyed by blood to all sites within the body, including the eliminating organs. Sites of administration include: *a*, artery; *b*, peripheral vein; *c*, muscle and subcutaneous tissue; *d*, lung; and *e*, gastrointestinal tract, the most common route (denoted by *open arrow*). When given intravenously into an arm vein, the opposite arm should then be used for blood sampling. The movement of virtually any drug can be followed from site of administration to site of elimination.

unaltered, or unchanged, drug. The liver is the usual organ for drug metabolism; however, the kidneys, the intestinal tissues, and other organs can also play an important metabolic role for certain drugs. The metabolites so formed are either further metabolized, or excreted unchanged, or both. The liver may also secrete (actively transport) unchanged drug into the bile. The lungs are, or may be, an important route for eliminating volatile substances, for example, gaseous anesthetics. Another potential route of elimination (not shown) is lactation. Although generally an insignificant route of elimination in the mother, drug in milk may be consumed in sufficient quantity to affect a suckling infant.

Drugs are rarely given alone as a pure substance. They are formulated into a product that is convenient for the patient and optimizes the drug's performance when administered. For example, tablets and capsules permit a fixed dose to be easily administered orally. The formulation of the product may result in rapid release of the active drug, or its release may be modified to diminish fluctuation in systemic exposure between doses or to allow less frequent dosing.

CHEMICAL PURITY AND ANALYTIC SPECIFICITY

A general statement needs to be made about the chemical purity of prescribed medicines and the specificity of chemical assays. Over the years, a major thrust of the pharmaceutical industry has been to produce therapeutic agents and products that are not only as safe and effective as possible, but well characterized to ensure reproducible qualities. The majority of administered drug products today are therefore prepared with essentially pure drugs and, together with specific analytic techniques for their determination in biologic fluids, definitive information about their pharmacokinetics is gained. However, a large number of drug substances are not single chemical entities but rather mixtures. This particularly applies to stereoisomers and protein drugs. The most common stereoisomers found together in medicines are optical isomers, or compounds for which their structures are mirror images; the drug substance is often a racemate, a 50:50 mixture of the *R*- and *S-isomers*. Some drug substances contain geometric isomers, such as *cis* and *trans*. Still others, especially proteins of high molecular weight derived from natural products or through fermentation, may be a mixture of structurally related, but chemically distinct, compounds. Each chemical entity within the drug product can have a different pharmacologic, toxicologic, and/or pharmacokinetic profile. Sometimes these differences are small and inconsequential; other times, the differences are therapeutically important. For example, dextroamphetamine (*S*-isomer) is a potent central nervous stimulant, whereas the *R*-isomer is almost devoid of such activity. To avoid possible misinterpretation, stereospecific assays are now commonly employed to measure individual isomers following administration of racemic mixtures, and many stereoisomers are increasingly developed and marketed as single chemical entities, such as *S*-naproxyn, a nonsteroidal anti-inflammatory agent, and tamsulosin (*R*-isomer: Flomax), an α-adrenergic blocking agent to treat benign prostatic hyperplasia. In contrast, many new protein and polypeptide drugs are large and complex that defy ready chemical analysis; for these drugs, the assay is often based on a measure of activity, which may not be specific to the administered compound and so require careful interpretation.

Some medicinal products contain several active compounds, an example being the combination of a thiazide diuretic and a β-adrenergic blocking agent to lower blood pressure—each acting by a different mechanism. Specific assays are therefore needed to follow the pharmacokinetics of each compound. Herbal preparations contain a myriad of compounds, some of which may be active, although firm evidence of clinical activity with many is lacking. Moreover, given the variable composition of such preparations and the uncertainty as to what might contribute to any observed effect, attempting to characterize the input–exposure-response relationships, if indeed there are any, for herbal products is highly problematic. An added concern exists following drug administration, namely, the formation of metabolites. To be of value, an analytic procedure must distinguish between drug and metabolite(s) that may have pharmacokinetic and pharmacodynamic properties very different from those of the parent compound. Today, most assays for small molecular weight drugs have this desired specificity.

During drug development, radiolabeled drugs are used to determine the complete fate of drug and related materials after administration, which presents a potential problem. Incorporation of one or more radionuclides, usually ^{14}C, into the molecular structure allows for simple and ready detection within a complex biologic milieu, but not necessarily of the administered drug. Complete recovery of all of a radiolabeled dose in urine following oral drug administration is useful in identifying the ultimate location of drug-related material, but may provide little to no kinetic information about the drug itself. Consider, for example, a case in which the entire dose of an orally administered drug is destroyed in the gastrointestinal tract; yet, degradation products enter the body and are ultimately excreted into the urine. Full recovery of radioactivity may suggest that the drug is completely available systemically when, in fact, it is not.

A basic lesson is learned here. Distinguish carefully between drug and metabolite(s). Many metabolites are of interest, especially if they are active or toxic. Each chemical entity must be considered separately for kinetic data to be meaningful.

DEFINITIONS

Although the processes of absorption, distribution, and elimination are descriptive and their meanings are apparent at first glance, it is only within the context of experimental observation that they can be quantified (Chapters 5, 7, and 11). General definitions of the processes follow.

Systemic Absorption

Systemic absorption is the process by which unchanged drug proceeds from site of administration to site of measurement within the body, usually plasma derived from an arm vein. To illustrate why systemic absorption is defined in this way, consider the events depicted in Fig. 2-3 as a drug, given orally, moves from the site of administration (mouth) to the general circulation.

Several possible sites of loss exist along the way. One site is the gastrointestinal lumen where decomposition may occur. Suppose, however, that a drug survives destruction in the lumen only to be completely metabolized by enzymes as it passes through the membranes of the gastrointestinal tract. One would ask—Is the drug absorbed? Even though the drug leaves the gastrointestinal tract, it would not be detected in the general circulation. Hence, the drug is not absorbed systematically. Taking this argument one step further—Is the drug absorbed if all of the orally administered drug were to pass through the membranes of the gastrointestinal tract into the portal vein (which collects all blood perfusing the stomach and intestines) only to be metabolized completely as the blood passes through the liver? If we were to sample the portal blood entering the liver, the answer would be positive. However, if blood or plasma in an arm vein is the site of measurement, as is common, the answer would be negative because no drug would be detected. Indeed, loss at any site prior to the site of measurement decreases systemic absorption. The gastrointestinal tissues and the liver, in particular, are often sites of loss. The requirement for an orally administered drug to pass through these tissues, before reaching the site of measurement, interconnects the extent of systemic absorption and elimination. This loss of drug as it passes through these tissues is called the **first-pass effect**. Drugs that show extensive first-pass loss may require much larger oral than intravenous doses to achieve the same therapeutic effect.

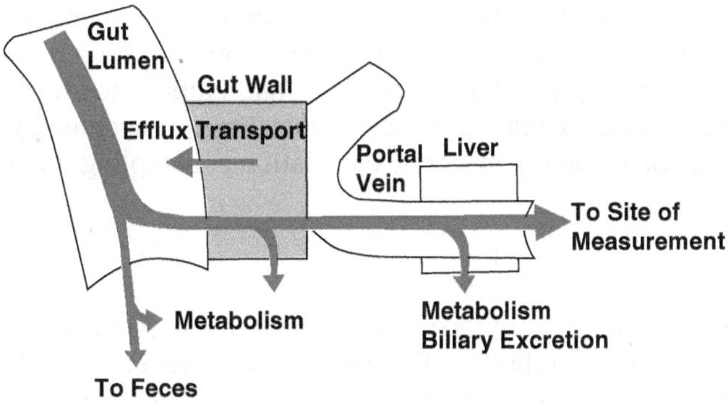

FIGURE 2-3 A drug, given as a solid, encounters several barriers and sites of loss in its sequential movement (colored arrows) through the gastrointestinal tissues and the liver. Incomplete dissolution, degradation in the gut lumen, metabolism by enzymes, and efflux by transporters, in the gut wall are causes of incomplete input into the systemic circulation. Removal of drug as it first passes through the liver may further reduce systemic input.

The movement of drug across the intestinal epithelium is often called absorption, or, more precisely, intestinal absorption. But it is extremely difficult to measure in vivo. As mentioned, assessment of intestinal absorption requires measurement of drug in the portal vein draining the intestine, a very invasive procedure. Moreover, in itself, intestinally absorbed drug is only of direct interest clinically if the drug acts directly on or within the liver. In most cases, and the ones of primary focus in this book, drugs act systemically and, to that extent, intestinal absorption is only one component of **systemic absorption** (hereafter simply called **absorption,** unless otherwise specified).

Absorption is not restricted to oral administration. The term also applies following intramuscular, subcutaneous, and all other extravascular routes of absorption, for which first-pass loss is also possible. Monitoring intact drug in plasma offers a useful means of assessing the entry of drug into the systemic circulation after administration by any extravascular route.

The term **bioavailability** is used as a measure of the extent of system absorption. It is defined as the fraction, or percentage, of the administered dose systematically absorbed intact. The oral bioavailability of drugs ranges from virtually zero, such as for the bisphosphonate drug alendronate (0.5%) used to strengthen bone to limit fractures in the elderly, to virtually 100% for caffeine.

Disposition

As absorption and elimination of drugs are connected for physiologic and anatomic reasons, so too are distribution and elimination. Once absorbed systematically, a drug is delivered simultaneously by arterial blood to all tissues, including organs of elimination. Distinguishing between elimination and distribution as a cause for a decline in concentration in plasma is sometimes difficult, especially during the earlier times following drug administration before tissue distribution is complete. Disposition is the term used to embrace both processes. **Disposition** may also be defined as all the kinetic processes that occur to a drug subsequent to its systemic absorption. By definition, the components of disposition are distribution and elimination.

Distribution

Distribution is the process of reversible transfer of a drug to and from the site of measurement and the peripheral tissues. An example is distribution between blood and muscle. The pathway for return of drug need not be the same as that leaving the circulation. For example, drug may be excreted in the bile, stored in and released from the gallbladder, transited into the small intestine via the common bile duct, and reabsorbed there back into the circulation. By doing so, the drug completes a cycle, the **enterohepatic cycle**, a component of distribution (Fig. 2-4). The situation is analogous to one in which water is pumped from one reservoir into another, only to drain back into the original one. Food causes the gallbladder to contract and empty the stored bile into the small intestine via the common bile duct, which exits there. Consequently, one sometimes observes multiple peaks in the systemic circulation at sampling times just following food ingestion.

Elimination

Elimination is the irreversible loss of drug from the site of measurement. Elimination occurs by two processes: excretion and metabolism. **Excretion** is the irreversible loss of chemically unchanged compound. **Metabolism** is the conversion of one chemical

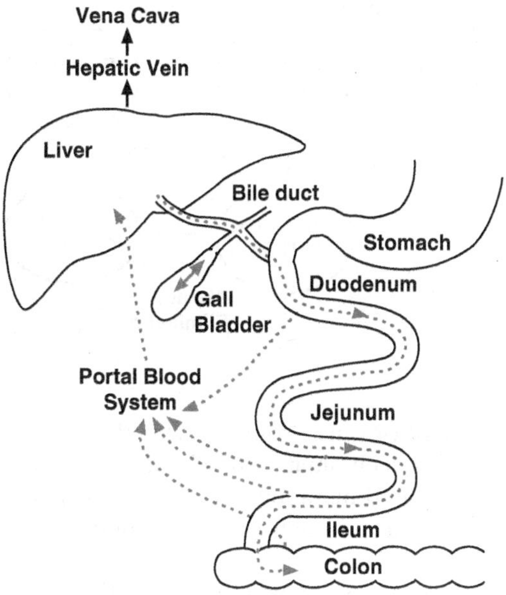

FIGURE 2-4 Drugs are sometimes excreted from the liver into the bile and stored in the gallbladder. Contraction of the gallbladder, particularly when induced by food, causes drug to pass via the common bile duct into the lumen of the small intestine, where it may be absorbed into a mesenteric vein draining the small or large intestine and conveyed by blood back to the liver via the portal vein. The drug has then completed a cycle, the **enterohepatic cycle**, as shown in color.

species to another and is usually mediated by enzymes. Occasionally, metabolites are converted back to the drug. For example, the anti-inflammatory steroid prednisolone is metabolized to inactive prednisone, which is converted, by a different enzyme, back to prednisolone. As with enterohepatic cycling, this **metabolic interconversion** becomes a route of drug elimination only to the extent that the metabolite is excreted or otherwise irreversibly lost from the body.

When a compound fails, partially or completely, to be reabsorbed from the gastrointestinal tract after biliary secretion, it is excreted from the body via the feces. For example, the hydroxylated metabolites of zafirlukast, an anti-asthmatic drug, are quantitatively excreted in the feces. Indeed, the metabolites in feces account for about 90% of an oral dose of this drug.

BASIC MODEL FOR DRUG ABSORPTION AND DISPOSITION

The complexities of human anatomy and physiology appear to make it difficult, if not impossible, to model how the body handles a drug. It is surprising then that simple pharmacokinetic models have proved useful in many applications and are emphasized throughout this book.

One conceptually useful model is that of accounting for drug both inside and outside the body. Such a model is depicted in Fig. 2-5 (next page).

Compartments

The ovals in Fig. 2-5 represent **compartments** that logically fall into two classes: transfer and chemical. The absorption site, the body, and excreta are clearly different places. Each place may be referred to as a location or transfer compartment. Sometimes, more complex models in which the body consists of two or more transfer compartments are used. In contrast to location, metabolism involves a chemical

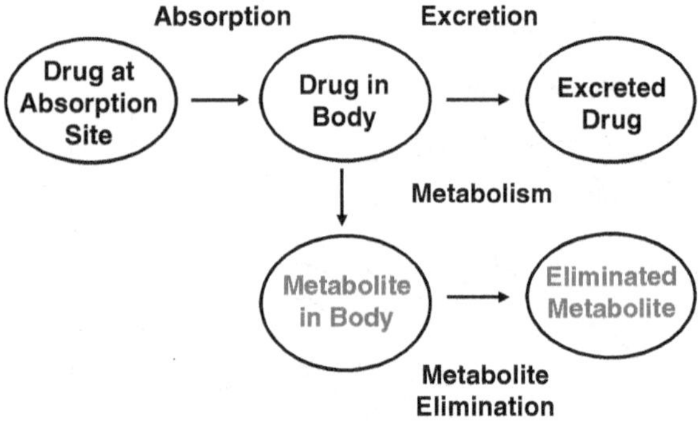

FIGURE 2-5 A drug is simultaneously absorbed into the body and eliminated from it by excretion and metabolism. The processes of absorption, excretion, and metabolism are indicated with arrows, and the compartments with ovals. The compartments represent different locations and different chemical species (color = metabolite). Metabolite elimination may occur by further metabolism (not shown) or excretion.

conversion. The metabolite in the body is therefore in a compartment that differs chemically from that of the drug. Excreted drug and eliminated metabolite are treated as separate compartments. In this model, eliminated metabolite includes renally excreted metabolite as well as all subsequent metabolic products of the metabolite in the body, bile, and urine.

The model in Fig. 2-5 is readily visualized from mass balance considerations. The dose is accounted for at any time by the molar amounts in each of the compartments:

$$\text{Dose} = \begin{array}{c}\text{Amount of}\\ \text{drug at}\\ \text{absorption site}\end{array} + \begin{array}{c}\text{Amount}\\ \text{of drug}\\ \text{in body}\end{array} + \begin{array}{c}\text{Amount}\\ \text{of drug}\\ \text{excreted}\end{array} + \begin{array}{c}\text{Amount of}\\ \text{metabolite}\\ \text{in body}\end{array} + \begin{array}{c}\text{Amount of}\\ \text{metabolite}\\ \text{eliminated}\end{array} \qquad \text{Eq. 2-1}$$

The mass balance of drug and related material with time is shown in Fig. 2-6. Because the sum of the molar amounts of drug in transfer and chemical components is equal to the dose, the sum of the rates of change of the drug in these compartments must be equal to zero so that:

$$\begin{array}{c}\text{Rate of change of}\\ \text{drug in body}\end{array} = \begin{array}{c}\text{Rate of drug}\\ \text{absorption}\end{array} - \begin{array}{c}\text{Rate of drug}\\ \text{elimination}\end{array} \qquad \text{Eq. 2-2}$$

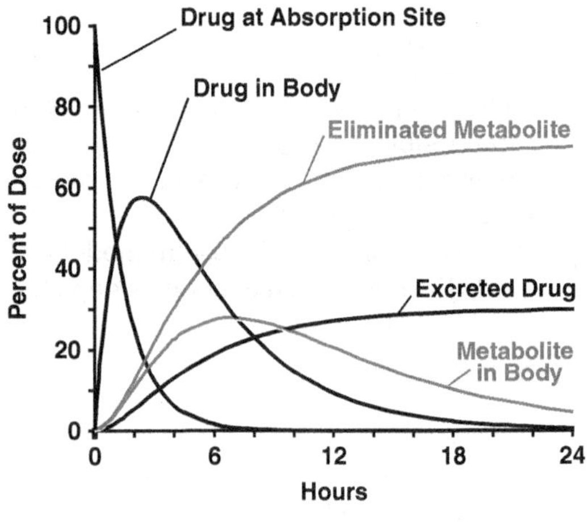

FIGURE 2-6 Time course of drug and metabolite in each of the compartments shown in Fig. 2-5. The amount in each compartment is expressed as a percentage of the dose administered. In this example, the dose is completely absorbed. At all times, the sum of the molar amounts in the five compartments equals the dose.

Metabolites

Metabolites are sometimes thought of as weakly active or inactive end-products. For many drugs, this is the case, but for many others it is not. Sometimes, the compound administered is an inactive **prodrug** that must be metabolized to the active compound. A prodrug is often developed intentionally to overcome an inherent problem with the active drug, such as poor or highly variable oral absorption. Examples of prodrugs include most of the angiotensin-converting enzyme (ACE) inhibitors, used to lower blood pressure; dolasetron mesylate, used to prevent chemotherapy-induced nausea and vomiting; pivampicillin, an ester that improves the oral bioavailability of ampicillin; and famciclovir, a prodrug of the antiviral agent penciclovir. Many drugs produce metabolites that augment the activity of the administered compound, as in the case with sildenafil, an agent used to treat erectile dysfunction. Some drugs form metabolites that produce other effects. For example, acyl glucuronides of a number of drugs (polar esters of the drug formed by its conjugation with glucuronic acid), including several nonsteroidal anti-inflammatory agents, react with some proteins and have been implicated in a wide range of adverse effects, including hypersensitivity reactions and cellular toxicity. The need to consider metabolites is clear.

SUMMARY

- Plasma is commonly used to measure systemic exposure to a drug.
- Intravascular administration refers to placing a drug directly into the systemic circulation (blood vessels). Extravascular administration refers to administration at all other sites.
- The terms pharmacokinetics, absorption, distribution, disposition, metabolism, excretion, first-pass loss, enterohepatic cycling, and compartment are all defined.
- Mass balance concepts can help in evaluating a drug's absorption and disposition.
- It is important to determine the contribution of metabolites to the activity seen with an administered compound.

KEY TERM REVIEW

Absorption
Area under the plasma concentration–time curve
Biliary excretion
Bioavailability
Blood drug concentration
Compartment
Disposition
Distribution
Early exposure
Enterohepatic cycling
Excretion
Extravascular administration
First-pass loss
Fraction unbound
Intramuscular route
Intravascular route
Local administration
Maximum concentration
Maximum systemic exposure
Metabolic interconversion
Metabolism
Oral route
Plasma drug concentration
Prodrug
Routes of administration
Serum concentration
Subcutaneous route
Sublingual administration
Systemic absorption
Systemic exposure
Time of maximum concentration
Time of maximum exposure

KEY RELATIONSHIPS

$$\text{Dose} = \begin{matrix}\text{Amount of}\\\text{drug at}\\\text{absorption site}\end{matrix} + \begin{matrix}\text{Amount}\\\text{of drug}\\\text{in body}\end{matrix} + \begin{matrix}\text{Amount}\\\text{of drug}\\\text{excreted}\end{matrix} + \begin{matrix}\text{Amount of}\\\text{metabolite}\\\text{in body}\end{matrix} + \begin{matrix}\text{Amount of}\\\text{metabolite}\\\text{eliminated}\end{matrix}$$

$$\begin{matrix}\text{Rate of change of}\\\text{drug in body}\end{matrix} = \begin{matrix}\text{Rate of drug}\\\text{absorption}\end{matrix} - \begin{matrix}\text{Rate of drug}\\\text{elimination}\end{matrix}$$

STUDY PROBLEMS

1. Which of the following reasons explain(s) why plasma, rather than whole blood or serum, is the most common site used to assess the systemic exposure of drugs?
   I. Constituents in whole blood interfere with the quantification of drugs in many assays.
   II. Serum is harder to obtain than plasma.
   III. Hemolysis of blood cells can be a problem.

A. I only	**E.** I and III
B. II only	**F.** II and III
C. III only	**G.** All
D. I and II	**H.** None

2. Which of the following conditions explain(s) why, for a given blood sample following drug administration, the concentration of a drug is likely to be higher in whole blood than in plasma?
   I. Drug readily enters blood cells and is extensively bound there, but not to plasma proteins. Acetazolamide is an example.
   II. Drug is not bound to plasma proteins or blood cells, and is unable to cross the membranes of blood cells. Gentamicin is an example.
   III. Drug is extensively bound to plasma proteins, but not within or to blood cells. Warfarin is an example.

A. I only	**E.** I and III
B. II only	**F.** II and III
C. III only	**G.** All
D. I and II	**H.** None

3. In which of the following conditions can the total concentration of drug in plasma serve as an alternative to the pharmacologically active unbound drug to track events in the body?
   I. When the drug is very highly bound to plasma proteins.
   II. When disease alters the degree of plasma protein binding.
   III. When the drug is displaced from its plasma binding site by other drugs.

A. I only	**E.** I and III
B. II only	**F.** II and III
C. III only	**G.** All
D. I and II	**H.** None

4. Which of the following statements explains why measurement of drug in plasma can be used for interpreting kinetic events in the body and relating concentration to response?

I. Drug in plasma reflects events at the site of action at all times.
II. Most sites of action are inaccessible for sampling.
III. Drug in plasma reflects what enters and leaves the body.

A. I only **E.** I and III
B. II only **F.** II and III
C. III only **G.** All
D. I and II **H.** None

5. Which *one* of the following statements is the most *incorrect*, after swallowing a single oral dose of a drug?
   a. Enterohepatic cycling is a component of drug distribution, not elimination.
   b. A drug, labeled with a radioactive atom, is given orally. Complete recovery of the radioactive dose in urine does not guarantee that the drug is completely absorbed systemically.
   c. A drug is completely recovered (100%) as a metabolite in the feces. Fecal excretion is therefore the primary route of elimination of this drug.
   d. Systemic absorption refers to the process by which unchanged drug proceeds from the site of administration (oral in this case) to the site of measurement within the body.
6. Fig. 2-7 shows the plasma concentration–time profiles of a drug (*black line*) and its major metabolite (*red line*) after a single intravenous dose of drug. Only the drug has activity.
   a. Draw a line on the graph to show the *measured* (by the analytical method used) concentration–time profile when a nonspecific assay, which equally measures drug and metabolite, is used.
   b. Briefly discuss problems that may be associated with the use of the measured concentration, using the nonspecific assay, in interpreting this drug's pharmacokinetics and response with time.
7. Identify which one or more of the following statements below is (are) correct after a single oral dose of drug. For the incorrect one(s), state the reason why, or supply a qualification.
   a. The maximum amount of drug in the body occurs when the rate of absorption and the rate of elimination are equal.
   b. The rate of change of amount of drug in the body equals the rate of elimination at all times after drug absorption is complete.

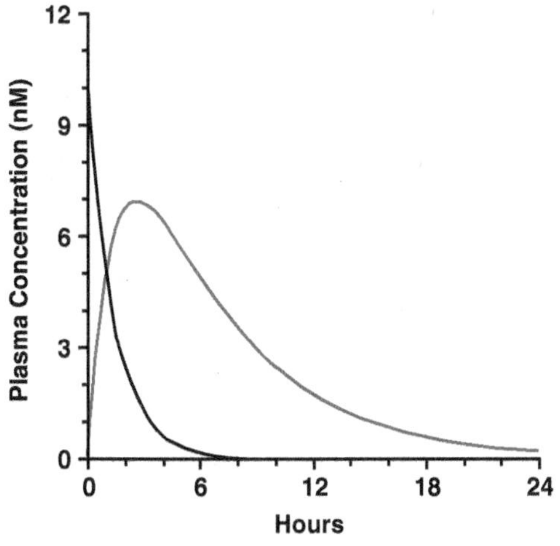

FIGURE 2–7 Plasma concentration-time profiles of a drug (*black line*) and its major metabolite (*red line*) after a single intravenous dose of drug.

c. The rate of change of drug in the body approaches the rate of absorption at the peak time.
d. The rate of drug absorption equals the rate of drug elimination minus the rate of change of drug in the body.

8. a. Midazolam exhibits a substantial "first-pass effect" after its oral administration. Explain what is meant by first-pass effect, and briefly discuss its impact on systemic exposure following an oral dose relative to an intravenous dose of drug.
   b. Do you think the terms "first-pass effect" or "first-pass loss" can be applied to routes of administration other than oral, such as intramuscular, subcutaneous, sublingual, if there is loss of drug before reaching the systemic circulation?
9. Would you consider transdermal (applied to skin) and intranasal (sprayed into nasal cavity) administrations to be forms of parenteral administration when systemic activity is intended? Briefly discuss.
10. An analytical method used to measure a given drug does not distinguish between *R*- and *S*-isomers. Discuss how this can lead to problems in interpreting plasma data following administration of a racemic mixture.

CHAPTER 3

Exposure–Response Relationships

OBJECTIVES

The reader will be able to:

- Explain why plasma drug concentration can serve as a useful correlate of response.
- Define the following terms: acquired resistance, agonist, all-or-none response, antagonist, baseline, biomarker, clinical response, cumulative frequency, disease progression, endogenous, exogenous, full agonist, full antagonist, graded response, inducer, inhibitor, maximum effect, maximum response, partial agonist, partial antagonist, pharmacodynamics, placebo, potency, quantal response, safety biomarker, specificity, steepness factor, surrogate end point.
- Briefly discuss issues involved in the assessment of drug effect.
- Describe, with examples, how the intensity of a graded response changes with drug concentration at the site of action.
- Describe the parameters of the model that often characterizes the relationship between a graded response and plasma drug concentration.
- Describe how to relate an all-or-none response to plasma drug concentration.
- Discuss the importance of potency, maximum effect, and specificity in drug therapy.
- Briefly discuss why the more important features of the exposure–time profile after a single dose of drug vary with the condition being treated.

Drugs produce a therapeutic effect when there is an adequate exposure–time profile at the target site, that is, the location where the therapeutic response is initiated. Often, the target is distant from the site of application, a common example being that of antidepressant drugs taken orally. For these drugs, exposure at the target site within the brain occurs through delivery of drug via the alimentary canal and the systemic circulation. And, because drug concentration cannot be or is rarely measured within the brain or indeed at any other site of action within the body, measurement of systemic drug exposure offers a generally useful substitute for exposure at the active site. Although, as mentioned in Chapter 2, the potential role of metabolites should always be kept in mind, the subsequent discussion is based on the assumption that it is the administered compound that drives the response.

Drugs interact with components within the body to produce a response. These components are commonly proteins, such as enzymes or receptors, or they may be genes or DNA itself. When acting on enzymes, drugs can be **inducers,** which increase synthesis, or activators, leading to an increase in the activity of the enzyme. They can also act as **inhibitors**, effectively decreasing enzyme activity. Similarly, other drugs produce their effects by causing **up- and down-regulation** of a protein responsible for the drug's effect by increasing or decreasing its concentration. Drugs that act on receptors are said to be either **agonists** or **antagonists,** depending on whether they increase or diminish the functional response of the receptor. When they produce the maximum possible effect, they are said to be **full agonists** or **full antagonists.** Compounds that fail to achieve the greatest effect, even at very high concentrations, are said to be **partial agonists** or **partial antagonists.**

In this chapter, we consider the relationship between response and systemic exposure of a drug, that is, its **pharmacodynamics**. In subsequent chapters, we integrate pharmacokinetics with response over time, in which case we speak of **pharmacokinetic–pharmacodynamic (PK/PD) modeling** in the sense that we are linking a model of the pharmacokinetics with a model of the pharmacodynamics of a drug to obtain a complete picture of the relationship between drug administration and response over time.

CLASSIFICATION OF RESPONSE

There are a variety of ways to classify response. Clinically, the most important is whether the effect produced is desired or adverse. However, this classification gives little insight into the mechanisms involved. For example, for some drugs, the adverse effect is simply an extension of the desired effect and is entirely predictable from its pharmacology. An example is the oral anticoagulant warfarin. It is used clinically to reduce the risk of developing an embolism by decreasing the tendency of blood to clot, whereas the adverse and potentially fatal effect is internal hemorrhage due to excessive anticoagulation. In many other cases, the adverse effect occurs via a completely different and often more unpredictable mechanism, such as the hepatic or cardiac toxicity caused by some antibiotics.

Another form of classification is whether the measured effect is a **clinical response,** a **surrogate end point,** or a **biomarker.** Clinical responses may be divided into subjective and objective measures. Subjective measures are personal judgments made by either the patient or the clinician (investigator) and include psychological evaluations, description of the degree of relief from pain, and assessment of ability to do daily chores, which may collectively form part of a global measure of "quality of life." Examples of objective measures are an increase in survival time, stroke prevention, or prevention of bone fracture. However, although these objective measures are clearly therapeutically relevant, the need for another measure arises in many cases because the clinical response may not be fully manifested for many years, and a more immediate measure is sought to guide therapy or simply to know that an effect has been produced. An example is the use of antihypertensive agents to reduce the risk of morbidity of several sequelae of prolonged hypertension, such as blindness and renal failure, as well as premature mortality. These outcomes are evident only after years of prolonged treatment. A more rapid, ready, and simple measure of effect, which correlates strongly with the clinical outcome, is needed. Measurement of blood pressure has been and continues to be used to achieve this goal. Because lowering of blood pressure has been shown through many large studies to correlate with the clinical effect, it is called a surrogate (or substitute) end point, in this case one that is on the causal pathway to the clinical effect.

The last category of response is the biomarker, which broadly may be considered as any measurable effect produced by a drug. It may be a change in a laboratory test, such as blood glucose when evaluating antidiabetic drug therapy, a change in a physiologic test, such as the response time in a simulated driving test when evaluating an antidepressant with concern about possible changes in motor reflex, or the binding of a positron-emitting (PET)–labeled drug to a specific brain receptor determined using positron emission tomography (PET), a noninvasive technique that measures externally the location and quantity of the labeled compound within the brain. These are examples of biomarkers that are intended to relate in some way to the desired action of the drug. Others, called **safety biomarkers,** are general measures not specifically related to the drug and are used to monitor for potential adverse effects. Examples are liver function tests, white cell count, erythrocyte sedimentation rate, and fecal blood loss. Drugs often produce multiple effects; the biomarker may therefore not be at all related to the clinical effect of the drug. In this sense, all pharmacodynamic responses are biomarkers unless they are either accepted as the clinical response, which is rarely the case, or they have been shown through rigorous evaluation to predict clinical response, in which case they are classified as surrogate end points. Clearly, biomarkers are most likely to serve as surrogate end points if they are on the causal pathway between drug action and clinical response.

Most drugs used clinically act reversibly in that the effect is reversed when the concentration at the site of action is reduced. An exception is the class of anticancer drugs known as alkylating agents, such as busulfan. These compounds covalently, and hence irreversibly, bind to DNA causing death of proliferating cells, taking advantage of the fact that cancer cells proliferate more rapidly than most healthy cells within the body. Many responses produced are **graded,** so called because the magnitude or intensity of the response can be scaled or graded within an individual. An example of a graded response, shown in Fig. 3-1, is anesthesia produced by ketamine given intravenously.

The intensity of a graded response varies continuously with the drug concentration in plasma within the individual. Many other pharmacologic and adverse responses do not occur on a continuous basis; these are known as **quantal** responses, for instance, when the response is placed in several levels or categories or when it is, by nature or by choice, **all-or-none**. An example of a categorized response is pain in

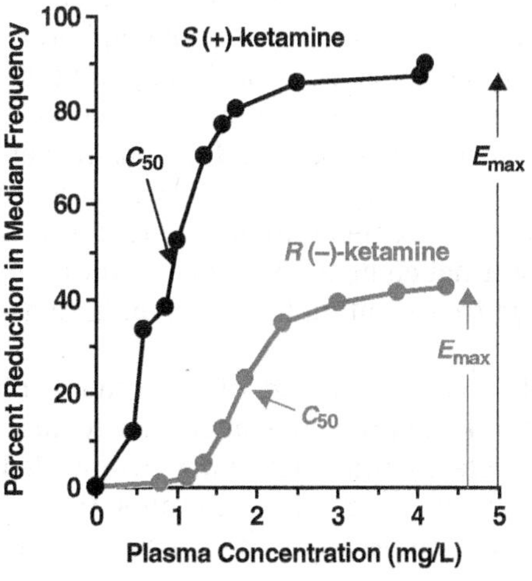

FIGURE 3-1 Changes in the electroencephalographic median frequency were followed to quantify the anesthetic effect of *R*(–)-ketamine and *S*(+)-ketamine in a subject who received an infusion of these two optical isomers on separate occasions. Shown is the percent reduction in the median frequencies versus plasma concentration. Although characteristic S-shaped, or sigmoidal, curves are seen with both compounds, they differ in both maximum effect achieved, E_{max}, and concentration needed to produce 50% of E_{max}, the C_{50}. *S*(+)-ketamine appears to be a partial antagonist (reduction in electroencephalographic measure) and less potent than the R(-) isomer. These relationships may be considered direct ones as no significant time delay was found between response and plasma concentration. (Redrawn from Schuttler J, Stoeckel H, Schweilden H, et al. Hypnotic drugs. In: Stoeckel H, ed. *Quantitation, Modeling and Control in Anesthesia.* Stuttgart, Germany: Georg Thieme Verlag, 1985:196–210.)

which a patient is asked to evaluate his/her pain as severe, strong, tolerable, or minor. Categorizing the symptoms of depression is another example. An obvious but extreme example of an adverse all-or-none event is death. Another is the statistical suppression of a cardiac arrhythmia. The measure is then all or none—there is or is not a statistically significant reduction. A graded (continuous) response can be made quantal by establishing limits, for example, by asking the question: Does a drug reduce blood pressure by 20 mm Hg or does it not?

ASSESSMENT OF DRUG EFFECT

Most drugs do not occur naturally within the body, so that when they are found in plasma, we can be confident that they have been taken. Exceptions are drugs that are normally produced within the body, that is, **endogenous** compounds, such as insulin, or are found in our diet, such as caffeine. There is always a basal plasma concentration of insulin, a protein secreted by the pancreas, and a correction is needed in its measured concentration if we wish to characterize the kinetics of externally, or **exogenously**, administered insulin. In contrast to drug concentration, a baseline almost always exists when attempting to assess drug effect. For example, antihypertensive drugs act by lowering blood pressure in hypertensive patients. Hence, the drug effect is the difference between the high baseline blood pressure in such a patient and the blood pressure when the patient is on antihypertensive therapy. For many drugs, there is an additional factor to consider, **the placebo effect**. A placebo effect, based on one's perception, is a deviation from the baseline value produced when the patient takes or receives what has all the appearances of drug treatment but lacks the active principle. This may take the form of giving the patient a tablet that looks and tastes identical to the one containing the drug. Thus, in general, when attempting to assess response following drug administration, we can write:

$$\begin{matrix}\text{Measured} \\ \text{response}\end{matrix} = \begin{matrix}\text{Drug} \\ \text{response}\end{matrix} + \begin{matrix}\text{Placebo} \\ \text{response}\end{matrix} + \text{Baseline} \qquad \textbf{Eq. 3-1}$$

An additional issue is that not only does drug response vary with time after drug administration but so, commonly, do both the placebo effect and the baseline. Hence, separating and characterizing the true drug effect requires careful attention to these other factors. This is equally true when assessing both the desired and the adverse effects of the drug. Let us examine several examples to illustrate these points.

Fig. 3-2 shows FEV_1 (the volume exhaled during the first second of a forced expiration started from the level of total lung capacity), a common measure of respiratory function with time following the oral administration of placebo and 10-mg montelukast, a specific leukotriene receptor antagonist that improves respiratory function in asthmatic patients. Notice both the appreciable placebo response and the positive effect of montelukast, seen as the difference in FEV_1 between the two treatments, which is sustained over the 24-hour period. In this study, and commonly in others, there is no specific and independent assessment of the normal changes in baseline over time; these are subsumed in the assessment after drug treatment and placebo and are assumed to be independent of treatment.

Sometimes the baseline is relatively stable over the period of assessment of drug effect, but this is not always so. Many physiologic processes undergo rhythmic changes with time. For some, the period of the cycle approximates a day (a so-called circadian rhythm), such as that seen with the hormone cortisol. For others, the period is much shorter or much longer than 1 day, sometimes being as long as 1 month,

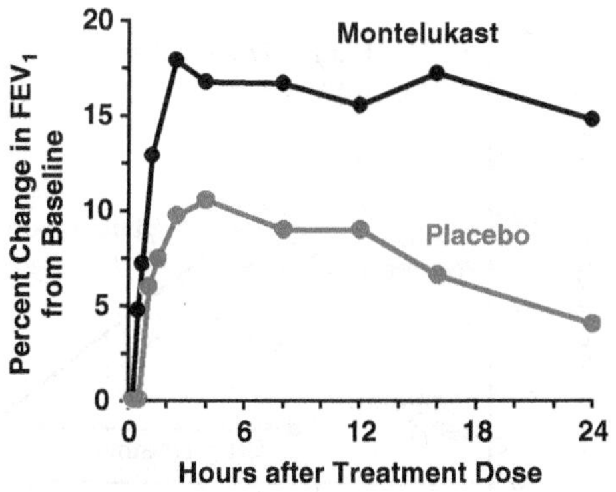

FIGURE 3-2 Figure showing changes in FEV_1, a measure of respiratory function, with time following administration of a single dose of a placebo (*color*) or montelukast (10 mg, *black*), a specific leukotriene receptor antagonist, in asthmatic patients. Notice both the appreciable difference in FEV_1 from baseline between the two treatments, which is sustained over the 24-hour period response and also the positive effect of montelukast seen as the difference in FEV_1 between the two treatments, which is sustained over the 24-hour period of study. (Redrawn from Dockendorf RJ, Baumgartner RA, Leff JA, et al. Comparison of the effects of intravenous and oral montelukast on airway function: a double blind, placebo controlled, three period, crossover study in asthmatic patients. *Thorax* 2000;55:260–265.)

such as with hormones associated with the estrus cycle. Correcting for the variable baseline is then more difficult. Returning to Fig. 3-2, we see that after placebo, FEV_1 first increases with time and then wanes (with a time course relatively similar to that observed following drug administration), although this is not always the case. However, without independent baseline data, it is not possible to know how much of the temporal change in FEV_1 is due to a change in the baseline function, and how much to the placebo. Placebo effects can be subtle even when using what are thought to be objective assessments, such as loss of weight. They are commonly extensive when assessing subjective effects, such as a feeling of well-being or depression, or a sense of nausea or dizziness. Indeed, the interaction between the mind and various physiologic processes can be very strong. Because placebo effects can be clinically significant, double-blind placebo-controlled trials, in which neither the clinician nor the patient knows whether placebo or active treatment has been given, are usually employed to assess drug effects; but there is still a potential for bias because both the clinician and the patient believe each patient *may* be taking the drug.

The clinical benefit of many drugs requires that drug treatment be continued for many months or years. During this time, the baseline itself often changes, reflecting the natural course of the disease or condition. Consider, for example, the data in Fig. 3-3 showing the change in average muscle strength in a group of boys with Duchenne dystrophy, a degenerating muscle disease associated with a gene defect. The aim of the study was to assess the potential benefit of the corticosteroid prednisone, which is converted in the body to the active prednisolone. The study was randomized and

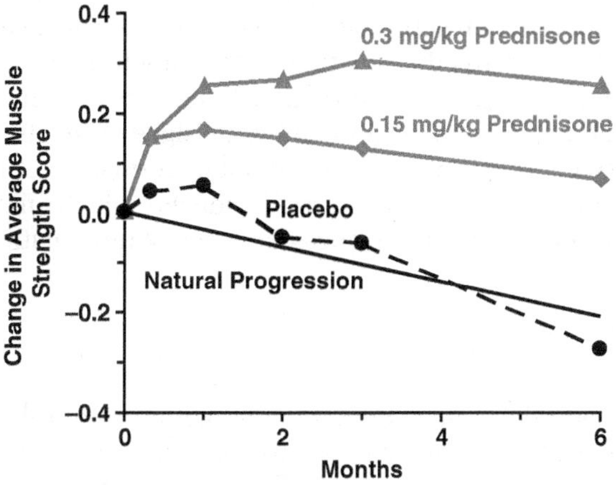

FIGURE 3-3 Mean changes in the score for average muscle strength in placebo- (*black circle*) and prednisone-treated groups (*colored diamond,* 0.3 mg/kg daily; *colored triangle,* 0.75 mg/kg daily) of male children suffering with Duchenne dystrophy after the initiation of treatments. The solid continuous straight black line represents the average natural course of the change in muscle strength score observed in another group of 177 such patients who received no treatment. (Redrawn from Griggs RC, Moxley RT, Mendell JR, et al. Prednisone in Duchenne dystrophy. *Arch Neurol* 1991;44:383–388.)

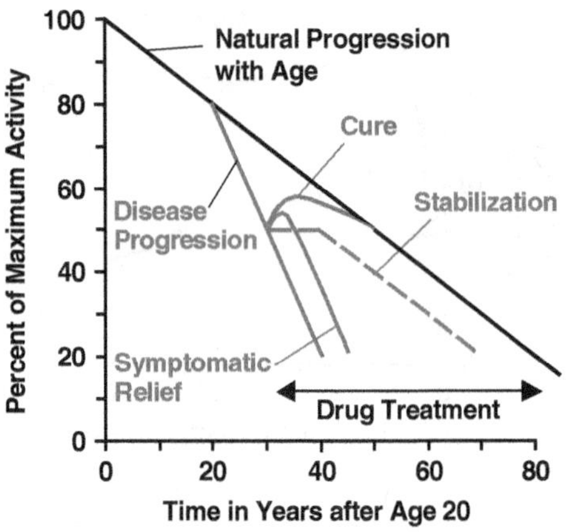

FIGURE 3-4 Schematic diagram illustrating various scenarios of effectiveness of a drug in the treatment of patients suffering from a disease that causes a faster rate of decline of a measured function than seen in otherwise healthy subjects. Treatment is symptomatic if after a period of initial benefit the measured function returns to a rate of decline seen in patients not receiving treatment. Treatment is stabilizing if it arrests the disease, returning the rate of function decline to that in otherwise healthy subjects; it may also temporarily stop further deterioration of function. Cure is achieved if the drug treatment returns the patient to the trend line for normal physiologic function with age. Drug effectiveness can, of course, lie anywhere between these various extremes.

double-blinded. Patients were assigned to one of three treatments: placebo, 0.3 mg/kg prednisone, or 0.75 mg/kg prednisone in the form of 1 capsule daily, with the study period extending over 6 months.

The data in Fig. 3-3 show several interesting points. First, at best the placebo appeared to produce an initial slight benefit when judged against the natural progression of the disease, but it was not statistically significant. Second, prednisone had a dose-dependent positive effect. For patients receiving 0.3 mg/kg prednisone daily, muscle strength increased to a maximum by the end of the first month of treatment and then declined in parallel with the natural course of the disease. A similar pattern was seen in the patient group receiving the 0.75 mg/kg daily dose, except that the improvement was greater and continued over approximately 3 months of treatment before declining once again in parallel with the natural progression of the disease. From these findings, we can conclude that prednisone provides relief of the symptoms but does not alter the course of the underlying disease.

Fig. 3-4 schematically generalizes the distinction between symptomatic relief and cure against the background of the natural course of a physiologic function. A characteristic of virtually all of our physiologic functions is that they tend to decline with advancing age beyond around 20 years. The rate of decline varies for different functions, but is commonly around 1% per year (see also Chapter 13). Many chronic diseases accelerate this rate of decline, as occurs in patients with chronic renal disease or Alzheimer's disease. Alternatively, a drug may arrest disease progression, thereby stabilizing the function, such that the measured function subsequently declines at the normal physiologic rate. A drug is curative if it restores the function in the patient back to within the normal range expected of an otherwise healthy person. For example, some drugs cure certain cancers in that such patients no longer exhibit the signs of the disease and go on to live a normal life span. This is an example of a long-term cure. An example of a short-term cure is the abolition of a severe "stress" headache, which fails to return. Obviously, there are many shades of effectiveness between symptomatic relief and long-term cure.

RELATING RESPONSE TO CONCENTRATION

Because most sites of action lie outside the vasculature, such as within the brain, delays often exist between plasma concentration and the response produced. Such delays can obscure underlying relationships between concentration and response. One potential solution is to measure concentration at the site of action. Although this may be possible in an isolated tissue system, it is rarely a practical possibility in humans. Apart from ethical and technical issues that often arise, an additional complexity is that many observed responses in vivo represent an integration of multiple drug effects and events at numerous sites within the body. Another approach to solving the relationship between plasma concentration and response is to develop a model that incorporates the time course of drug movement between plasma and site of action, thereby predicting "effect site" concentrations that can then be related to response. Still another approach is to relate plasma concentration to response under conditions whereby a constant concentration is maintained using a constant rate of drug input, which obviates consideration of the time course of its distribution. Whatever the approach adopted, the resulting concentration–response relationships for most drugs have features in common.

Graded Response

Response increases with concentration at low concentrations and tends to approach a maximum at high values. Such an effect is seen for the anesthetic ketamine, as illustrated in Fig. 3-1. *R*(−)-ketamine and *S*(+)-ketamine are optical isomers that, as the racemate (50%/50% mixture of the isomers), constitute the commercially available intravenous (IV) anesthetic agent, ketamine. Although both compounds have an anesthetic effect, they clearly differ from each other. Not only is the maximum response (E_{max}) with *R*(−)-ketamine less than that with *S*(+)-ketamine, but the plasma concentration required to produce 50% of E_{max}, referred to as the C_{50} value, is also greater (1.8 mg/L vs. 0.7 mg/L). Although the reason for the differences is unclear, these observations stress the importance that stereochemistry can have in drug response, and that drugs acting on even the same receptor do not necessarily produce the same maximal response.

An equation to describe the response ***E*** associated with the types of observations seen in Fig. 3-1 for ketamine is:

$$E = \frac{E_{max} \cdot C^{\gamma}}{C_{50}^{\gamma} + C^{\gamma}} \qquad \text{Eq. 3-2}$$

where E_{max} and C_{50} are as defined above and γ is a **steepness factor** that accommodates for the steepness of the curve around the C_{50} value. The intensity of response is usually a change in a measurement from its basal value expressed as either an absolute difference or a percent change. Examples are an increase in blood pressure and a decrease in blood glucose, expressed as a percentage of the baseline. One should always keep in mind that unbound drug drives response, and therefore the unbound concentration should be used when relating response to systemic exposure, particularly when plasma protein binding varies extensively. In the case of ketamine, the extent of plasma protein binding of (+)- and (−)-isomers is the same, so this is not the explanation for the difference in measured potency.

Although empirical, Equation 3-2 has found wide application. Certainly, it has the right properties; when $C = 0$, E is zero, and when C greatly exceeds C_{50}, response approaches E_{max}. Fig. 3-5A (next page) shows the influence of γ on the steepness of the concentration–response relationship.

The larger the value of γ, the greater is the change in response with concentration around the C_{50} value. For example, if $\gamma = 1$, then, by appropriate substitution

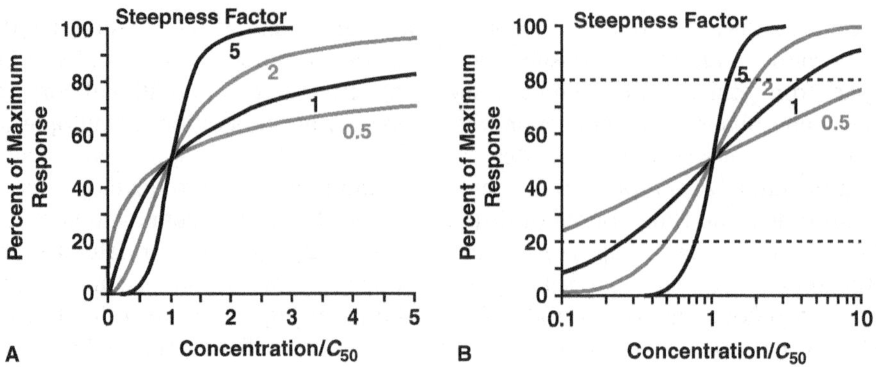

FIGURE 3-5 Linear (**A**) and semilogarithmic (**B**) concentration–response plots, predicted according to Equation 3-2, for three hypothetical drugs that have the same C_{50}, the concentration at which the response is one-half the maximum value, but different values of the steepness factor, γ. At low concentrations, the effect increases almost linearly with concentration (**A**), when $\gamma = 1$, approaching a maximal value at high concentrations. The greater the value of γ, the steeper is the change in response around the C_{50} value. Between 20% and 80% of maximal effect, the response appears to be proportional to the logarithm of the concentration (**B**) for all values of γ. Concentrations are expressed relative to C_{50}.

into Equation 3-2, the concentrations corresponding to 20% and 80% of maximal response are 0.25 and 4 times C_{50}, respectively, a 16-fold range. Whereas, if $\gamma = 2$, the corresponding concentrations are 0.5 and 2 times C_{50}, only a 4-fold range. Using the percent decrease in heart rate during a standard exercise as a measure of response to propranolol, the average value of γ is close to 1 (Fig. 3-6). Generally, the value of γ for drugs lies between 1 and 3. Occasionally, it is much greater, in which case the effect appears almost as an all-or-none response because the range of concentrations associated with minimal and maximal responses becomes so narrow.

A common form of representing concentration–response data is a plot of the intensity of response against the *logarithm* of concentration. Fig. 3-5B shows this transformation of the curves in Fig. 3-5A. This transformation is popular because it expands the initial part of the curve, where response is changing markedly with a small change in concentration, and contracts the latter part, where a large change in concentration produces only a slight change in response. It also shows that between approximately 20% and 80% of the maximum value, response appears to be proportional to the logarithm of concentration, regardless of the value of the steepness factor, γ. This relationship occurs with propranolol within the range of unbound concentrations of 1 and 10 μg/L, as shown in Fig. 3-6B after transformation of the data in Fig. 3-6A.

The greatest response produced clinically for some drugs may be less than that pharmacologically possible. For example, for a drug stimulating heart rate, the entire cardiovascular system may deteriorate, and the patient may die long before the heart rate approaches its maximum value. Other adverse effects of the drug or metabolite(s) may further limit the maximally tolerated concentration in vivo. As a general rule, it is more difficult to define the E_{max} of an agonist than of an antagonist. For an antagonist, such as a neuromuscular blocking agent used to prevent muscle movement during surgery, the maximum possible effect is easy to identify; it is the absence of a measurable response. That is, total muscle paralysis. For an agonist, it is not always certain how great the response produced can be.

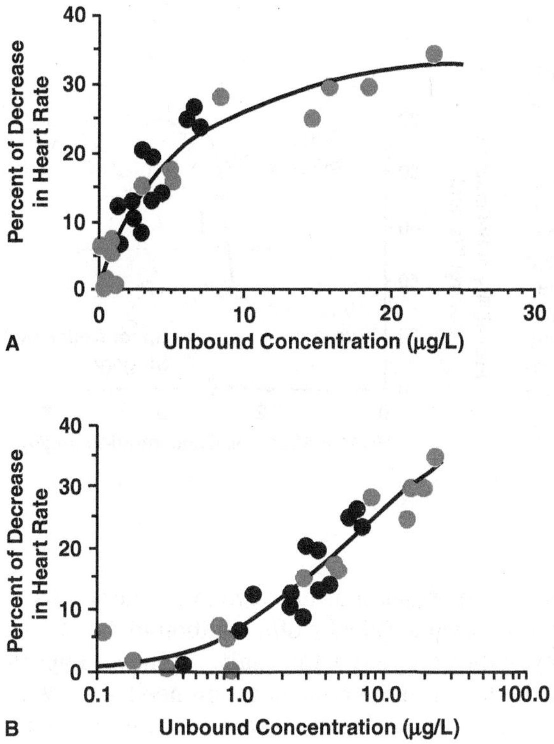

FIGURE 3-6 **A.** Response, measured by the percent decrease in exercise-induced tachycardia, to propranolol increases with an increase in the unbound concentration of the drug in plasma. **B.** The same data as in **(A)**, except that now concentration is plotted on a logarithmic scale. The data points represent measurements after single and multiple (daily) oral doses of two 80-mg tablets of propranolol (*black circle*) or a 160-mg modified-release capsule (*color*) in an individual subject. The solid line is the fit of Equation 3-2 to the data. The response appears to follow the E_{max} model with a γ of 1, an E_{max} of 40%, and a C_{50} of 5.3 μg/L. (Redrawn from Lalonde RL, Straka RJ, Pieper JA, et al. Propranolol pharmacodynamic modeling using unbound and total concentrations in healthy volunteers. *J Pharmacokinet Pharmacodyn* 1987;15:569–582.)

Quantal Response

All the preceding examples are graded responses. Unlike a graded response, a quantal response cannot be correlated continuously with concentration. Instead, the overall response is evaluated from the **cumulative frequency** or **likelihood** of the event with concentration. This is illustrated in Fig. 3-7 (next page) by a plot of cumulative frequency of satisfactory control in patients receiving the opioid analgesic alfentanil to supplement nitrous oxide anesthesia during surgery. In such cases, C_{50} refers to the concentration that produces the predetermined response in 50% of the patients, and the shape of the cumulative probability–concentration curve is determined by the distribution of values in the patient population. Fig. 3-7 also shows that the concentration needed to produce an effect may vary with the specific application. In this case, the mean C_{50} values for the three procedures were in the order: upper abdominal surgery > lower abdominal surgery > breast surgery. In common with other opioids, the cumulative frequency of the response vs. concentration curve is very steep in all three procedures. These data show that there is a narrow range of alfentanil concentrations between that which just begins to produce a satisfactory response in some patients and that which produces a satisfactory response in all patients for each type of surgery.

It should also be noted that when the quantal response is categorical, within the patient population, at any given drug concentration the sum of the probabilities of finding patients in each of the categories, for example of pain relief (no relief, mild, moderate, or full relief), always adds up to 100%. What changes with drug concentration is the probability in each category, with a shift toward a higher probability of patients experiencing full pain relief and a lower probability of no pain relief as drug concentration increases.

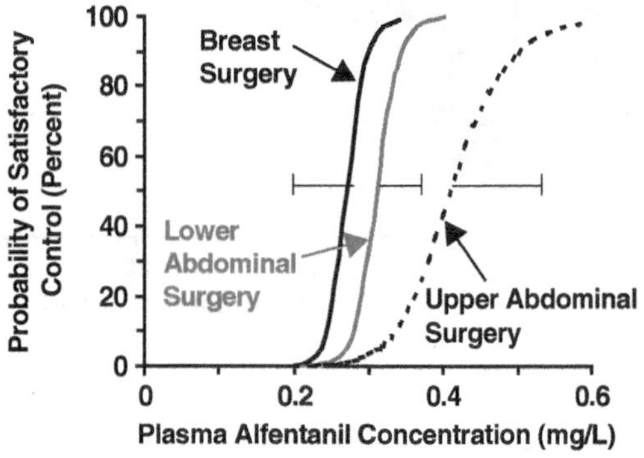

FIGURE 3-7 The relationship between the cumulative frequency in satisfactory response versus the mean arterial concentration obtained for alfentanil, an opioid analgesic, during the intraoperative period in each of three surgical groups of patients receiving nitrous oxide anesthesia. Notice, for any group, the narrow range of alfentanil concentrations between that which just begins to produce a satisfactory response in some patients to that which produces a satisfactory response in all patients. Notice also that the concentration needed to produce 50% satisfactory response is in the order: breast (0.27) < lower abdomen (0.31) < upper abdomen (0.42) surgery. (Redrawn from Ausems ME, Hug CC, Stanski DR, et al. Plasma concentrations of alfentanil required to supplement nitrous oxide anesthesia for general surgery. *Anesthesiology* 1986;65:362–373. Reproduced by permission of JB Lippincott.)

Desirable Characteristics

There is a tendency to think that the most important pharmacodynamic characteristic of a drug is its **potency**, expressed by its C_{50} value (ideally of the unbound drug). The lower the C_{50}, the greater is the potency of the compound. Certainly, potency is important, as generally the higher its value, the lower is the concentration needed to drive a therapeutic response. However, several other factors are also equally, if not more, important. One is the **selectivity** of the drug, that is, a greater therapeutic response relative to its adverse responses.

One way of increasing potency is to increase lipophilicity, for example, by adding lipophilic groups onto the molecule that increase binding to the specific target site. However, this approach also tends to increase its binding to many other nonspecific sites within the body, which may result in an increase in its side effects, relative to the desired effect, and therefore a decrease in its overall specificity, or the converse. Another very important factor is the **maximum effect** of the drug. That is, the greatest possible effect, E_{max}, that can be achieved with the compound. Returning to the example of ketamine (Fig. 3-1), it is apparent that however high we increase the concentration of *R*(−)-ketamine, we can never achieve the same maximum response as can be achieved with the *S*(+)-isomer. Clearly, if the desired therapeutic response demands that the effect be greater than can be achieved with *R*(−)-ketamine then, no matter how potent this compound, it would be of little therapeutic value when given alone. The last important pharmacodynamic factor is the steepness factor, γ. If it is very high, it may be difficult to manage the use of the drug because only a small shift in concentration around the C_{50} causes the response to change from zero to full effect, and vice versa.

EXPOSURE–RESPONSE RELATIONSHIPS

So far, relationships between response and measures of drug exposure have been explored. In clinical practice, decisions have to be made as to the dosage regimen needed to ensure optimal benefit within the confines of the conditions in which the patient receives a drug. This is a complex decision involving consideration of many factors, including not only the pharmacokinetics and pharmacodynamics of the drug but also the nature of the disease being treated, as well as a host of patient factors, both clinical and social. Some of these aspects are considered in the remainder of the book. However, at this point some broad issues centered around exposure–response relationships are worth considering.

Drugs are given to achieve therapeutic objectives; the practical question is, how best to do so? One approach is to examine the pharmacokinetics of a drug. In Fig. 3-8 are typical plots of plasma drug concentration with time following oral administration of a single dose.

One may then ask: What feature of the exposure profile is most important in the context of the desired therapeutic objective? One may argue that attention should always be placed on unbound drug, as this is the active component because bound drug is too large to cross membranes and interact with many target sites. But as discussed in Chapter 2, as long as the fraction unbound in plasma does not vary that much, as is often the case, then relating response to total drug in plasma is reasonable. In Fig. 3-8A are displayed the concentration–time profiles for two drugs achieving the same maximum concentration (C_{max}) and the same time to reach C_{max} (t_{max}) but differing in the kinetics of decline in their concentrations beyond the peak. For some drugs intended to be given chronically, it is important to only maintain the plasma concentration above a defined minimum, below which little clinical benefit is derived, even though a pharmacologic response may be measurable at still lower concentrations. Then a distinct advantage exists for the drug with the slower decline in exposure because the duration of clinical effect is clearly longer. For other drugs, however, such as those taken for the relief of a headache, the critical factor is the rapid achievement of an adequate concentration, after which maintenance of exposure becomes less important. Then C_{max} and t_{max} become the important determinants of efficacy, in which case there may be little difference between the two drugs in Fig. 3-8A. However, there may be benefit in having a rapid fall in plasma concentration, if prolonged exposure to the drug leads to an increased risk of adverse effects.

Now consider the kinetic events depicted in Fig. 3-8B in which total exposure (AUC) is the same for a drug but input is slower in one case than the other, leading to a slower decline in concentration. A slowed input may be a disadvantage if response is related directly to concentration because C_{max} would be lower and t_{max} would occur later, with the possibility of failing to achieve a sufficiently adequate clinical response. Speed of input would be of limited importance, however, if the clinical benefit for the drug were

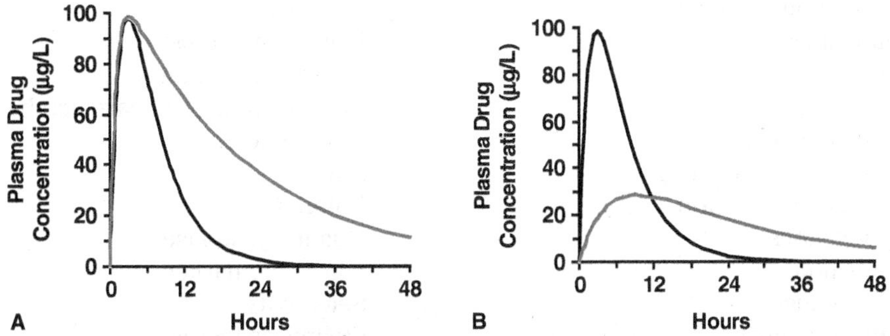

FIGURE 3-8 Schematic representations of the plasma concentration–time profiles after a single oral dose. **A.** For two drugs that produce similar peak concentrations and time to peak are shown, but one (colored line) declines more slowly than the other, thereby creating a greater total exposure (AUC) and higher concentrations at later times. **B.** For a drug that produces the same total AUC when given in two different dosage forms, the peak concentration is lower and later for the one (colored line) with the slower absorption.

determined by the total exposure (total AUC) rather than a particular concentration. These simple scenarios, as sometimes occur, clearly demonstrate that the relative therapeutic importance of different parts of the exposure–time profile of a drug depends on the clinical application and the nature of the exposure–response relationship.

Armed with the basic concepts of input–exposure and exposure–response, we now need to turn our attention in Section II, to a more in-depth consideration of the determinants of these relationships after a single dose before moving on further in Section III, to the application of this information to the design of dosage regimens. We begin by examining the critical role played by membranes.

SUMMARY

- Drugs act to provide symptomatic relief or to arrest or cure a disease or condition.
- When assessing drug effects, both the baseline and the placebo effect need to be taken into account.
- The measure of drug response may be a biomarker, a surrogate end point, or a clinical response, and may be either a measure of its effectiveness or its safety.
- Drug response may be quantal or graded. Those that are quantal may be categorical or all-or-none in nature.
- On increasing drug concentration, a graded response increases toward a maximal value, E_{max}.
- For graded responses, the concentration–response relationship may be characterized by C_{50}, E_{max}, and γ.
- Between 20% and 80% of the maximum response, the intensity of a graded response varies approximately linearly with the logarithm of the plasma concentration.
- For a quantal response, the relationship with concentration is best seen by plotting the cumulative frequency or likelihood of response against concentration, or its logarithm.
- The relative therapeutic importance of different parts of the exposure–time profile of a drug depends on the clinical application, and the nature of the concentration–response relationship.

KEY TERM REVIEW

Agonist
All-or-none response
Antagonist
Baseline
Biomarker
Clinical response
Cumulative frequency
Disease progression
Endogenous
Exogenous
Full agonist
Full antagonist
Inducer
Inhibitor
Maximum response
Partial agonist
Partial antagonist
Pharmacodynamics
Pharmacokinetic/pharmacodynamic modeling
Placebo
Potency
Quantal response
Safety biomarker
Selectivity
Steepness factor
Surrogate end point

KEY RELATIONSHIPS

$$\text{Measured response} = \text{Drug response} + \text{Placebo response} + \text{Baseline}$$

$$E = \frac{E_{max} \cdot C^{\gamma}}{C_{50}^{\gamma} + C^{\gamma}}$$

STUDY PROBLEMS

1. Which, if any, of the following terms used in classifying drug response is (are) correctly described?
   - I. Surrogate end point refers to any response that a drug produces without regard to its relationship to the clinical effect.
   - II. A safety biomarker is a response that is safe to use.
   - III. Clinical responses can be divided into subjective and objective categories. An objective measure of drug response is one in which quantitative information is obtained.

A. I only	**E.** I and III
B. II only	**F.** II and III
C. III only	**G.** All
D. I and II	**H.** None

2. The potencies of two drugs are compared in three different ways below. The two drugs act on the same receptor. Which of the statements below is (are) good description(s) of the outcome of the comparison?
   - I. The drug given in the lower dose to achieve the same response is the most potent.
   - II. When the intensity of response is the same, it is the drug with the lower C_{max} after a single dose that is the more potent.
   - III. The unbound concentration of the more potent of the two drugs during chronic therapy is lower than that of the less potent drug when the intensity of response is the same.

A. I only	**E.** I and III
B. II only	**F.** II and III
C. III only	**G.** All
D. I and II	**H.** None

3. Which *one* of the following statements assessing drug response is the *most* accurate?
   - a. The placebo response is just the difference between the measured response to a drug and the baseline.
   - b. The baseline is the difference between the measured response and the placebo response.
   - c. The drug response is the difference between the measured response and the baseline.
   - d. The measured response is the sum of the drug response, the placebo response, and the baseline.
   - e. The drug response is the difference between the measured response and the placebo response.

4. The general model for a graded drug response is

$$E = \frac{E_{\max} \cdot C^{\gamma}}{C_{50}^{\gamma} + C^{\gamma}}$$

Which of the following statements is (are) likely to be true:

I. When the value of γ, the steepness factor, is much greater than one in a mean"response versus concentration" plot, the response has the appearance of an "all-or-none" one.

II. The value of C_{50} is the concentration at which the response is one-half the maximum ($E_{max}/2$) regardless of the γ value of the steepness factor.

III. On comparing two drugs that are equally bound to plasma proteins, the one with the lower C_{50} on chronic therapy is the more potent one.

A. I only **E.** I and III
B. II only **F.** II and III
C. III only **G.** All
D. I and II **H.** None

5. What is meant by the words "agonist and antagonist" when referring to drug response?

6. a. What is a placebo effect, and why is it so important to determine it when assessing the effect of drugs?

b. Blood CD4 count is used as a measure of the strength of the immune system and to gain an estimate of the beneficial effect of drug therapy in the treatment of patients with AIDS or HIV infection. Changes in blood CD4 count during treatment with placebo and zidovudine, a nucleoside reverse transcriptase inhibitor, are displayed in Fig. 3-9. Discuss what effect zidovudine has on CD4 count in light of these observations.

7. Fig. 3-10 (next page) displays the relationship between the percent increase in the β-electroencephalographic (EEG) amplitude, expressed as a change from baseline, a measure of the central nervous system effect, and the plasma concentration of the benzodiazepine alprazolam.

a. Is the measured effect graded or quantal?

b. Estimate the E_{max}.

c. Estimate the C_{50}.

d. Is the value of the slope factor approximately one, or significantly greater?

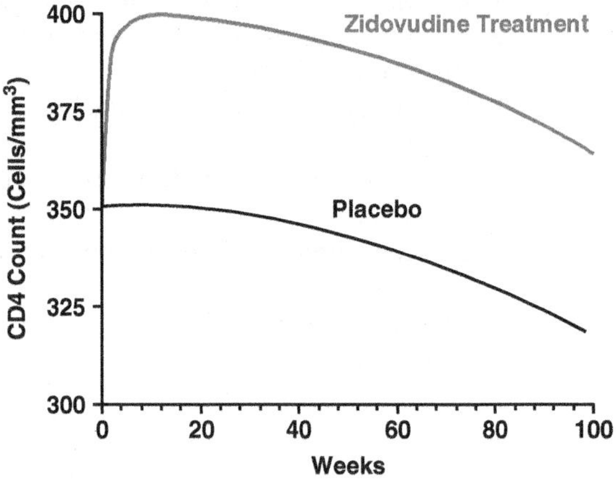

FIGURE 3-9 Changes in the blood CD4 count in HIV patients receiving either placebo (black line) or zidovudine treatment (colored line). (From Sale M, Sheiner LB, Volberding P, et al. Zidovudine response relationships in early human immunodeficiency virus infection. *Clin Pharmacol Ther* 1993;54:556–566.)

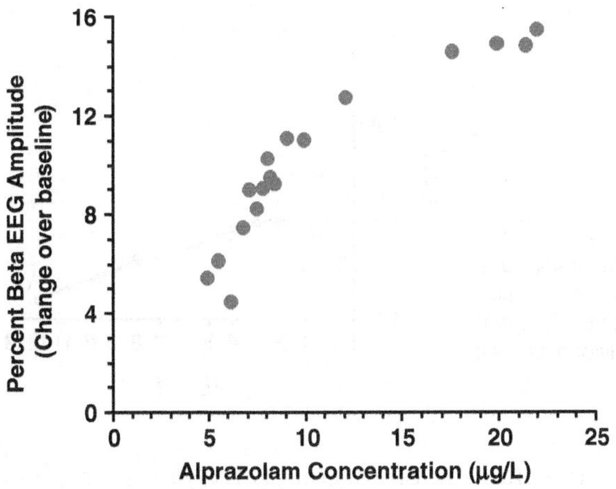

FIGURE 3-10 Mean change over baseline in the β-electroencephalographic (EEG) amplitude against alprazolam concentration in subjects receiving 1 mg alprazolam intravenously. (From Venkatakrishnan K, Culm KE, Ehrenberg BL, et al. Kinetics and dynamics of intravenous adinazolam, *N*-desmethyladinazolam, and alprazolam in healthy volunteers. *J Clin Pharmacol* 2005;45: 529–537.)

8. Fig. 3-11 is a plot of the cumulative incidence of hepatic toxicity (taken to be greater than a threefold increase in serum alanine aminotransferase [ALT], a measure of inflammation of the liver) and the total AUC of a drug in the patient population following chronic therapy. Corresponding plots against the maximum plasma concentration, or concentration at any particular time after administration of the drug, failed to show as significant a relationship as seen with AUC.
   a. Is the measured effect graded or quantal?
   b. Why might hepatic toxicity be better correlated with AUC than any particular concentration of the drug?

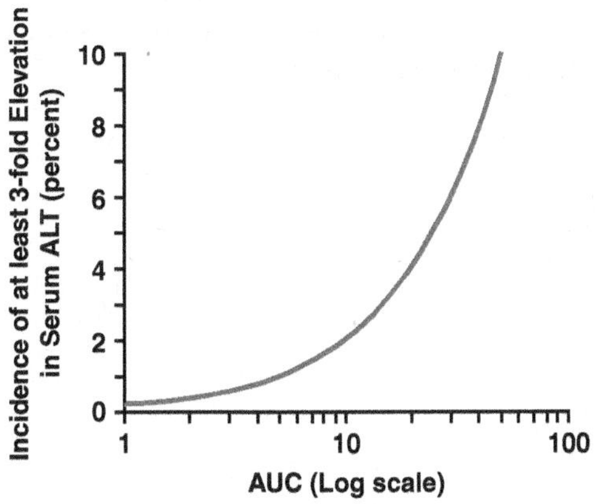

FIGURE 3-11 Incidence of hepatic toxicity (expressed as percentage of the patient population with at least a threefold increase in serum ALT) against the AUC of a drug.

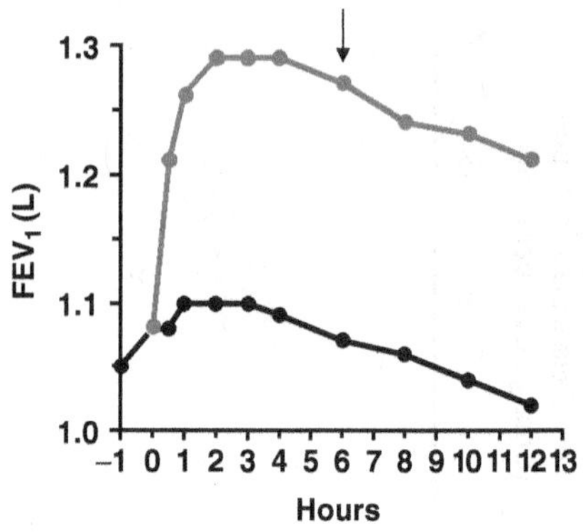

FIGURE 3-12 Time course of the FEV_1 after administration of a placebo Handihaler (*black circle*) and a Spiriva Handihaler (*colored circle*) after a single dose of tiotropium bromide. (Adapted from data in *Physician's Desk Reference*. 60th Ed. Montvale, NJ: Medical Economics Co.; 2006;900.)

9. Fig. 3-12 shows the forced expiratory volume in one second (FEV_1) for tiotropium bromide inhalation powder (Spiriva). Complete the table below to show the measured response, drug response, and placebo response to the drug ***at the 6-hour time point*** (shown by arrow). Use the value at time −1 in the graph for the baseline, and assume that the baseline does not change with time.

Measured, drug, and placebo responses to Spiriva 6 hours after its inhalation.

Measure	Measured Response	Drug Response	Placebo Response
FEV_1 (L)			
FEV_1 (% of baseline)			

10. The concentration–response relationship in a patient population for a drug that is measured by an all-or-none response is characterized by a C_{50} of 100 μg/L and a γ value of 2. Calculate the range of concentrations that are needed to achieve responses in 20% and 80% of the total population. To address this question assume that the model of Equation 3-2 can be applied to a quantal response.

SECTION II

Exposure and Response After a Single Dose

CHAPTER 4

Membranes: A Determining Factor

OBJECTIVES

The reader will be able to:

- Define the following terms: active transport, hydrophilic, hydrophobic, lipophilic, lipophobic, paracellular permeation, passive diffusion, passive facilitated transport, permeability, transcellular permeation, and transporter.
- List two examples of transporters involved in systemic absorption after oral administration, and three involved in the distribution of drugs into and out of tissues, including eliminating organs.
- Distinguish between perfusion rate–limited and permeability rate–limited passage of drugs through membranes.
- Describe the role of pH in the movement of drugs through membranes.
- Describe the consequences of the reversible nature of movement of drugs through membranes.

So far in this book, emphasis has been placed on input–response and exposure–response relationships. This section focuses primarily on factors controlling the input–exposure relationship, particularly their influence on a drug's pharmacokinetic parameters. In this chapter, we discuss the role and function of membranes primarily in the context of drug absorption and disposition, although many aspects are equally important in pharmacodynamics. We do so because essentially all drugs must pass through one or more membranes between the site of administration and the site of action to elicit a systemic response. This is followed in Chapter 5 by a discussion of the kinetics of drug disposition after intravenous administration, and in Chapter 6 by a consideration of the physiologic and physicochemical determinants of drug disposition. The next two chapters of this section cover the kinetics of drug absorption and disposition following extravascular administration (Chapter 7), and the physiologic and physicochemical determinants of drug absorption (Chapter 8). The last chapter in this section deals with response following a single dose (Chapter 9).

The order of the chapters within this section is worth commenting on. Although extravascular administration, and particularly oral dosing, is much more common than intravenous administration and therefore might reasonably be expected to be discussed first, a problem arises; namely, observations in the systemic circulation after an extravascular dose depend on both input and disposition, with no way to view or readily interpret drug input alone from such data. It is therefore helpful to first appreciate disposition principles gained following intravenous administration before analyzing observations after extravascular administration.

Before examining membranes as a determinant of drug absorption and disposition, a few terms commonly applied to the physicochemical properties of drugs need to be defined. **Hydrophilic** and **hydrophobic** are adjectives that refer to water (hydro-)-loving (-philic) and -fearing (-phobic) properties. Similarly, **lipophilic** and **lipophobic** are adjectives that relate to lipid (lipo-) -loving and lipid-fearing properties. In general, the terms hydrophilic and lipophobic are interchangeable and imply that a substance is soluble in water, but very poorly soluble in nonpolar lipids. Similarly, the terms lipophilic and hydrophobic are interchangeable and refer to substances that are soluble in lipids, but very poorly soluble in water. A common measure of lipophilicity (or hydrophobicity) of a substance is its partition between *n*-octanol (an organic solvent with hydrogen bonding properties aimed at mimicking the physicochemical properties of tissue membranes) and water. The higher the **partition coefficient,** the ratio of drug concentrations in the two phases at equilibrium, the greater is the lipophilicity. Some compounds, such as alcohol, are readily soluble in both water and many lipids. Others, such as digoxin, are poorly soluble in both water and lipids. Thus, both solubility and partition coefficient are important in absorption and disposition.

MEMBRANES

Movement through membranes is required for absorption into the body, for distribution to the various tissues of the body, including the active site, and for elimination from the body. This movement is known as **drug permeation,** a term that is often used more specifically to describe the processes and transport systems (transporters) that facilitate movement across membranes. The physicochemical, anatomic, and physiologic factors that determine the rapidity of drug permeation are the focus of this chapter. Understanding these processes is a prerequisite for an appreciation of factors controlling the pharmacokinetics and pharmacodynamics of drugs.

Cellular membranes are composed of an inner, predominantly lipoidal, matrix covered on each surface by either a continuous layer or a lattice of protein (Fig. 4-1, upper section of drawing). The hydrophobic portions of the lipid molecules are oriented toward the center of the membrane, and the outer hydrophilic regions face the surrounding aqueous environment. For some drugs, facilitative mechanisms are embedded in the protein lattice. Narrow aqueous-filled channels exist between some cells, such as blood capillary membranes, the glomerulus of the kidney, and intestinal epithelia.

The permeation or passage of drugs is often viewed as movement across a series of membranes and spaces, which, in aggregate, serve as a "functional" macroscopic membrane. The cells and interstitial spaces that lie between the intestinal lumen and the capillary blood perfusing the intestine, those that separate the brain from the blood, and the skin (Fig. 4-1) are examples. Each of the interposing cellular membranes and spaces impede drug transport to varying degrees, and any one of them can be the slowest step, rate-controlling the overall process. In the small intestine, it is the apical side of the epithelial cells, that is, the side facing the lumen. In the brain, it is the cells of, and those surrounding, the capillaries, while in the skin, the stratum corneum is the major site of impedance. These complexities of structure make it difficult to accurately extrapolate the quantitative features of drug transport from one membrane to another. Nonetheless, much can be gained by considering the general qualitative features governing drug movement across these "functional" membranes.

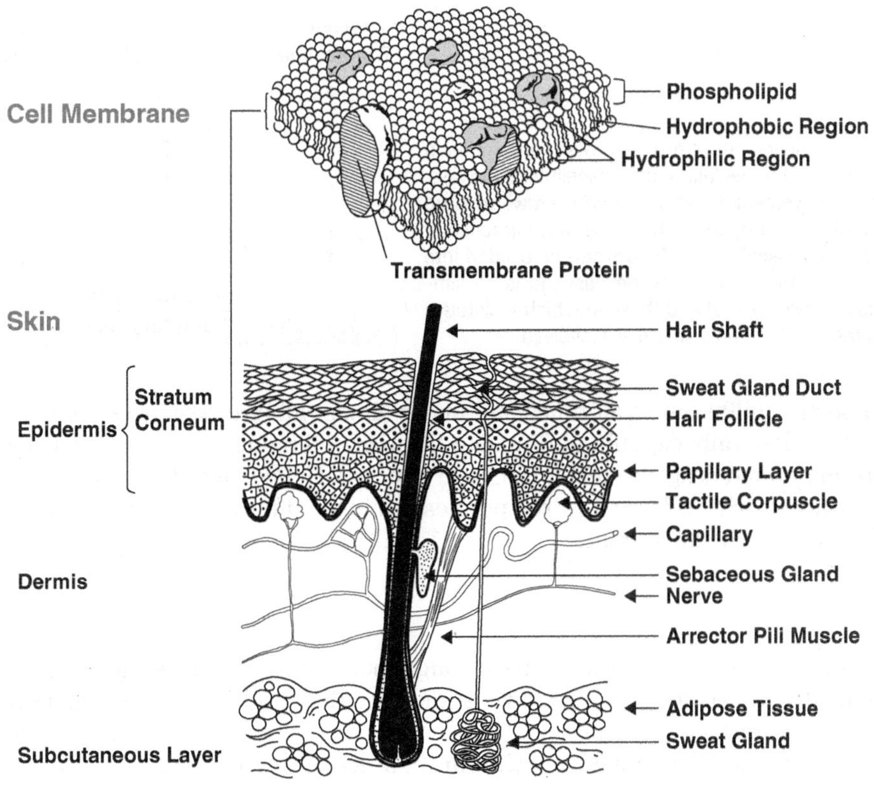

FIGURE 4-1 Functional membranes vary enormously in structure and thickness. They can be as thin as a single-cell membrane of approximately 1×10^{-6} cm thickness (*top*) to as thick as the multicellular barrier of the skin (*bottom*). This multicellular barrier extends from the stratum corneum to the upper part of the papillary layer of the dermis, adjacent to the capillaries of the microcirculation, a distance of approximately 2×10^{-2} cm. The cell membrane consists of a bimolecular leaflet, with a lipid interior and a polar exterior, dispersed through which are globular proteins, depicted as large solid irregular-shaped bodies. (Cell membrane reproduced from Singer SJ, Nicolson GL. The fluid mosaic model of the structure of cell membranes. *Science* 1972;175:720; copyright 1982 by the AAS; skin was kindly drawn by Mandy North.)

THE PROCESSES OF DRUG PERMEATION

Drug permeation can be broadly divided into **transcellular** and **paracellular** processes, as shown in Fig. 4-2 (next page). Transcellular movement, which involves the passage of drug through cells, is the most common route of drug permeation. Some drugs, however, are too polar to pass across a lipoidal cell membrane; for these, generally only the paracellular pathway through aqueous channels between the cells is available. Other drugs move across some cells by facilitative mechanisms, also called carrier-mediated transport, a topic covered later in this chapter.

Protein Binding

Before considering the determinants of the movement of drug across membranes, a comment needs to be made about protein binding. Many drugs bind to plasma proteins and tissue components (discussed in Chapter 6). Such binding is generally reversible and usually so rapid that equilibrium is established within milliseconds. In such cases, the associated (bound) and dissociated (unbound) forms of the drug can be assumed

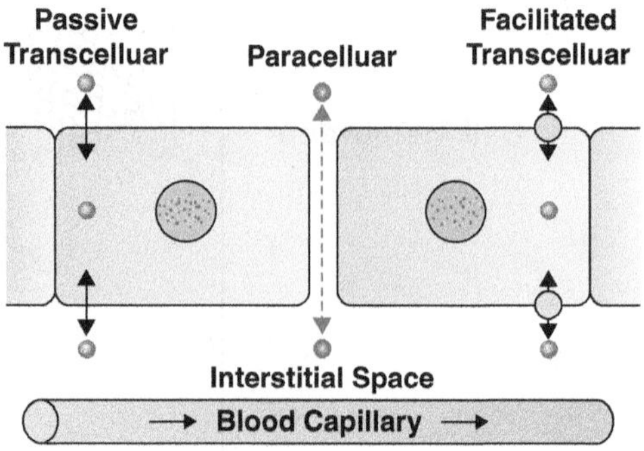

FIGURE 4-2 Movement of drugs across membranes in tissues occurs by paracellular and transcellular pathways. Paracellular movement (*dashed colored arrow*) of drug (*circle*) is influenced by the tightness of the intercellular junctions. The transcellular pathways can be divided into two categories: those in which the passage is by simple diffusion (*solid arrows*) and those in which facilitative mechanisms (*arrows with a circle*) are involved.

to be at equilibrium at all times and under almost all circumstances. Only **unbound drug** is generally capable of diffusing through cell membranes. Proteins, and hence protein-bound drug, are much too large to do so. Hence, one of the factors determining the net driving force for drug permeation is the difference in unbound concentrations across the membrane.

Diffusion

One process by which drugs pass through membranes is **diffusion,** the natural tendency for molecules to move down a concentration gradient. Movement results from the kinetic energy of the molecules. Because no work is expended by the system, the process is known as **passive diffusion.** Paracellular passage is always passive; so, too, is the transcellular permeation of many, particularly lipophilic, drugs.

To appreciate the properties of passive diffusion across a membrane, consider a simple system in which a membrane separates two well-stirred aqueous compartments. The driving force for drug transfer is the difference between the unbound concentrations in compartment 1, Cu_1, and compartment 2, Cu_2. The net rate of permeation is:

$$\text{Net rate of permeation} = P \times \text{SA} \times (Cu_1 - Cu_2) \quad \textbf{Eq. 4-1}$$

where P = permeability, SA = surface area, and $Cu_1 - Cu_2$ = the concentration difference.

The importance of the surface area of the membrane is readily apparent. For example, doubling the surface area for the same volume of fluid doubles the probability of collision with the membrane and thereby increases the permeation rate twofold. Some drugs readily pass through a membrane; others do not. This difference in ease of penetration is quantitatively expressed in terms of the **permeability, *P*,** of the drug with units of velocity (e.g., μm/min). Note that the product $P \times$ SA has the units typical of flow, volume/time.

Drug Properties Determining Passive Permeability

Three major molecular properties affecting, and sometimes limiting, the passive diffusion of a drug across a given membrane are: size, lipophilicity, and charge (or degree of ionization). These properties, together with the nature of the membrane and the medium on either side, determine the overall speed of movement of a compound across the membrane.

Molecular size has only a small impact on diffusion of substances in water. However, it has a major impact on movement through membranes. This sensitivity to size is due to the relative rigidity of cell membranes, which sterically impedes drug movement. To appreciate the impact of molecular size on the (paracellular) movement between cells, consider, for example, the passage of three water-soluble drugs, atenolol, oxytocin, and calcitonin-salmon, across two membranes, the relatively loosely knit nasal membranes and the more tightly knit gastrointestinal membranes. Atenolol, used in the treatment of hypertension, is a small stable molecule (246 g/mol) that readily passes across the nasal membranes and is even reasonably well absorbed across the gastrointestinal membranes with an oral bioavailability of 50%, facilitating its oral dosing. Oxytocin, a moderate-sized cyclic nanopeptide (1007 g/mol) used to induce labor, also rapidly crosses the nasal membranes paracellularly, but is almost totally unable to cross the gastrointestinal membranes because of its size. On the other hand, calcitonin-salmon, a synthetic polypeptide of 32 amino acids (3432 g/mol) used in the treatment of postmenopausal osteoporosis, is so large that it is only 3% absorbed from a nasal spray and cannot pass across the intestinal epithelium. Furthermore, the majority of the nasally applied oxytocin and calcitonin runs down the nasal cavity into the throat and is swallowed. The swallowed peptide then undergoes extensive degradation (digestion) by peptidases in the gastrointestinal tract such that these two drugs, and other drugs with these properties, are not prescribed for oral dosing.

A second determinant of permeability is lipophilicity. Generally, the more lipophilic a molecule the greater is its permeability, but, as mentioned, size is also important. Small lipid-soluble un-ionized drugs tend to traverse lipid membranes transcellularly with ease. This tendency and the effect of molecular size are shown in Fig. 4-3 for transdermal passage of a variety of uncharged molecules. Notice, as mentioned above, that as size increases, permeability drops sharply. For example, for only a doubling of molecular weight from 400 to 800 g/mol for molecules with the same lipophilicity, permeability decreases by a factor of almost 2.5 log units, or 300-fold.

The importance of lipophilicity and molecular size is also supported by observations of the movement of various drugs into the central nervous system (CNS), as shown in Fig. 4-4 (next page). The brain and spinal cord are protected from exposure to a variety of substances. The protective mechanism was observed many years ago

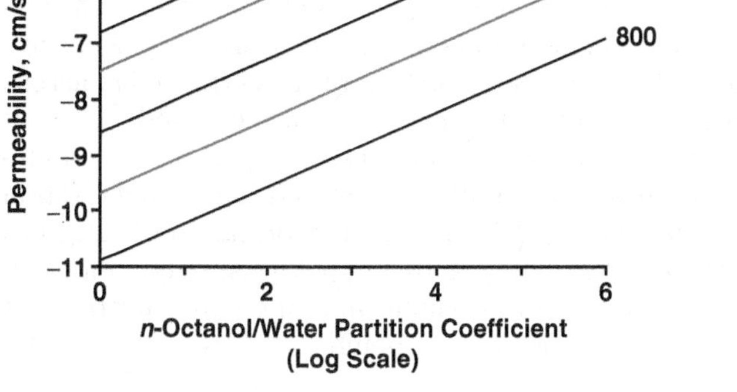

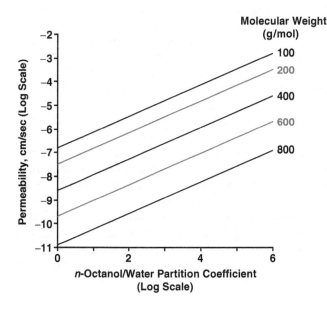

FIGURE 4-3 Permeability across skin as a function of molecular size and lipophilicity of neutral molecules. Lipophilicity is expressed as the *n*-octanol/water partition coefficient. Each line represents substances of the same molecular weight but different lipophilicity. Note that to offset the effect of reducing permeability on doubling of molecular weight from 400 to 800 g/mol, lipophilicity has to increase by four log units, from two to six, equivalent to a 10,000-fold increase in the partition coefficient. (Modified from Potts RO, Guy RH. Predicting skin permeability. *Pharm Res* 1992;9:633–669. Reproduced with permission of Plenum Publishing Corporation.)

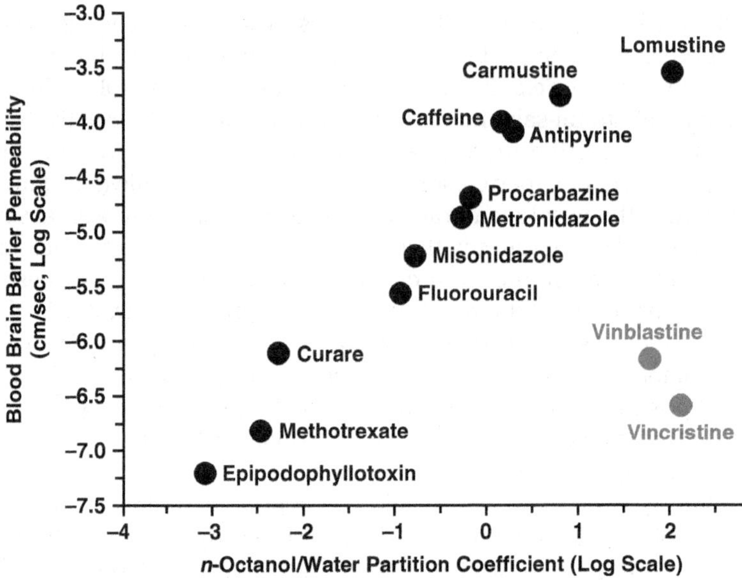

FIGURE 4-4 Relationship between permeability of a drug across the blood-brain barrier and its *n*-octanol/water partition coefficient, a measure of lipophilicity. Generally, permeability increases progressively with increasing lipophilicity (*black circles*), but not always. For compounds such as vinblastine and vincristine (*color*), the permeability is lower than expected, owing in large part to their being substrates for the efflux transporter, P-glycoprotein, which pumps these compounds out of the brain back into cerebral blood. Both axes are logarithmic. (Adapted from a chapter by Greig N. Drug delivery to the brain by blood-brain barrier circumvention and drug modification. In: Neuwelt E, ed. *Implication of the Blood-Brain Barrier and Its Manipulation.* New York, NY: Plenum Publishing Company; 1989:311-367. *Basic Science Aspects;* vol 1.)

when various hydrophilic dyes, injected intravenously into animals, stained most tissues of the body, but not the CNS, which appeared to exclude them. Thus, the concept of high impedance to the movement of these substances into the brain arose, namely, the **blood–brain barrier.** The barrier exists because of very tight junctions between the endothelial capillary cells as well as highly resistant glial processes surrounding the capillaries. Fig. 4-4 clearly shows that lipophilicity, as measured by the *n*-octanol/water partition coefficient, is a major correlate of permeability of drugs across the blood–brain barrier. The two major exceptions, the anticancer drugs vinblastine and vincristine, are large molecules (molecular masses of 814 and 824 g/mol, respectively), and, as stated above, size is a major determinant of passage across membranes. The drugs are also good substrates of efflux transporters, a topic of the next section.

Charge is the third major constraint to transmembrane passage. Again, there is considerable variation in the impedance of different membranes to charged molecules, but with a few exceptions (e.g., those involving paracellular permeation across the blood capillary membranes and renal glomerulus), the effect of charge is always large. The larger and more hydrophilic a molecule, the lower is its permeability across membranes. Permeability is further reduced if the molecule is also charged.

Most drugs are weak acids or weak bases and exist in solution with their un-ionized and ionized forms in equilibrium with each other. Increased total concentration of drug on the side of a membrane where pH favors greater ionization of drug has led to the **pH partition hypothesis.** According to this hypothesis, only un-ionized nonpolar drug penetrates the membrane, and at equilibrium, the concentrations of the un-ionized species are equal on both sides of the membrane. However, the total

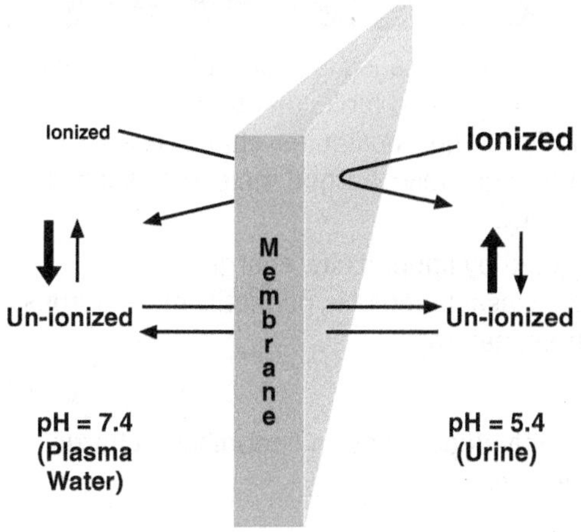

FIGURE 4-5 When a drug is a weak acid or weak base, its total concentration on one side of a lipid membrane may be very different from that on the other side at equilibrium, if the pH values of the two aqueous phases are different. One mechanism producing this concentration difference is the **pH partition hypothesis,** which states that only the un-ionized form can cross the membrane and be equal on both sides at equilibrium. The total concentration on each side at equilibrium depends on the degree of ionization. The side with greater ionization has the higher total concentration. For weak bases, in the example shown, the total concentration is greater on the side with the lower pH; the opposite applies to weak acids. The relative concentrations of un-ionized and ionized drug on both sides of the membrane are shown by the font sizes and the direction of the heavy arrows. The weak base has a p*Ka* of 6.4.

concentrations may be very different because of the differences in degree of ionization, as shown in Fig. 4-5. The topic of ionization and the pH partition hypothesis is expanded upon in Appendix C.

The majority of evidence supporting the pH partition hypothesis stems from studies of gastric secretion, intestinal absorption, and renal excretion—all anatomic locations where pH is highly variable and different. The pH of gastric fluid varies between 1.5 and 7.0; that of intestinal fluids varies between 6.2 and 7.5, whereas urine pH varies between 4.5 and 7.5. Elsewhere in the body, changes in pH tend to be much smaller and to show less deviation from the pH of blood, 7.4. An exception is the acidic (pH 5) lysosomal region of cells where digestion of intracellular material takes place.

Despite its general appeal, the pH partition hypothesis fails to explain certain observations. Some small quaternary ammonium compounds (e.g., bethanachol chloride), which are always ionized, elicit systemic effects when given orally. These and the ionized form of other compounds move through the gastrointestinal membranes, although at a slow and unpredictable rate. For some small compounds, permeation is paracellular, whereas for many others permeating transcellularly, influx and efflux transporters are involved. For these reasons, although the trend is for greater accumulation on the side that favors ionization, quantitative prediction of the influence of pH on the movement of drugs across a membrane is often inaccurate.

Membrane Characteristics

Although molecular size, lipophilicity, and charge are generally key determinants of passage of compounds across membranes, properties of the membrane itself are also important. Some membranes, such as the renal glomerulus and blood capillaries of most tissues, are highly permeable to molecules up to 5000 g/mol in size with little effect of charge or lipophilicity. In these cases, drug transfer occurs paracellularly by movement through large fenestrations (windows) in the membrane. Movement of plasma water through the fenestrations (a convective process) augments the transport. Table 4-1 lists membranes in general ascending order (from blood capillaries to blood–brain barrier) with regard to the influence of size, lipophilicity, and charge on drug permeation.

Another determinant of permeability is membrane thickness, the distance a molecule has to traverse from the site of interest (e.g., an absorption surface) to a blood

TABLE 4-1 | Properties of Different Membranes

Blood capillaries (except in testes, placenta, and most of the CNS) Renal glomerulus	Transport through membranes is basically independent of lipophilicity, charge, and molecular size (up to ~5000 g/mol). For larger molecules, charge is also important, with negatively charged molecules showing lower permeability.
Nasal mucosa Buccal mucosa Gastrointestinal tract Lung	Transport affected by lipophilicity, charge, and molecular size. Nasal mucosa is generally more porous than gastrointestinal tract.
Hepatocyte Renal tubule Blood-brain barrier	Transport is highly dependent on lipophilicity, charge, and molecular size.

capillary. The shorter the distance, the higher is the permeability. This distance can vary from about 0.005 to 0.01 μm (for cell membranes) to several millimeters (at some skin sites, Fig. 4-1, lower part of figure).

Movement across membranes continues toward equilibrium, a condition in which the concentrations of the diffusing (generally unbound and uncharged) species are the same in the aqueous phases on both sides of the membrane. Movement of drug between these phases still continues at equilibrium, but the net flux is zero. Equilibrium is achieved more rapidly with highly permeable drugs, and when there is a large surface area of contact with the membrane, that is when the $P \times SA$ product is high.

Initially, when drug is placed on one side of the membrane, it follows from Equation 4-1 that the rate of its movement across the membrane is directly proportional to concentration (Fig. 4-6). For example, the rate of its passage is increased twofold when the concentration of drug is doubled. Stated differently, each molecule diffuses independently of the other, and there is no upper limit to the rate of transport unless the drug alters the nature of the membrane or one reaches the solubility of the drug. Both absence of competition between molecules and lack of an upper limit to the rate of passage are characteristics of passive diffusion.

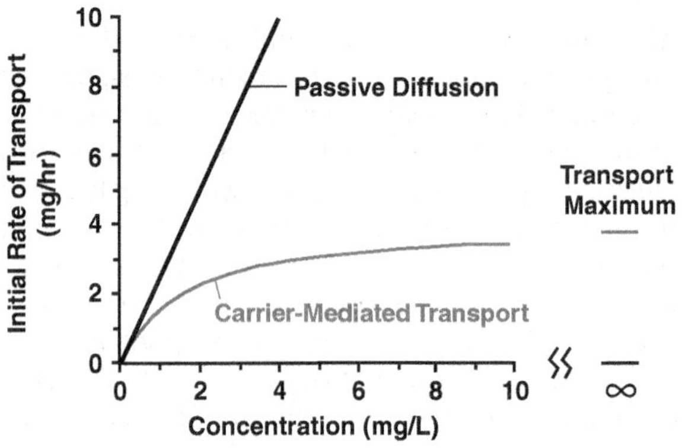

FIGURE 4-6 Initial rate of drug transport is plotted against the concentration of drug placed on one side of a membrane. With passive diffusion, the rate of transport increases linearly with concentration. With carrier-mediated transport, the rate of transport approaches a limiting value at high concentrations, the transport maximum.

Carrier-Mediated Transport

Although many drugs passively move through cells, for many others, the movement is facilitated; that is, their passage across a membrane is facilitated or faster than expected from their physicochemical properties assuming passive diffusion alone. Fig. 4-7 shows several types of facilitated processes. The first example is **passive facilitated diffusion,** in which movement is facilitated by a **transporter,** or transport system, which aids in speeding up the bidirectional process but does not change the condition at equilibrium. Such transporters are sometimes known as **equilibrating transporters.**

Passive facilitated diffusion is exemplified by the gastrointestinal absorption of many nucleosides and nucleobases, and their transmembrane passage into and out of tissue cells. It is a passive process; the nucleosides and nucleobases move down a concentration gradient without expenditure of energy, and, at equilibrium, the concentrations across the membrane are equal. At high plasma drug concentrations, however, the rate of transport reaches a limiting value or **transport maximum.** This is a characteristic of facilitated transport processes, as shown schematically in Fig. 4-6, and these processes are therefore commonly said to show **capacity-limited transport**. Furthermore, in common with other carrier-mediated systems, passive facilitated transport is reasonably specific and is inhibited by other substrates of the same carrier. Drugs, so handled, include cytarabine, used to treat hairy cell leukemia, and gemcitabine, used in treating pancreatic cancer.

Additional types of facilitated transport, shown in Fig. 4-7 for intestinal transport, require energy and are capable of moving drug against an opposing concentration gradient. They are ATP (adenosine triphosphate)-dependent, the source of the energy on conversion of ATP to ADP (adenosine diphosphate), and are examples of **active transport** systems, sometimes known as **concentrating transporters.** The direction of net movement may be either into the cell (**influx** or **uptake transporter**) or out of the cell (**efflux transporter**) and may occur on either the apical (lumen) or basolateral (blood) side of the membrane. Intracellular metabolizing enzymes may

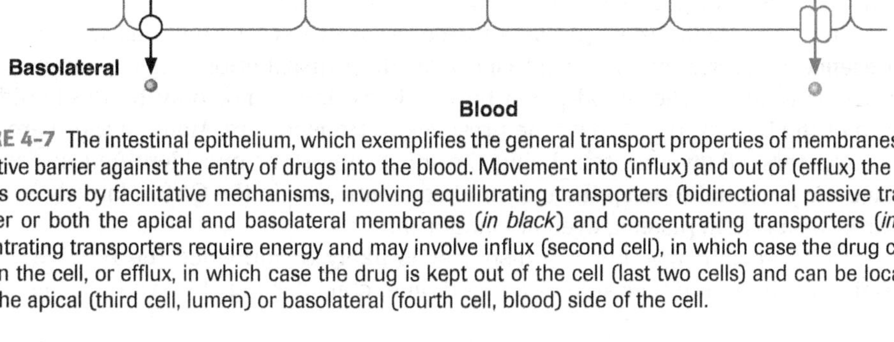

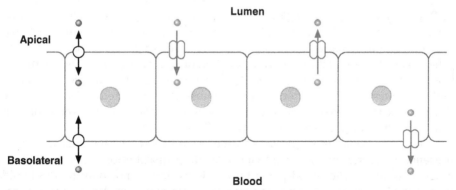

FIGURE 4-7 The intestinal epithelium, which exemplifies the general transport properties of membranes, forms a selective barrier against the entry of drugs into the blood. Movement into (influx) and out of (efflux) the epithelial cells occurs by facilitative mechanisms, involving equilibrating transporters (bidirectional passive transport at either or both the apical and basolateral membranes (*in black*) and concentrating transporters (*in color*). Concentrating transporters require energy and may involve influx (second cell), in which case the drug concentrates in the cell, or efflux, in which case the drug is kept out of the cell (last two cells) and can be located on either the apical (third cell, lumen) or basolateral (fourth cell, blood) side of the cell.

TABLE 4-2 | Examples of Transporters and Their Substrates

Human Gene	Common Name	Other Names	Substrates	Cellular Transport Direction
Concentrating Transporters				
ABCB1	MDRI	P-glycoprotein	Cationic or neutral drugs	Efflux
ABCC2	MRP2	cMOAT	Anionic drug conjugates, Methotrexate	Efflux
ABCG2	BCRP[a]	MXRI	Doxorubicin	Efflux
SLCO1B1	OATP1B1		Atorvastatin	Influx
SLC21A6	OATP-C[b]	LST-1	Benzylpenicillin	Influx
		OATP2	Digoxin	
		OATP6	Pravastatin, Rifampicin	
SLC22A8	OAT3		Methotrexate	Influx
Equilibrating Transporters				
SLC29A1	ENT1		Purine and pyrimidine	Both
SLC29A2	ENT2		Nucleosides	Both

[a]Breast cancer resistance protein.
[b]Organic anion-transporting polypeptide.
Adapted from information kindly provided by Jash Unadkat, University of Washington.

convert the drug to another substance before they both reach the blood. Apical efflux transporters and intracellular enzymes in the intestines can, by concerted action, materially reduce systemic absorption of some drugs given orally.

Efflux transporters also play a major role in removing metabolic end products and xenobiotic (foreign) substances from cells and organs. Our awareness of the therapeutic importance of efflux transporters began when certain tumor cells were observed to be resistant to specific anticancer drugs. A transporter appeared to exclude many drugs from the cell—the multiple drug-resistant receptor (MDR1). A specific glycoprotein, which resides in the cell membrane and is called *permeability* glycoprotein, or **P-glycoprotein** (170,000 g/mol), was found to be responsible. This ATP-dependent transporter is located in the cell membrane of many organs and tissues. It also plays a major role in the hepatic secretion into bile of many drugs, the renal secretion of many others, and the rate and extent of absorption of some drugs from the gastrointestinal tract. Many other drug transporters have been identified. Examples of equilibrating and concentrating transporters and their substrates are listed in Table 4-2. The location of these transporters and the processes in which they are involved in drug absorption and disposition are shown schematically in Fig. 4-8.

The CNS exemplifies, perhaps to the greatest extent, the consequences of the presence of carrier-mediated transport on drug distribution. The apparent lack of movement across the blood–brain barrier is explained not only by the lipoidal nature of the barrier, but also by the presence of transporters. Many of these are efflux transporters—P-glycoprotein being the most important one identified so far—that have the potential to keep the unbound concentration in the CNS relatively low compared with that in plasma, even at equilibrium.

To appreciate whether a transporter is likely to influence the relative concentration of drug on either side of a membrane, consider Fig. 4-9, which schematically

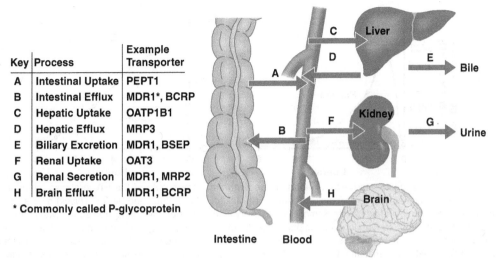

Key	Process	Example Transporter
A	Intestinal Uptake	PEPT1
B	Intestinal Efflux	MDR1*, BCRP
C	Hepatic Uptake	OATP1B1
D	Hepatic Efflux	MRP3
E	Biliary Excretion	MDR1, BSEP
F	Renal Uptake	OAT3
G	Renal Secretion	MDR1, MRP2
H	Brain Efflux	MDR1, BCRP

* Commonly called P-glycoprotein

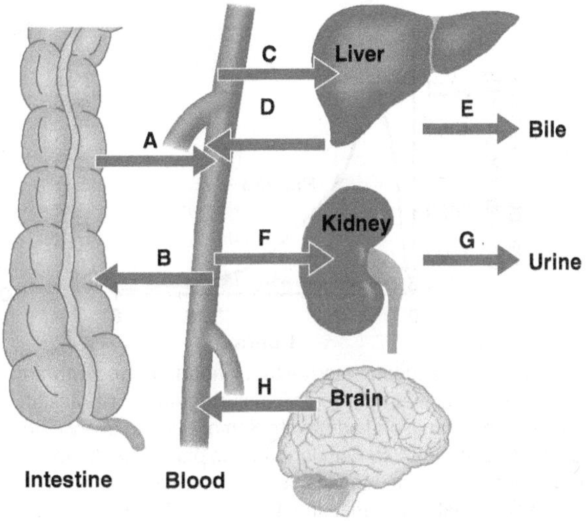

FIGURE 4-8 Selected transporters involved in intestinal absorption and in disposition of drugs within the liver, kidney, and brain. The names of these transporters and their general transport function within each of these tissues are identified. The arrows point in the direction of the transport process.

shows three permeation processes in the brain; passive diffusion, passive facilitated diffusion, and active efflux transport. In Fig. 4-9A, the passive processes are fast, and active efflux transport is relatively slow or absent. As a consequence, the unbound concentration in the brain is virtually the same as that in plasma at equilibrium. In Fig. 4-9B, the passive processes are slow compared with the efflux process, so that

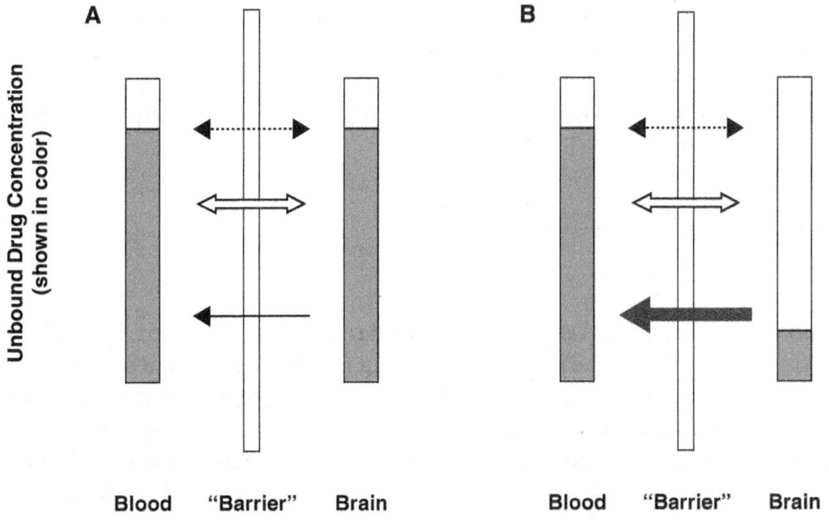

FIGURE 4-9 Substances enter the brain by simple diffusion (*dashed arrow*) and facilitated diffusion (*open arrow*). **A**: Even when active efflux transporters (*solid arrow*) are also involved, the equilibrium ratio of unbound concentrations, brain to blood, can be close to one if the passive processes are inherently faster than the efflux transport (*fine arrow*), or close to zero if the opposite is true (**B**; thick efflux arrow). For substances whose physicochemical properties (small in size, lipophilic, no charge) make them diffuse quickly, equilibrium tends to be rapidly achieved.

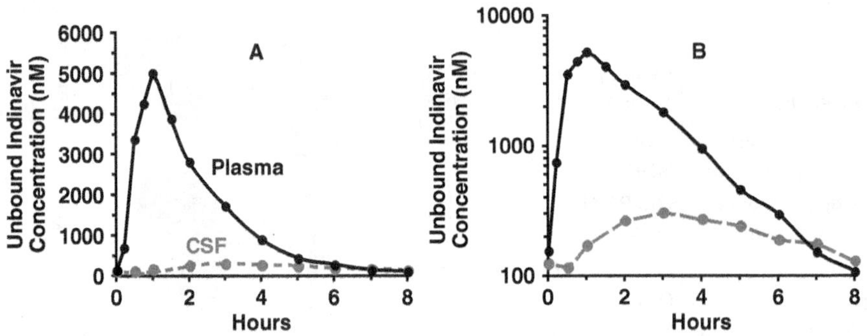

FIGURE 4-10 The mean steady-state unbound concentration–time profile of the HIV protease inhibitor indinavir in cerebrospinal fluid (*color*), a surrogate for extracellular brain fluid, and plasma (*black*) over a dosing interval during chronic oral administration of 800 mg every 8 hours in eight symptom-free adults with HIV type 1 infection. **A.** Linear plot. **B.** Semilogarithmic plot. Note the much lower average unbound indinavir concentration in cerebrospinal fluid than in plasma. Also, note that the unbound cerebrospinal fluid concentration peaks much later than does that of plasma, and it has a greatly reduced fluctuation. These observations are consequences of the drug being actively transported out, resulting in a slow and incomplete movement of drug into the cerebrospinal fluid. (Data from Haas DW, Stone J, Clough LA, et al. Steady-state pharmacokinetics of indinavir in cerebrospinal fluid and plasma among adults with human immunodeficiency virus type 1 infection. *Clin Pharmacol Ther* 2000;68:367–374.)

the unbound concentration within the brain always remains low compared with that in plasma. The apparent lack of entry into the CNS is shown in Fig. 4-10 for indinavir, a relatively large compound (MW = 712 g/mol) that has been used for treating HIV infections. Such concentration gradients are also found for vinblastine and vincristine, mentioned previously.

Antihistamines demonstrate the importance of drug transport and lipophilicity in drug action. Unlike the first-generation antihistamines, which caused drowsiness, the second-generation antihistamines are essentially devoid of sedative properties, not because they interact at a different receptor or have a stimulating effect, but because they penetrate the blood–brain barrier poorly. This poor penetration is a consequence of their being good substrates for the efflux transporter, P-glycoprotein, as well as being more hydrophilic (Fig. 4-9B).

BLOOD FLOW VERSUS PERMEABILITY

Perfusion-Rate Limitation

Blood, while perfusing tissues, delivers and removes substances. Accordingly, viewing any tissue as a whole, the movement of drug through membranes cannot be separated from perfusion considerations. Perfusion is usually expressed in units of milliliters per minute (mL/min) per gram of tissue. When movement through a membrane readily occurs, the slowest or rate-limiting step in the entire process is perfusion, not permeability, as shown in Fig. 4-11A. The initial rate of movement of drug into a tissue is determined by the rate of its delivery, which depends on blood flow.

Similarly, the concentration of a highly permeable drug in blood leaving a tissue is at equilibrium with that in the tissue. Thus, blood flow determines how quickly drug is both taken up by, and removed from, the tissue. Such a **perfusion-rate limitation** is exemplified in Fig. 4-12 (on p 62) for the passage of selected hydrophilic substances across the jejunal membranes of a rat, from lumen to blood. The blood acts as a sink

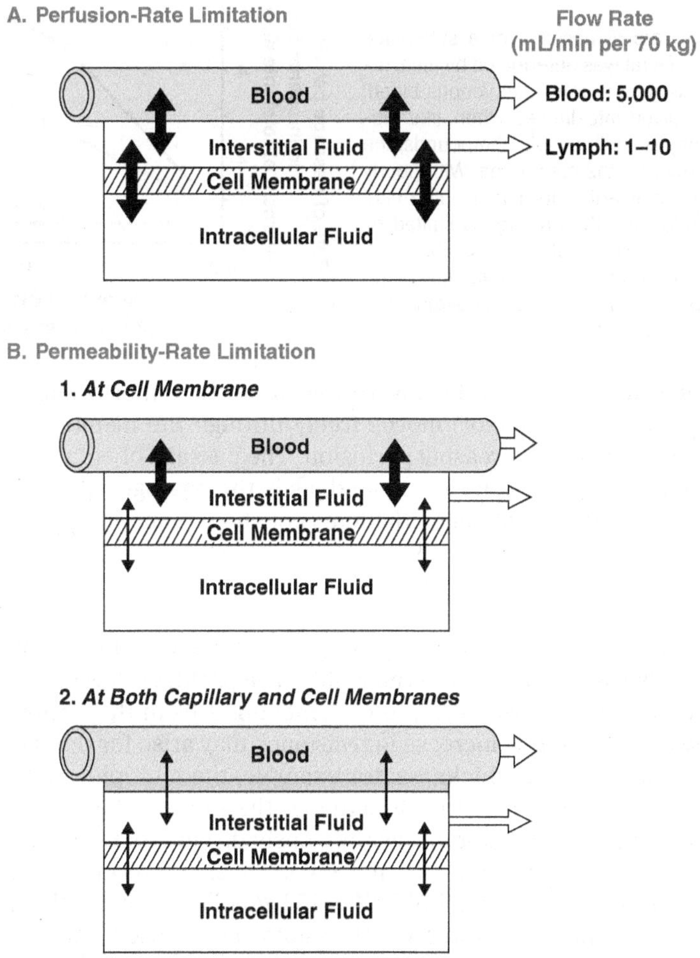

FIGURE 4-11 The limiting step controlling rate of movement of drug across membranes, from blood to tissue or the converse, varies. **A.** If membranes offer no resistance (noted by *large arrows*), drug in the blood leaving the tissue is in virtual equilibrium with that within the interstitial fluids and cells; blood and tissue may be viewed as one compartment. Here, movement of drug is limited by blood flow, a perfusion-rate limitation. **B.** A permeability-rate limitation exists if membrane resistance to drug movement becomes high (noted by *small arrows*); movement into such tissues is both slow and insensitive to changes in perfusion. Also, equilibrium is not achieved between cells and blood by the time the blood leaves the tissue; blood and tissue cells must now be viewed as separate drug compartments. For some tissues, such as muscle, kidneys and heart, the permeability limitation is at the cell membrane (**B1**). For others, such as the CNS, an additional permeability limitation occurs at the capillary membrane (**B2**). Interstitial fluid also flows into the lymphatic system. Although low at 1–10 mL/min/70 kg, compared with a blood flow of 5000 mL/min/70 kg, lymph flow plays a major role in keeping the concentration of slowly diffusing molecules, especially proteins, low in the interstitial fluid, relative to that in the blood. The lymphatic pathway is also important for the systemic absorption of macromolecules after intramuscular and subcutaneous administration (see Chapter 7). These large molecules move through the capillary membranes so slowly that by default they mostly reach the systemic blood by moving through the lymphatic vessels, which in turn empty into the systemic blood via the vena cava. For macromolecules, then, the arrows in the lower graph become thin ones, and movement into lymph predominates.

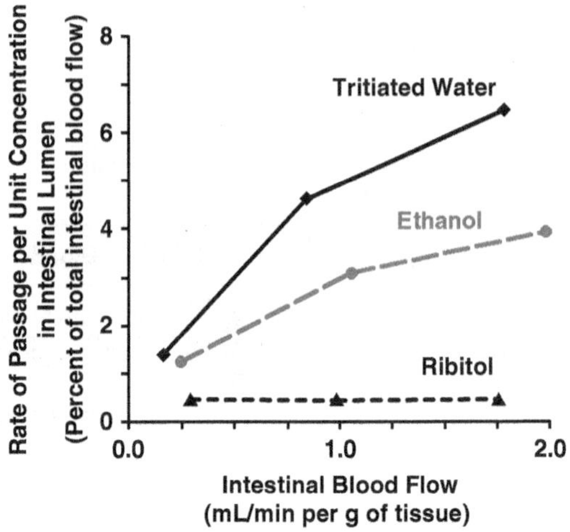

FIGURE 4-12 The rate of passage of a substance across the jejunum of a rat was determined by measuring its rate of appearance in intestinal venous blood. The passage is perfusion rate–limited when, like tritiated water and many small lipophilic compounds, the molecule freely permeates the membrane. With poorly permeable substances, like the polar molecule ribitol and many polar antibiotics, the passage is limited by transmembrane permeability, not by perfusion. (Redrawn from Winne D, Remischovsky J. Intestinal blood flow and absorption of non-dissociable substances. *J Pharm Pharmacol* 1970;22:640–641.)

by carrying drug away from the absorption site to the other tissues of the body. Tritiated water (MW = 18 g/mol) moves freely through the membrane, and its rate of passage increases with increasing perfusion. The passage of ethanol (MW = 46 g/mol) is similarly mostly perfusion rate–limited, as is the passage of many small lipophilic molecules across the intestinal epithelium (not shown) and many other membranes.

Permeability-Rate Limitation

As cell membrane resistance to drug passage increases, the rate limitation moves away from one of perfusion to one of permeability. The problem now lies in penetrating the membrane, not in delivering drug to or removing it from the tissue (Fig. 4-11B). As mentioned previously, this increase in resistance may arise for the same drug crossing membranes of increasing thickness; for example, the multiple cell layers of the skin epidermis are less permeable to a drug than is the single-cell layer of the capillary epithelium. For the same membrane, as previously discussed, resistance increases with increasing size and polarity of the molecule. Thus, transport across the jejunum is slower for the pentose sugar ribitol (MW = 152 g/mol) and many other large polar compounds than for ethanol or water, which results in decreased sensitivity to changes in perfusion (Fig. 4-12).

With large differences in perfusion and permeability of various tissues, it would appear to be impossible to predict tissue distribution of a drug. However, either of these two factors may limit the rate of **extravasation,** movement out of the vasculature, thereby simplifying the situation and allowing some conclusion to be drawn. Consider, for example, the following question: "Why, on measuring total tissue concentration, does the intravenous anesthetic propofol enter the brain much more rapidly than it does muscle tissue; yet for penicillin, the opposite is true?" The explanation lies in both the physicochemical properties of these drugs and the anatomic features of these tissues.

Propofol is a small (178 g/mol), nonpolar, highly lipophilic, very weak acid (pK_a = 11) that is insignificantly ionized at plasma pH (7.4). As such, its entry into both brain and muscle occurs readily and is perfusion-rate limited. Because perfusion of the brain, at an average of 0.5 mL/min/g of tissue, is much greater than that of muscle, at 0.025 mL/min/g of tissue, entry of propofol into the brain is the more rapid process, which explains its use in rapidly inducing anesthesia.

Penicillin, a polar, relatively strong, acid (pK_a = 2.7), MW 334 g/mol, is essentially fully ionized at pH 7.4 and does not readily pass through cell membranes. The faster rate of entry of penicillin into muscle than into the brain arises from the greater porosity of blood capillaries in muscle. As depicted in Fig. 4-11B1, for many tissues such as muscle and subcutaneous tissue, capillary membranes are very porous and have little influence on the entry of drugs of usual molecular weight (100–400 g/mol), and even larger molecules up to 5,000 g/mol, into the interstitial fluids between cells, regardless of the drug's physicochemical properties. There may well be a permeability limitation at the tissue cell membrane, but in terms of measurement of drug in the *whole* tissue, there appears to be minimal impedance to entry of either ionized or polar compounds, or both. Other tissues (Fig. 4-11B2), such as much of the CNS, anatomically have a permeability limitation at the capillary level that impedes movement of drug into the tissue as a whole, as observed with penicillin. As mentioned previously, this observation, especially with a number of polar organic dyes, led to the concept of the blood–brain barrier.

For macromolecules (>10,000 g/mol), especially charged or polar ones, movement across the capillary membrane is slow (permeability rate–limited). As a consequence, molecules that do slowly move from blood to the intestinal space tend not to return by this same route but rather, by default, move into the lymphatic system, which drains interstitial fluid from virtually all tissues. There is also a slow convective flow of water in the direction of the lymph, which may impede the back diffusion. The average flow of interstitial fluid into the lymph capillaries within the body is about 10 mL/min, whereas the rate of return of lymph to the blood is about 1 mL/min. The difference is accounted for by reabsorption of water from the lymphatic vessels and lymph nodes. As shown in Fig. 4-11, the flow of interstitial fluid into lymph capillaries and the return of lymph to the blood are much slower than the flow of blood to and from the body's tissues (~5000 mL/min). Nevertheless, the lymphatic system plays a major role in keeping the concentration of such large molecules lower in the interstitial fluids than in plasma. It is also important in determining the rate and extent of systemic absorption of macromolecules after their intramuscular or subcutaneous administration, a topic covered in Chapter 8.

REVERSIBLE NATURE OF DRUG PERMEATION

It is important to remember that drug permeation across membranes is generally bidirectional. One tends to think of the movement between gastrointestinal lumen and blood as unidirectional, resulting in drug absorption. Normally, with very high initial concentrations of drug in the gastrointestinal lumen after oral administration, relative to the unbound drug concentration in blood, the net rate of movement is indeed toward the systemic circulation. However, important applications can be made of movement in the opposite direction. For example, repeated oral administration of charcoal or the ion-exchange resin cholestyramine can hasten removal from the body of drugs such as digoxin, phenobarbital, and the active immunomodulatory metabolite of the prodrug leflunomide in cases of overdose. Data for the leflunomide metabolite are given in Table 4-3 (next page). Because of repeated administration of charcoal and extensive adsorption of the drug on to charcoal, the lumen of the gastrointestinal tract acts as a sink. The metabolite is removed both directly from blood via the intestinal membranes and by preventing its reabsorption after its biliary excretion. In general, to optimize removal, it is important to maintain distribution of adsorbent along the entire gastrointestinal tract by administering it repeatedly. Even with proper distribution of

TABLE 4-3 | Time to Reduce the Plasma Concentration of the Active Metabolite of the Prodrug Leflunomide by 50% in the Presence and Absence of Activated Charcoal Treatment

	No Charcoal Treatment	Charcoal Treatment[a]
Time for plasma concentration to drop in half	14–18 days	1–2 days

Suspension of activated charcoal was given (orally or by nasogastric tube) in a dosage of 50 g every 6 hours.
[a]Rozman B. Clinical pharmacokinetics of leflunomide. *Clin Pharmacokinet* 2002;41:421–430.

the adsorbent, the overall rate of transfer into the intestinal lumen depends on the permeability of the functional membranes along the length of the gut, as well as on blood flow to these various sites. When elimination primarily occurs by biliary excretion, as with the leflunomide metabolite, then it may be particularly important for the adsorbent to be in the duodenum in sufficient amounts to adsorb drug when the gallbladder empties, that is, after eating.

Adsorbents such as charcoal and cholestyramine are also administered (often by nasogastric tube) to decrease the rate and extent of absorption of drugs and other substances after their oral intake in cases of acute intoxication. One key to the success of these procedures is to administer the adsorbent while much of the substance still resides in the stomach to prevent or slow its intestinal absorption. Even if most of the dose has been systemically absorbed, the adsorbent may still help remove the substance from the body by the processes discussed in the previous paragraph.

The concepts of this chapter on passage of drugs across membranes are important to an understanding of movement of drugs into, within, and out of the body. In the following chapters these concepts are incorporated with other principles dealing with drug distribution, elimination, and absorption.

SUMMARY

- Molecular size, lipophilicity, charge, degree of ionization, blood flow, and protein binding play major roles in determining the permeation of drugs across membranes.
- Drug movement across membranes can be classified as transcellular and paracellular.
- Paracellular movement is always passive.
- Transcellular movement occurs by both passive diffusion and facilitated processes.
- Facilitated transport can be passive or active (requiring energy). The transport systems are called transporters.
- Both influx (uptake) and efflux transporters are involved in the absorption of many drugs in the gastrointestinal tract. They also contribute to movement into and out of various tissue cells, including those of organs of elimination, thus influencing drug disposition.
- In general, movement across membranes is bidirectional. For example, after a single dose, drug that distributes from blood to most tissues subsequently fully returns to the systemic circulation to be eliminated in the liver, kidneys, or other organ(s). Sometimes, drug movement can be virtually unidirectional when an efficient active transport process is present, as with the P-glycoprotein efflux transporter.
- Efflux transporters are particularly important in excluding many drugs from the brain and in reducing the systemic absorption of many drugs after their oral administration.

- Oral administration of charcoal or cholestyramine is sometimes useful to treat overdosed patients. These adsorbents act to reduce systemic absorption (if recently taken) and to hasten drug removal from the body.

KEY TERM REVIEW

Active transport
Blood–brain barrier
Capacity-limited transport
Capillary membranes
Carrier-mediated transport
Charcoal
Cholestyramine
Concentrating transporters
Diffusion
Drug overdose
Drug permeation
Efflux transporter
Equilibrating transporters
Extravasation
Facilitated transport
Hydrophilic
Hydrophobic
Influx (uptake) transporter
Ionization
Lipophilic
Lipophobic
Membranes
n-Octanol/water partition coefficient
Paracellular permeation
Partition coefficient
Passive diffusion
Passive facilitated diffusion
Perfusion rate–limited
Permeability
Permeability rate–limited
P-glycoprotein
pH partition hypothesis
Protein binding
Transcellular permeation
Transporter
Transport maximum
Unbound drug

STUDY PROBLEMS

1. Which of the following statements is (are) correct?
   I. Cell membranes comprise a hydrophilic interior and lipid exterior with globular proteins protruding from the surface.
   II. In vivo, membranes within the liver always limit the rate of movement of molecules from blood to the interior of hepatic cells.
   III. The rate of passive diffusion of a molecule across a membrane is directly proportional to the difference in its concentrations on the two sides of the membrane.
   A. I only
   B. II only
   C. III only
   D. I and II
   E. I and III
   F. II and III
   G. All
   H. None
2. Which of the following statements apply (ies) to active transport?
   I. Active transport exhibits concentration dependence.
   II. Equilibrium of compound across the membrane is achieved when the concentrations of the diffusing species on both sides of the membrane are equal.
   III. Active transport requires energy.
   A. I only
   B. II only
   C. III only
   D. I and II
   E. I and III
   F. II and III
   G. All
   H. None

3. Rank, from high to low, the expected order of decreasing resistance of the following membranes to permeation of a compound.
   a. Cerebral capillary
   b. Renal glomerulus
   c. Muscle capillary
   d. Intestinal epithelium
4. Which of the following statements accurately characterize(s) P-glycoprotein?
   I. It is a glycoprotein found in the interior of cells in many parts of the body.
   II. It is typically an influx transporter for many drugs.
   III. It is an equilibrating (passive) transporter.
   A. I only **E.** I and III
   B. II only **F.** II and III
   C. III only **G.** All
   D. I and II **H.** None
5. Which *one* of the following statements correctly describes the effect of pH on the passive movement of drugs across intestinal membranes?
   I. Lipophilic weak acids generally cross intestinal membranes faster at higher than lower pH values.
   II. At equilibrium in a system in which there is a pH gradient across a membrane, the total concentration of a lipophilic weak acid is higher on the side with the higher pH.
   III. For a given total concentration, a lipophilic weak base is expected to cross a membrane more quickly at a pH below than at one above its p*K*a.
   A. I only **E.** I and III
   B. II only **F.** II and III
   C. III only **G.** All
   D. I and II **H.** None
6. Which of the following statements is (are) true?
   I. When the surface area of a membrane is doubled, so is its permeability to a drug.
   II. Protein binding in the aqueous phases on either side of a membrane diminishes the permeability of the membrane to a drug.
   III. The thinner a membrane, the higher is its expected permeability.
   A. I only **E.** I and III
   B. II only **F.** II and III
   C. III only **G.** All
   D. I and II **H.** None
7. Charcoal can be given to help detoxify a patient who has absorbed and overdosed on some drugs, such as the active metabolite of the prodrug leflunomide. How should the charcoal be administered to treat a patient who has overdosed several hours before on leflunomide?
   a. As a single 10-g intravenous dose.
   b. As a single 50-g dose by nasogastric tube.
   c. As a 50-g dose given repeatedly by the oral or nasogastric routes every 6 hours until the patient has adequately responded or too many doses have been given.
   d. It should not be given for this drug.
   e. As a single 50-g dose by the oral route.
8. Briefly discuss the meaning of the following properties and how they are commonly assessed: hydrophilic, hydrophobic, lipophilic, and lipophobic.

9. State how transporters are involved in the systemic absorption, distribution, and elimination of drugs, and give an example of each.
10. For each of the following statements, indicate whether it is true or false. If false or ambiguous, provide an explanation for why it is so.
    a. The difference between equilibrating and concentrating transporters is that drug only reaches equilibrium across a membrane in the case of the former kind of transporter.
    b. When the initial rate of distribution of a drug into a tissue fails to increase with an increase in the rate of blood perfusion, the distribution to that tissue is said to be *permeability-rate limited.*
    c. All other factors being the same, absorption from solution within a given region of the small intestine where the pH is 6.4 is expected to be faster for a weak acid with a pK_a of 10.0 than for a weak base with a pK_a of 10.0.

CHAPTER 5

Quantifying Events Following an Intravenous Bolus

OBJECTIVES

The reader will be able to:

- Define the meaning of the key terms listed in the Key Term Review at the end of the chapter.
- Explain why plasma concentration often tends to fall exponentially following an IV bolus dose of drug.
- Calculate the elimination rate constant when the half-life is known, and vice versa.
- Explain why clearance is additive and how hepatic clearance is usually measured.
- Estimate from plasma and urine data after an intravenous dose of a drug: half-life, elimination rate constant, volume of distribution, total clearance, fraction excreted unchanged, and renal clearance.
- Calculate the concentration of drug in the plasma and the amount of drug in the body with time after an intravenous dose, given values for the pertinent pharmacokinetic parameters.
- Explain the statement "Half-life, and elimination rate constant, depend upon clearance and volume of distribution, and not vice versa."
- Discuss the kinetic consequences of it often taking some time to establish distribution equilibrium between drug in plasma with that in tissues.

Intravascular administration ensures that the entire dose of a drug enters the systemic circulation. By rapid injection, elevated concentrations of drug can be promptly achieved; by infusion at a controlled rate, a constant concentration, and often response, can be maintained. With no other route of administration can plasma concentration be as promptly and efficiently controlled. Intra-arterial administration is used less frequently than intravenous (IV) administration because it has greater inherent manipulative dangers. It is generally reserved for situations in which a higher exposure in a specific tissue, relative to others, is desired and is achieved by injecting drug into the artery directly perfusing the target tissue.

The disposition characteristics of a drug are defined by analyzing the temporal changes of drug in plasma and urine following IV administration. How this information is obtained after rapid injection of a drug is the topic of this chapter. The underlying processes controlling or determining distribution and elimination form the basis of Chapter 6.

APPRECIATION OF KINETIC CONCEPTS

In the last topic of Chapter 3, we considered the impact that various shapes of the exposure profile after an oral dose may have on the clinical utility of a drug. Figs. 5-1 and 5-2 provide a similar set of exposure–time profiles except that the drugs are now given as an IV bolus.

Several methods are used for graphically displaying plasma concentration–time data. One common method that has been mostly used in the preceding chapters, and shown on the left-hand side of Figs. 5-1 and 5-2, is to plot concentration against time. Depicted in this way, the plasma concentration is seen to fall in a curvilinear manner. Another method of display is a semilogarithmic plot of the same data (right-hand graphs in Figs. 5-1 and 5-2). The time scale is the same as before, but now the ordinate (concentration) scale is logarithmic. Notice now that all the profiles decline linearly and, being straight lines, it is much easier in many ways to predict the concentration at

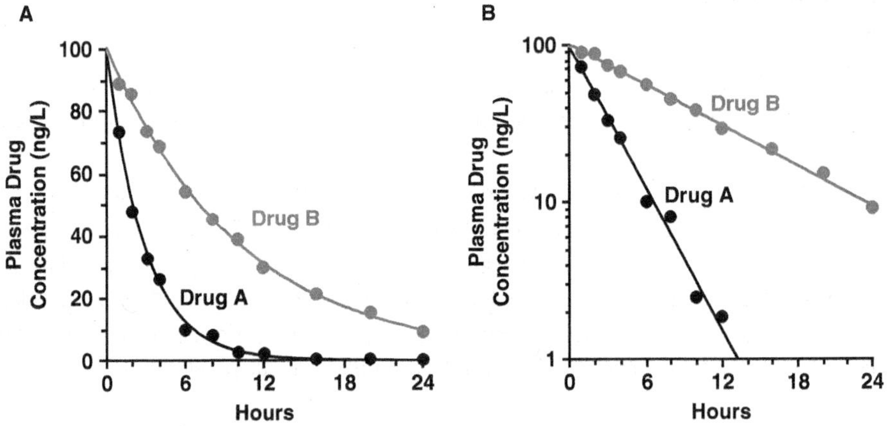

FIGURE 5-1 Drugs A (*black circle*) and B (*colored circle*) show the same initial (peak) exposure, but have different half-lives and total exposure-time profiles (AUC). Regular (cartesian) plot (*left*). Semilogarithmic plot (*right*). Doses of both drugs are the same.

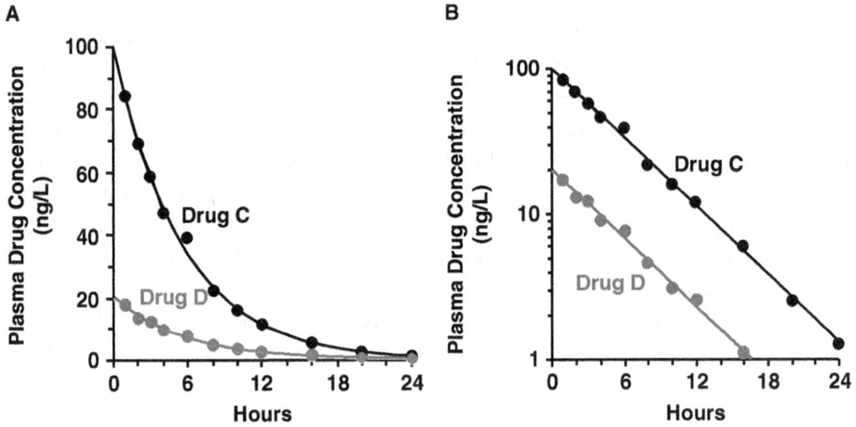

FIGURE 5-2 Drugs C (*black circle*) and D (*colored circle*) have the same half-life but different initial and total exposure-time (AUC) profiles. Regular (cartesian) plot (*left*). Semilogarithmic plot (*right*). Doses of both drugs are the same.

any time. But why do we get a **linear decline** with time when plotting the concentration data on a semilogarithmic scale, and what determines the large differences seen in the profiles of the four drugs?

Volume of Distribution and Clearance

To start to answer these questions, consider the simple scheme depicted in Fig. 5-3. Here, the drug is placed in a well-stirred reservoir with its contents continuously recirculated through an extractor that removes some drug on each passage through it. The scheme applies to a person as well, in which case the reservoir is the body and the extractor is the liver or kidneys. The drug concentrations in the reservoir, C, and that coming out of the extractor, C_{out}, can be measured. The initial concentration in the reservoir, $C(0)$, depends on the amount introduced, **Dose**, and the volume of the reservoir, V. Therefore,

$$C(0) = \frac{\text{Dose}}{V} \qquad \text{Eq. 5-1}$$

Fluid passes through the extractor at a flow rate, Q. With the concentration of drug entering the extractor being the same as that in the reservoir, C, it follows that the rate of input into the extractor is $Q \cdot C$. Of the drug entering the extractor, a fraction, E, is extracted (by elimination processes) on each passage through the extractor, never to return to the reservoir. The corresponding rate of drug leaving the extractor and returning to the reservoir is therefore $Q \cdot C_{out}$, which is less than the rate of entry. The rate of elimination (or rate of extraction) is then:

$$\text{Rate of elimination} = Q \cdot C \cdot E = Q(C - C_{out}) \qquad \text{Eq. 5-2}$$

from which it follows that the **extraction ratio, *E***, of the drug by the extractor is given by:

$$E = \frac{Q \cdot (C - C_{out})}{Q \cdot C} = \frac{(C - C_{out})}{C} \qquad \text{Eq. 5-3}$$

Thus, we see that the extraction ratio can be determined experimentally by measuring the concentrations entering and leaving the extractor and normalizing the difference between them by the entering concentration.

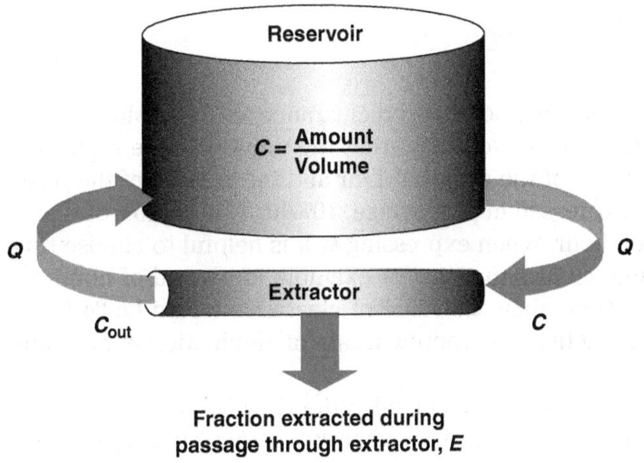

FIGURE 5-3 Schematic diagram of a perfused organ system. Drug is placed into a well-stirred reservoir, volume V, from which fluid perfuses an extractor at flow rate Q. A fraction of that presented to the extractor, E, is removed on each passage through it; the remainder, $1 - E$, returns to the reservoir. C and C_{out} are the concentrations of drug in the reservoir (and entering the extractor) and leaving the extractor, respectively. For modeling purposes, the amount of drug in the extractor is negligible compared with the amount of drug contained in the reservoir.

Conceptually, it is useful to relate the rate of elimination to the measured concentration. This parameter is called **clearance, *CL***. Therefore,

$$\text{Rate of elimination} = CL \cdot C \qquad \text{Eq. 5-4}$$

Note that the units of clearance are those of flow, which can be expressed in milliliters per minute (mL/min) or liters per hour (L/hr). This conclusion follows because rate of elimination is expressed in units of mass per unit time, such as μg/min or mg/hr, and concentration is expressed in units of mass per unit volume, such as μg/L or mg/L.

An important relationship is also obtained by comparing the equalities in Equations 5-2 and 5-4, yielding

$$CL = Q \cdot E \qquad \text{Eq. 5-5}$$

This equation provides a physical interpretation of clearance. Namely, clearance is the volume of the fluid presented to the eliminating organ (extractor) that is effectively completely cleared of drug per unit time. For example, if $Q = 1$ L/min and $E = 0.5$, then effectively 500 mL of the fluid entering the extractor from the reservoir is completely cleared of drug each minute. Also, it is seen that in the case of a perfect extractor ($E = 1$), CL equals Q, and the rate of extraction ($CL \cdot C$) is equal to, and cannot exceed, the rate of delivery ($Q \cdot C$). Under these circumstances, clearance is limited by, and therefore sensitive to, flow to the extractor.

Two very useful parameters in pharmacokinetics have now been introduced, **volume of distribution** (volume of the reservoir in this example) and **clearance** (the parameter relating rate of elimination to the concentration in the systemic [reservoir] circulation). The first parameter predicts the plasma concentration for a given amount in the body. The second provides an estimate of the rate of elimination at any concentration.

First-Order Elimination

The question that remains is: How quickly does drug decline from the reservoir? This may be answered by considering the rate of elimination ($CL \cdot C$) relative to the amount present in the reservoir (A), a ratio commonly referred to as the **fractional rate of elimination, *k***

$$k = \frac{\text{Rate of elimination}}{\text{Amount in the reservoir}} = \frac{CL \cdot C}{A} = \frac{CL \cdot C}{V \cdot C} \qquad \text{Eq. 5-6}$$

or

$$k = \frac{CL}{V} \qquad \text{Eq. 5-7}$$

This important relationship shows that k depends on clearance and the volume of the reservoir, two independent parameters. Note also that the units of k are reciprocal time. For example, if the clearance of the drug is 1 L/hr and the volume of the reservoir is 10 L, then $k = 0.1$/hr or, expressed in percentage, 10%/hr. That is, 10% of that in the reservoir is eliminated each hour. When expressing k, it is helpful to choose time units so that the value of k is much less than 1. For example, if instead of hours we had chosen days as the unit of time, then the value of clearance would be 24 L/day, and therefore $k = 2.4$/day, implying that the fractional rate of elimination is 240%/day, a number that is misleading.

To further appreciate the meaning of k, consider the data in Table 5-1, which shows the loss of drug in the reservoir with time when $k = 0.1$/hr. Starting with 100 mg, in 1 hour 10% has been eliminated, so that 90 mg remains. In the next hour, 10% of

TABLE 5-1 | Amount Remaining in the Reservoir Over a 5-Hour Period (After Introduction of a 100-mg Dose of a Drug With an Elimination Rate Constant of 0.1 /hr)

Time Interval (hr)	Amount Lost During Interval (mg)	Amount Remaining in Reservoir at the End of the Interval (mg)[a]
0	—	100
0–1	10	90.0
1–2	9	81.0
2–3	8.1	72.9
3–4	7.3	65.6
4–5	6.36	59.0

[a]If the time unit of k had been made smaller than hours, the amount lost (hence remaining in the reservoir) with time would be slightly different. This is because in this calculation, the assumption is made that the loss occurs at the initial rate throughout the interval, when in reality it falls exponentially. In the limiting case, the fraction remaining at time t is e^{-kt} (Equation 5-10), which in the above example is 60.63% at 5 hr.

90 mg, or 9 mg, is eliminated, leaving 81 mg remaining at 2 hours, and so on. Although this method illustrates the application of k in determining the time course of drug elimination, and hence drug remaining in the body, it is rather laborious and has some error associated with it. A simpler and more accurate way of calculating these values at any time is used (see *Fraction of Dose Remaining* below).

Considering further the rate of elimination, there are two ways of determining it experimentally. One method mentioned previously is to measure the rates entering and leaving the eliminating organ, although in practice this is inherently difficult. The other method is to determine the rate of loss of drug from the reservoir, since the only reason for the loss from the system is elimination in the extractor. Hence, by reference to Equation 5-6, it follows that

$$\text{Rate of elimination} = -\frac{dA}{dt} = k \cdot A \qquad \text{Eq. 5-8}$$

where $-dA$ is the small amount of drug lost (hence the negative sign) from the reservoir during a small interval of time dt. Processes, such as those represented by Equation 5-8, in which the rate of the process is directly proportional to the amount present, are known as **first-order processes** in that the rate varies in direct proportion to the amount there raised to the power of one ($A^1 = A$). For this reason, the parameter k is frequently called the **first-order elimination rate constant**. Then, substituting $A = V \cdot C$ on both sides of Equation 5-8, and dividing by V gives:

$$-\frac{dC}{dt} = k \cdot C \qquad \text{Eq. 5-9}$$

which, on integration, yields:

$$C = C(0) \cdot e^{-k \cdot t} \qquad \text{Eq. 5-10}$$

where e is the natural base with a value of 2.71828. Equation 5-10 is known as a **mono-exponential equation** in that it involves a single exponential term. Examination of this equation shows that it has the right properties. At time zero, $e^{-k \cdot t} = e^{-0} = 1$, so that $C = C(0)$ and, as time approaches infinity, $e^{-k \cdot t}$ approaches zero and so, therefore, does concentration. Equation 5-10 describes the curvilinear plots in Figs. 5-1 and 5-2.

To see why such curves become linear when reservoir concentration is plotted on a logarithmic scale, take the logarithms of both sides of Equation 5-10.

$$\ln C = \ln C(0) - k \cdot t \qquad \text{Eq. 5-11}$$

where ln is the natural logarithm. Thus, we see from Equation 5-11 that ln C is a linear function of time with a slope of $-k$, as indeed observed in Figs. 5-1 and 5-2. Moreover, the slope of the line determines how fast the concentration declines, which in turn is governed by V and CL, independent parameters. The larger the elimination rate constant k, the more rapid is drug elimination.

Half-Life

Commonly, the kinetics of a drug is characterized by a **half-life** ($t_{½}$), the time for the concentration (and amount in the reservoir) to fall by one half, rather than by an elimination rate constant. These two parameters are of course interrelated. This is seen from Equation 5-10. In one half-life, $C = 0.5 \times C(0)$; therefore,

$$0.5 \times C(0) = C(0) \cdot e^{-k \cdot t_{½}} \qquad \text{Eq. 5-12}$$

or

$$e^{-k \cdot t_{½}} = 0.5 \qquad \text{Eq. 5-13}$$

which, on inverting and taking logarithms on both sides, gives

$$t_{1/2} = \frac{\ln (2)}{k} \qquad \text{Eq. 5-14}$$

Further, given that ln (2) = 0.693,

$$t_{1/2} = \frac{0.693}{k} \qquad \text{Eq. 5-15}$$

or, on substituting CL/V for k, leads to another very important equation

$$t_{1/2} = \frac{0.693 \cdot V}{CL} \qquad \text{Eq. 5-16}$$

From Equation 5-16, it should be evident that half-life is controlled by and directly proportional to V and inversely proportional to CL.

To appreciate the application of Equation 5-16, consider creatinine, a product of muscle catabolism and used to assess renal function. For a 70-kg, 20-year-old male patient, creatinine has a clearance of 7.2 L/hr and is evenly distributed throughout the 42 L of total body water. As expected by calculation using Equation 5-16, its half-life is 4 hours. Inulin, a polysaccharide also used to assess renal function, has the same clearance as creatinine in such a patient, but a half-life of only 1.5 hours. This compound is too large (molecular weight is approximately 5000 g/mol) and polar to enter cells, and consequently, it is restricted in its distribution to the 16 L of extracellular water; that is, its "reservoir" size is smaller than that of creatinine, which explains its shorter half-life.

Fraction of Dose Remaining

Another view of the kinetics of drug elimination may be gained by examining how the fraction of the dose remaining in the reservoir (*A/Dose*) varies with time. By reference to Equation 5-10, and multiplying both sides by V

$$\text{Fraction of dose remaining} = \frac{A}{\text{Dose}} = e^{-k \cdot t} \qquad \text{Eq. 5-17}$$

Sometimes, it is useful to express time relative to the half-life of the drug. The benefit in doing so is seen by letting n be the number of half-lives elapsed after a bolus dose ($n = t/t_{½}$). Then, as $k = 0.693/t_{1/2}$, one obtains

$$\text{Fraction of dose remaining} = e^{-k \cdot t} = e^{-0.693n} \qquad \text{Eq. 5-18}$$

Since $e^{-0.693} = ½$, it follows that

$$\text{Fraction of dose remaining} = \left(\frac{1}{2}\right)^{n} \qquad \text{Eq. 5-19}$$

Thus, ½ or 50% of the dose remains after 1 half-life, and ¼ (½ × ½) or 25% remains after 2 half-lives, and so on. Satisfy yourself that by 4 half-lives only 6.25% of the dose remains to be eliminated. You might also prove to yourself that 10% remains at 3.32 half-lives.

If one uses 10% as a value for the percent remaining when the drug has been essentially eliminated, then 3.32 half-lives is the time. Some prefer a more conservative value and use 5 half-lives as the time to practically eliminate a drug. For a drug like esmolol (used in patients during surgery to prevent or treat tachycardia), with a 9-minute half-life, 5 half-lives is close to 45 minutes, whereas for a drug like dutasteride (used to treat benign prostatic hyperplasia), with a 5-week half-life, the corresponding time is nearly 6 months. Because of the long half-life and the effects of dutasteride on the formation of the potent androgen dihydrotestosterone, patients are told not to donate blood for at least 6 months after discontinuing therapy with this drug.

Clearance, Area, and Volume of Distribution

We are now in a position to fully explain the different curves seen in Figs. 5-1 and 5-2, which were simulated applying the simple scheme in Fig. 5-3. Drugs A and B in Fig. 5-1A have the same initial (peak) concentration after administration of the same dose. Therefore, they must have the same volume of distribution, V, which follows from Equation 5-1. However, Drug A has a shorter half-life, and hence a larger value of k, from which we conclude that, since $k = CL/V$, it must have a higher clearance. The lower total exposure (AUC) seen with Drug A follows from its higher clearance. This is seen from Equation 5-4, repeated here,

$$\text{Rate of elimination} = CL \cdot C$$

By rearranging this equation, it can be seen that during a small interval of time dt

$$\text{Amount eliminated in interval } dt = CL \cdot C \cdot dt \qquad \text{Eq. 5-20}$$

where the product $C \cdot dt$ is the corresponding small area under the concentration–time curve within the time interval dt. For example, if the clearance of a drug is 1 L/min and the area under the curve between 60 and 61 minutes is 1 mg-min/L, then the amount of drug eliminated in that minute is 1 mg. The total amount of drug eventually eliminated, which for an IV bolus equals the dose administered, is assessed by adding up or integrating the amounts eliminated in each time interval, from time zero to time infinity, and therefore,

$$\text{Dose} = CL \cdot \text{AUC} \qquad \text{Eq. 5-21}$$

where AUC is the total exposure. Thus, returning to the drugs depicted in Fig. 5-1, since the clearance of Drug A is higher, its AUC must be lower than that of Drug B for a given dose. On passing, it is worth noting that in practice once AUC is known, clearance is readily calculated. Furthermore, if this is the only parameter of interest, there is no need to know the half-life or volume of distribution to calculate clearance.

Finally, Equation 5-21 is independent of the shape of the concentration–time profile. The critical factor is to obtain a good estimate of AUC (See Appendix D).

Now consider the two drugs, C and D, in Fig. 5-2 in which, once again, the same dose of drug was administered. From the regular plot, it is apparent that as the initial concentration of Drug C is higher, it has a smaller *V*. And, as the total exposure (AUC) of Drug C is the greater, it has the lower clearance. However, from the semilogarithmic plot, it is apparent that because the slopes of the two lines are parallel, they must have the same value of the elimination rate constant, *k* (Equation 5-11), and hence the same value of half-life (Equation 5-15). These equalities can arise only because the ratio *CL/V* is the same for both drugs. The lesson is clear: *The important determinants of the kinetics of a drug following an IV bolus dose are clearance and volume of distribution.* These parameters determine the secondary parameters, *k* and $t_{1/2}$, and the resultant kinetic process.

A CASE STUDY

In reality, the body is more complex than depicted in the simple reservoir model. The body comprises many different types of tissues and organs. The eliminating organs, such as the liver and kidneys, are much more complex than a simple extractor. To gain a better appreciation of how drugs are handled by the body, consider the data in Fig. 5-4 showing the decline in the plasma concentration of diazepam displayed as both regular and semilogarithmic plots, following a 10-mg IV bolus dose to a young male adult. This drug is administered intravenously for the treatment of muscle spasms. As expected, the decline in concentration displayed on the regular plot is curvilinear. However, contrary to the expectation of the simple reservoir model of a monoexponential decline, the decline in the semilogarithmic plot is clearly biphasic, a phase with a rapid decline followed by one with a slower decline, with the rapid phase lasting for about 1 hour. The early phase is commonly called the **distribution phase,** and the latter the **terminal** or **elimination phase**.

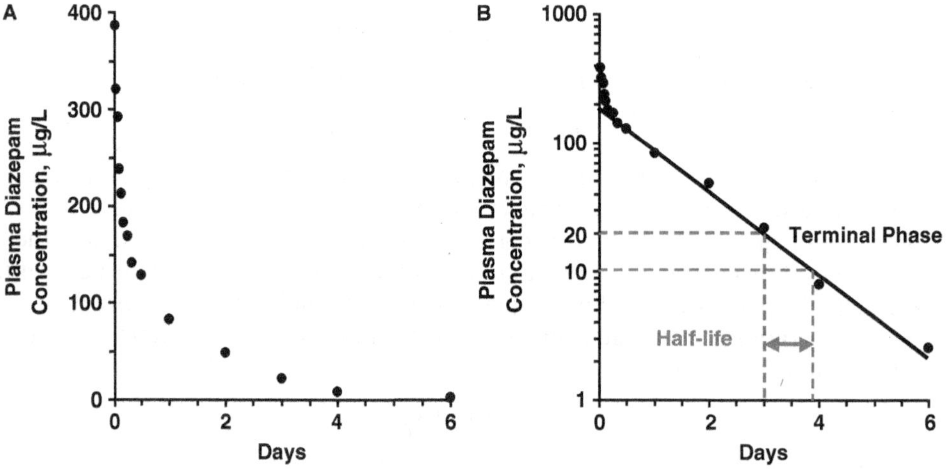

FIGURE 5-4 A. Plasma concentration of diazepam with time after a 10-mg IV bolus dose of diazepam in a young male adult. **B.** The data in **(A)** are redisplayed as a semilogarithmic plot. Note the short distribution phase and that the time taken for the concentration to decrease from 20 μg/L to 10 μg/L (colored lines), the half-life, is about 22 hours. (Figure adapted from the data of Greenblatt DJ, Allen MD, Harmatz JS, et al. Diazepam disposition determinants. *Clin Pharmacol Ther* 1980;27:301–312.)

Distribution Phase

The distribution phase is so called because distribution into tissues primarily determines the early rapid decline in plasma concentration. For diazepam, distribution is rapid and occurs significantly even by the time of the first measurement in Fig. 5-4, 15 minutes. This must be so because the amount of diazepam in plasma at this time is only 1.2 mg. This value is calculated by multiplying the plasma concentration at 15 minutes, 0.40 mg/L, by the physical volume of the plasma, 3 L, in an average adult. The majority, 8.8 mg or 88% of the total (10 mg) dose, must have already left the plasma and been distributed into other tissues. An **initial dilution space** of approximately 25 L (10 mg/0.4 mg/L) is needed to account for the initial concentration. Among the tissues that account for this space are the well-perfused liver and kidneys, which also eliminate drug from the body. However, although some drug is eliminated during the early moments, the fraction of the administered dose eliminated during the distribution phase is small for diazepam, and for many other drugs. This statement is based on exposure considerations and is discussed more fully later in this chapter. Nonetheless, because both distribution and elimination are occurring simultaneously, it is appropriate to apply the term **disposition kinetics** when characterizing the entire plasma concentration–time profile following an IV bolus dose.

Terminal Phase

During the distribution phase, changes in the concentration of drug in plasma reflect primarily movement of drug within, rather than loss from, the body. However, with time, distribution equilibrium of drug in tissue with that in plasma is established in more and more tissues, and eventually, changes in plasma concentration reflect a proportional change in the concentrations of drug in all other tissues and therefore in the amount of drug in the body. During this proportionality phase, the body acts kinetically as a single container or compartment, much like in the reservoir model. Because decline of the plasma concentration is now associated solely with elimination of drug from the body, this phase is often called the **elimination phase**, and parameters associated with it, such as k and $t_{1/2}$, are called the **elimination rate constant** and **elimination half-life**.

Elimination Half-Life

The elimination half-life, also called the **terminal half-life** as it is the half-life of the terminal phase, is the time taken for the plasma concentration, as well as the amount of the drug in the body, to fall by one-half. The terminal half-life of diazepam determined by the time taken to fall from 20 to 10 μg/L, for example, is 0.9 days, or 22 hours for this subject (Fig. 5-4B). This is the same time that it takes for the concentration to fall from 10 to 5 μg/L. In other words, the elimination half-life of diazepam is independent of the amount of drug in the body. It follows, therefore, that less drug is eliminated in each succeeding half-life. Initially, there is 10 mg, the dose, in the body. After 1 half-life (22 hours), 5 mg remains in the body, assuming that distribution equilibrium was virtually spontaneous (a reasonable approximation in the case of diazepam because distribution is so much faster than elimination). After 2 half-lives (44 hours), 2.5 mg remains, and after 3 half-lives (66 hours, or 2.7 days), 1.25 mg remains. For practical purposes, all of the drug (97%) may be regarded as having been eliminated by 5 half-lives (4.5 days).

Clearance

This parameter is obtained by calculating total exposure, since CL = Dose/AUC. For diazepam, total AUC in this subject is 6.60 mg-hr/L, and so CL =10 mg/6.60 mg-hr/L, or 1.5 L/hr. That is, 1.5 L of plasma is effectively cleared completely of drug each hour.

Volume of Distribution

The concentration in plasma achieved after distribution is complete is a function of dose and extent of distribution of drug into the tissues. This extent of distribution can be determined by relating the concentration obtained with a known amount of drug in the body. This is analogous to the determination of the volume of the reservoir in Fig. 5-3 by dividing the amount of compound added to it by the resultant concentration after thorough mixing. The volume measured is, in effect, a dilution space but, unlike the reservoir, this volume is not a physical space but rather an apparent one.

The apparent volume into which a drug distributes in the body at equilibrium is called the **(apparent) volume of distribution**. Plasma, rather than blood, is usually measured. Consequently, the volume of distribution, V, is the volume of plasma at the drug concentration, C, required to account for all drug in the body at equilibrium, A.

$$V = \frac{A}{C}$$

$$\text{Volume of distribution} = \frac{\text{Amount of drug in body}}{\text{Plasma drug concentration}} \qquad \textbf{Eq. 5-22}$$

Volume of distribution is useful in estimating the dose required to achieve a given plasma concentration or, conversely, in estimating the amount of drug in the body when the plasma concentration is known.

Calculation of volume of distribution requires that distribution equilibrium be achieved between drug in tissues and that in plasma. The amount of drug in the body is known immediately after an IV bolus; it is the dose administered. However, distribution equilibrium has not yet been achieved, so, unlike the reservoir model we cannot use, with any confidence, the concentration obtained by extrapolating to zero time to obtain an estimate of V. To overcome this problem, use is made of a previously derived important relationship $k = CL/V$, which on rearrangement gives

$$V = \frac{CL}{k} \qquad \textbf{Eq. 5-23}$$

or, since $k = 0.693/t_{1/2}$, and the reciprocal of 0.693 is 1.44

$$V = 1.44 \cdot CL \cdot t_{1/2} \qquad \textbf{Eq. 5-24}$$

So, although half-life is known, we need an estimate of clearance to estimate V. Substituting CL = 1.5 L/hr and $t_{1/2}$ = 22 hours into Equation 5-24 gives a value for the volume of distribution of diazepam in the subject of 48 L.

Volume of distribution is a direct measure of the extent of distribution. It rarely, however, corresponds to a physical volume (values for a 70-kg adult), such as plasma volume (3 L), extracellular water (16 L), or total body water (42 L). Drug distribution may be to any one or a combination of tissues and fluids of the body. Furthermore, binding to tissue components may be so great that the volume of distribution is many times the total body size.

To appreciate the effect of tissue binding, consider the distribution of 100 mg of a drug in a 1-L system composed of water and 10 g of activated charcoal, and where 99%

of drug is adsorbed onto the charcoal. When the charcoal has settled, the concentration of drug in the aqueous phase would be 1 mg/L; thus, 100 L of the aqueous phase, a volume 100 times greater than that of the entire system, would be required to account for the entire amount in the system.

Clearance and Elimination

Knowing clearance allows calculation of the rate of elimination for any plasma concentration. Using Equation 5-4, since CL = 1.5 L/hr, the rate of elimination of diazepam from the body is 0.15 mg/hr at a plasma concentration of 0.1 mg/L (100 μg/L). One can also calculate the amount eliminated during any time interval, as illustrated in Fig. 5-5. Thus, it follows from Equation 5-20 that multiplying the area up to a given time [AUC(*0, t*)] by clearance gives the amount of drug that has been eliminated up to that time.

Alternatively, when the area is expressed as a fraction of the total AUC, one obtains the fraction of the dose eliminated. The fraction of the total area beyond a given time is a measure of the fraction of dose remaining to be eliminated. For example, in the case of diazepam, by the end of day 1 the area is 53% of the total AUC. Therefore, 53% of the administered 10-mg dose, or 5.3 mg, has been eliminated from the body; 4.7 mg has yet to be eliminated.

Distribution and Elimination: Competing Processes

Previously, it was stated that little diazepam is eliminated before the attainment of distribution equilibrium. This conclusion is based on the finding that the area under the concentration–time profile during the distribution phase (up to 6 hours; see Fig. 5-4B) represents only a small fraction of the total AUC, and hence a small fraction of the total amount eliminated. This occurs because the speed of tissue distribution of this and many other drugs is much faster than that of elimination. These competing events of distribution and elimination, which determine the disposition kinetics of a drug, are shown schematically in Fig. 5-6. Here, the body is portrayed as a **compartmental model**, comprising two body pools, or compartments, with exchange of drug between them and with elimination from the first pool. One can think of the blood,

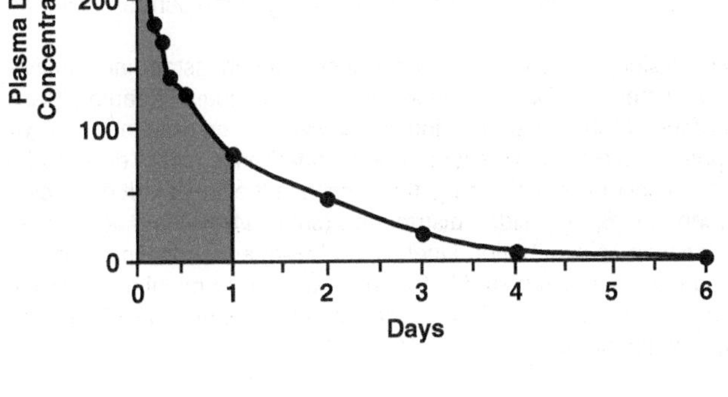

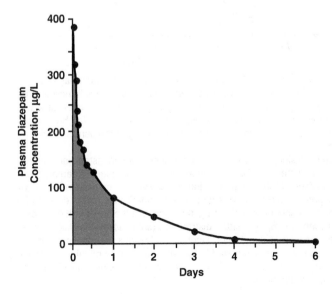

FIGURE 5-5 A linear plot of the same plasma concentration–time data for diazepam as displayed in Fig. 5-4A. The area up to 1 day is 53% of the total AUC, indicating that 53% of the dose administered has been eliminated by then. The area beyond 1 day represents the 47% of the administered drug remaining to be eliminated.

liver, kidneys, and other well-perfused organs into which drug equilibrates rapidly as being part of this central pool where elimination and input of drug occurs, and one can think of the more slowly equilibrating poorly perfused tissues, such as muscle and fat, as the other pool. The size of each arrow represents the speed of the process; the larger the arrow, the faster the process. Two scenarios are depicted. The first, and the most common, scenario, depicted in Fig. 5-6A, is one in which distribution is much faster than elimination. Displayed is a semilogarithmic plot of the fraction of an IV bolus dose within each of the pools, as well as the sum of the two (total fraction remaining in the body), as a function of time. Notice that, as with diazepam, a biphasic

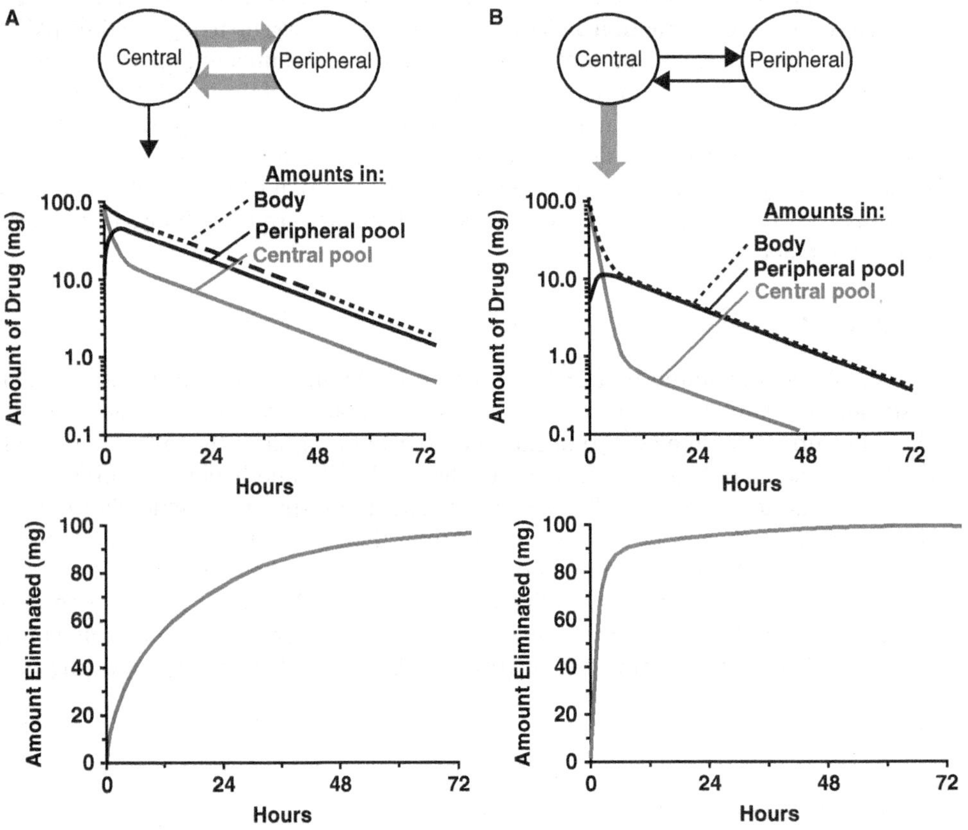

FIGURE 5-6 The events occurring within the body after an IV bolus dose are the result of interplay between the kinetics of distribution and elimination. Distribution is depicted here (*top* of figure) as an exchange of drug between a central pool (comprising blood and rapidly equilibrating tissues, including the eliminating organs, liver and kidneys) and a pool containing the more slowly equilibrating tissues, such as muscle and fat. Because of distribution kinetics, a biexponential decline is seen in the semilogarithmic plot of drug in the central pool (and hence plasma).

Two scenarios are considered. The first (**A**, *left* side) is one in which distribution is much faster than elimination, shown by large arrows for distribution and a small one for elimination. Distribution occurs so rapidly (*seen as large colored arrows*) that little drug is lost before distribution equilibrium is achieved, when drug in the slowly equilibrating pool parallels that in the central pool, as is clearly evident in the semilogarithmic plot of events with time. Most drug elimination occurs during the terminal phase of the drug; this is seen in the linear plot of percent of dose eliminated with time. In the second scenario (**B**, *right* side), distribution (*small arrows*) is much slower than elimination (*large colored arrow*). Then, because of distribution kinetics, a biexponential decline from the central pool is still evident, but most of the drug has been eliminated before reaching the terminal phase when distribution equilibration has been achieved. In this scenario, the phase associated with the majority of elimination is the first phase, and not the terminal exponential phase.

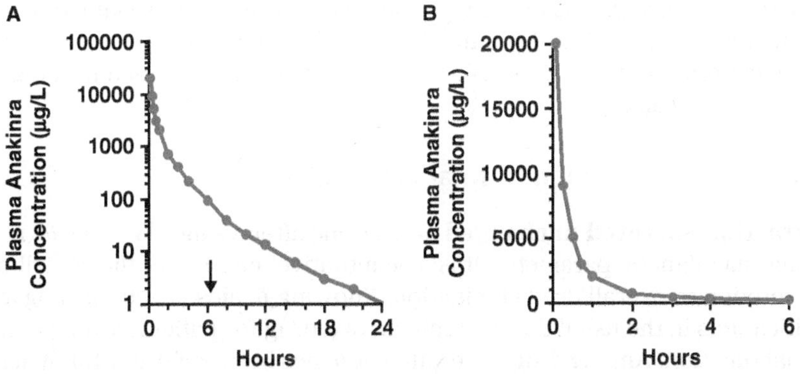

FIGURE 5-7 Semilogarithmic (**A**, to 24 hours) and linear (**B**, to 6 hours as noted in **A**) plots of the decline in the mean concentration of anakinra after the intravenous administration of a bolus of 82 mg in healthy subjects. Notice that, although a multiexponential decline is seen in the semilogarithmic plot with a terminal phase reached soon after 6 hours (indicated by *arrow*), based on analysis of the linear plot, essentially all the area, and hence elimination, have occurred before reaching the terminal phase. This is a result of elimination being much faster than tissue distribution. (Redraw from data in Yang B-B, Baughman S, Sullivan JT, Pharmacokinetics of anakinra in subjects with different levels of renal function. *Clin Pharmacol Ther* 2003;74:85–94.)

curve is seen and that little drug is eliminated from the body before distribution equilibrium is achieved; thereafter, during the terminal phase, drug in the two pools is in a pseudoequilibrium, and the only reason for the subsequent decline is elimination of drug from the body. The decline (half-life) of drug in plasma then reflects the decline of the total amount of drug in the body.

Next, consider the situation, albeit less common, depicted in Fig. 5-6B. Here, distribution of drug between the two pools is slow, and elimination from the central pool is rapid. Once again, a biphasic curve is seen. Also, during the terminal phase, at which time distribution equilibrium has been achieved between the two pools, the only reason for decline is, again, elimination of drug from the body, and events in plasma reflect the decline in the rest of the body. There the similarity ends. Now, most of the drug has been eliminated from the body *before distribution equilibrium is achieved,* so there is little drug left to be eliminated during the terminal phase, and the amount in the peripheral compartment, although small, is much greater than that in the central compartment. An example of this latter situation is shown in Fig. 5-7 for anakinra, a drug used to treat rheumatoid arthritis. This protein (17,258 g/mol) is rapidly cleared from the body by the kidneys and permeates very slowly into many cells of the body. Most of an intravenous dose of this protein drug is eliminated before distribution equilibrium is reached. Hence, with respect to drug elimination, it is the first phase and not the terminal phase that predominates. In conclusion, assigning the terminal phase to be the elimination phase during which the majority of elimination occurs is generally reasonable and, unless mentioned otherwise, is assumed to be the case for the rest of this book. However, keep in mind, there are exceptions.

PATHWAYS OF ELIMINATION

The aminoglycoside antibiotic gentamicin is almost totally excreted unchanged in urine. Other drugs are extensively metabolized usually within the liver with little renally excreted. Knowing the relative proportions eliminated by each pathway is important as it helps to predict the sensitivity of clearance of a given drug in patients with diseases of these organs, or who are concurrently receiving other drugs that affect these pathways, particularly metabolism. Of the two, renal excretion and hepatic metabolism, the former is much the easier to quantify, achieved by collecting unchanged drug in urine; there is no comparable method for determining the rate of hepatic metabolism.

Renal Excretion as a Fraction of Total Elimination

The **fraction excreted unchanged** in the urine after a single IV dose, *fe*, is an important pharmacokinetic parameter. It is a quantitative measure of the contribution of renal excretion to overall drug elimination. Knowing *fe* aids in establishing appropriate modifications in the usual dosage regimen of a drug for patients with varying degrees of renal function. Among drugs, the value of *fe* lies between 0 and 1.0. When the value is low, which is common for many highly lipophilic drugs that are extensively metabolized, excretion is a minor pathway of drug elimination. Occasionally, as in the case of gentamicin and the β-adrenergic blocking agent atenolol used to lower blood pressure, renal excretion is virtually the sole route of elimination, in which case the value of *fe* is close to 1.0. By definition, the complement, 1 − *fe*, is the fraction of the IV dose that is eliminated by other mechanisms, usually hepatic metabolism.

An estimate of *fe* is most readily obtained from cumulative urinary excretion data following IV administration of a single dose, since, by definition,

$$fe = \frac{\text{Total amount excreted unchanged}}{\text{Dose}} \quad \textbf{Eq. 5-25}$$

In practice, care should be taken to ensure that all of the excreted urine is collected, that is, over a sufficient period of time (usually 4–5 half-lives) so that a good estimate of total amount excreted unchanged is obtained. This does make it particularly demanding for drugs with long half-lives.

Additivity of Clearance

The clearance of a drug by one organ adds to clearance by another. This is a consequence of the anatomy of the circulatory system. Consider, for example, a drug that is eliminated only by renal excretion and hepatic metabolism. Then,

$$\text{Rate of elimination} = \text{Rate of renal excretion} + \text{Rate of hepatic metabolism} \quad \textbf{Eq. 5-26}$$

Dividing the rate of removal associated with each process by the incoming drug concentration (blood or plasma), which for both organs is the same (C), gives the clearance associated with that process:

$$\frac{\text{Rate of elimination}}{C} = \frac{\text{Rate of renal excretion}}{C} + \frac{\text{Rate of hepatic metabolism}}{C} \quad \textbf{Eq. 5-27}$$

Analogous to total clearance, renal clearance (CL_R) is defined as the proportionality term between urinary excretion rate of unchanged drug and plasma concentration. Similarly, hepatic clearance (CL_H) is the proportionality term between rate of hepatic metabolism and plasma concentration. Therefore,

$$\underset{\text{Total clearance}}{CL} = \underset{\text{Renal clearance}}{CL_R} + \underset{\text{Hepatic clearance}}{CL_H} \quad \textbf{Eq. 5-28}$$

Recall, total clearance is determined from the total exposure following an IV dose (Equation 5-21). Renal clearance can be determined experimentally from urinary excretion data and total clearance. This is readily seen by noting that *fe* is the ratio of renal to total clearance, so that,

$$\text{Renal clearance} = fe \cdot CL \quad \textbf{Eq. 5-29}$$

In contrast, rate and extent of metabolism can rarely be measured directly, but by taking advantage of the additivity of clearance, hepatic clearance (nonrenal clearance if there are other eliminating organs) is readily estimated as the difference between total and renal clearance, that is: $CL_H = (1 - fe) \cdot CL$.

HALF-LIFE, CLEARANCE, AND DISTRIBUTION

Fig. 5-8 summarizes the half-lives of a variety of prescribed drugs for various combinations of clearance and volume of distribution in adults. One striking feature is the enormous range of values for all three parameters with half-lives of 0.2 to 1000 hours, volumes of distribution ranging 2000-fold, from 3 to 7000 L, and clearance values from 0.01 to close to 100 L/hr, a 10,000-fold range. Even so, note that there are many drugs with half-lives of a similar value, such as 10 hours. This similarity arises because despite differences in clearance and volume of distribution, their ratio is almost the same. To appreciate the reason for these very wide ranges in clearance and volume of distribution, and also the factors likely to influence them, we need to examine more closely the processes involved, the subject of Chapter 6, where we first consider distribution and then elimination.

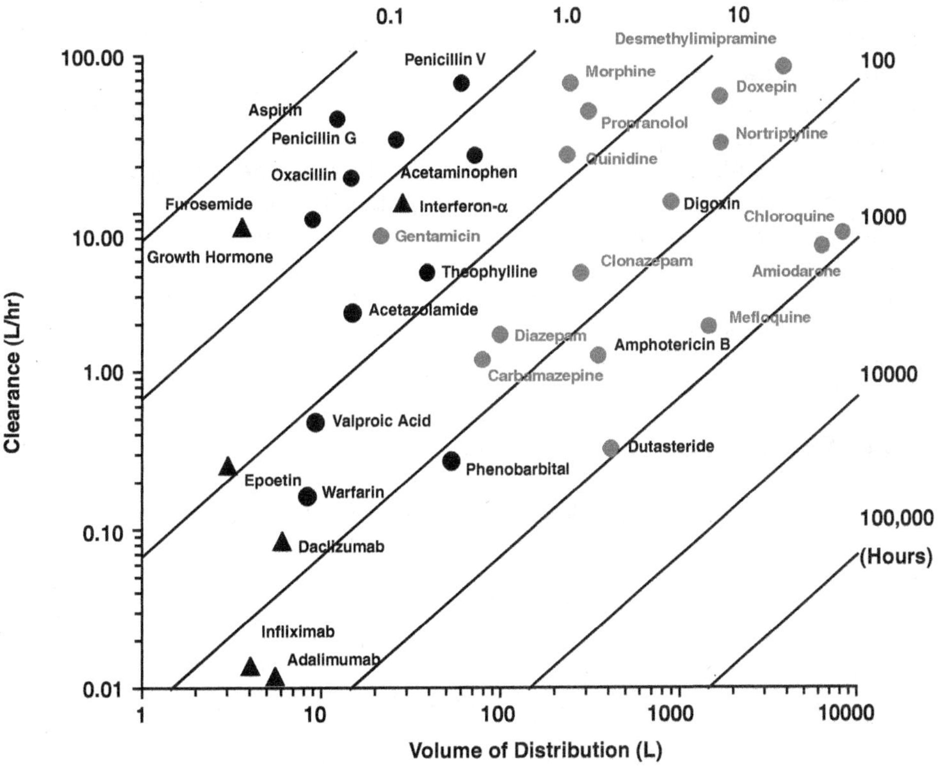

FIGURE 5-8 Clearance (*ordinate*) and volume of distribution (*abscissa*) of selected acidic (*black circle*) and basic (*colored names*), as well as protein (*black triangle*), drugs vary widely. Diagonal lines on the fully logarithmic plot show the combinations of clearance and volume values with the same half-lives (hours). Note that drugs with very low clearance and very large volumes (*lower right-hand quadrant*) are uncommon; their half-lives are often too long for these drugs to be used practically in drug therapy. Note also that large protein drugs have volumes of distribution close to plasma volume (3 L) and that basic compounds tend to have larger volumes of distribution than acids. Digoxin and dutasteride are neutral compounds, while amphotericin B is both a weak acid and a weak base.

SUMMARY

Estimation of Disposition Parameters

- Total clearance is estimated by dividing the administered IV dose by the total systemic exposure–time profile (AUC).
- Terminal half-life, and hence the elimination rate constant, are estimated from the terminal linear slope of a semilogarithmic plot of the plasma concentration–time profile.
- Volume of distribution is calculated knowing clearance and terminal half-life.
- Renal clearance is obtained from the product of the total fraction excreted in urine unchanged and total clearance.
- Total clearance is the sum of the clearances by eliminating organs.
- Because the liver and kidneys are often the major organs of elimination, total clearance is the sum of renal and hepatic clearances.
- As total and renal clearances are readily measured, the difference between them is nonrenal clearance, which can reflect elimination in several organs, but is usually assumed to occur in the liver.

KEY TERM REVIEW

Clearance
Compartmental model
Disposition kinetics
Distribution phase
Elimination half-life
Elimination phase
Elimination rate constant
Extraction ratio
First-order process
Fractional rate of elimination
Fraction excreted unchanged
Half-life
Hepatic clearance
Initial volume of distribution
Loglinear decline
Monoexponential equation
Renal clearance
Terminal half-life
Terminal phase
Total clearance
Volume of distribution

KEY RELATIONSHIPS

$$E = \frac{Q \cdot (C - C_{out})}{Q \cdot C} = \frac{(C - C_{out})}{C}$$

$$\text{Rate of elimination} = CL \cdot C$$

$$CL = Q \cdot E$$

$$k = \frac{CL}{V}$$

$$\text{Rate of elimination} = -\frac{dA}{dt} = k \cdot A$$

$$C = C(0) \cdot e^{-k \cdot t}$$

$$\ln C = \ln C(0) - k \cdot t$$

$$t_{1/2} = \frac{0.693}{k}$$

$$t_{1/2} = \frac{0.693 \cdot V}{CL}$$

$$\text{Fraction of dose remaining} = \frac{A}{\text{Dose}} = e^{-k \cdot t}$$

$$\text{Fraction of dose remaining} = \left(\tfrac{1}{2}\right)^n$$

$$\text{Dose} = CL \cdot \text{AUC}$$

$$V = \frac{A}{C}$$

$$\text{Volume of distribution} = \frac{\text{Amount of drug in body}}{\text{Plasma drug concentration}}$$

$$V = 1\ 44 \cdot CL \cdot t_{1/2}$$

$$fe = \frac{\text{Total amount excreted unchanged}}{\text{Dose}}$$

$$\underset{\text{Total clearance}}{CL} = \underset{\text{Renal clearance}}{CL_R} + \underset{\text{Hepatic clearance}}{CL_H}$$

$$\text{Renal clearance} = fe \cdot CL$$

STUDY PROBLEMS

1. Which of the statements below is (are) correct?
   - I. Drug A has a clearance that is twice as great as that of Drug B, but they both have the same volume of distribution. Therefore, Drug A has the longer half-life.
   - II. Drug A and Drug B have the same half-life, but very different volumes of distribution. The AUC values of both drugs are expected, therefore, to be the same when the same intravenous dose is given.
   - III. Drugs A and B have different clearance values and half-lives, so they cannot have the same initial concentrations when given the same dose intravenously.

   A. I only　　**E.** I and III
   B. II only　　**F.** II and III
   C. III only　　**G.** All
   D. I and II　　**H.** None
2. After an intravenous bolus of diazepam, the kinetics of the drug exhibits the characteristics of a two-compartment model. Which of the following statements is (are) correct for diazepam and other drugs showing this kinetic behavior?
   - I. Diazepam exhibits a rapid initial distribution phase followed by a slower elimination phase.
   - II. The plasma concentration–time curve of diazepam can be simulated by the sum of two exponential terms.

III. Diazepam shows an almost immediate equilibration of drug in plasma with that in highly perfused tissues (central compartment) followed by a slower distribution to other peripheral tissues (tissue compartment).

A. I only **E.** I and III
B. II only **F.** II and III
C. III only **G.** All
D. I and II **H.** None

3. Which *one* of the following statements below is correct for a drug whose disposition kinetics is described by a one-compartment model and a half-life of 10 hours?
   a. The elimination rate constant (fractional rate of loss) of this drug is 0.00693/hr.
   b. It takes 40 hours for 87.5% of an intravenous bolus dose to be eliminated from the body.
   c. The fraction of the dose remaining in the body at 20 hours following an intravenous bolus dose is 0.125.
   d. It takes twice as long to eliminate 37.5 mg following a 50-mg intravenous bolus dose as it does to eliminate 50 mg after a 100-mg dose.
4. Piroxicam, a nonsteroidal anti-inflammatory drug (NSAID), demonstrates first-order elimination kinetics. It has a half-life of 48 hours in a specific male patient. Roughly what percentage of an absorbed dose (absorption is finished in about 2 hours) would you expect to remain in the body of the patient 6 days after he took a single 60-mg dose, instead of the usual 20-mg dose?
   a. 6.25% b. 12.5% c. 25% d. 50% e. 75%
5. On Fig. 5-9, a semilogarithmic graph scaled to 24 hours, draw the time course of each of the following two drugs as it would appear after an intravenous bolus dose. Both drugs show one-compartment distribution characteristics and are given in a dose of 10 mg.
   Drug A: V = 100 L; Half-life = 4 hours Drug B: V = 500 L; Half-life = 12 hours
6. When 2 mg of lorazepam, a drug used orally in the management of anxiety disorders or for the short-term relief of the symptoms of anxiety or anxiety associated with depressive symptoms, was administered intravenously as a bolus to a patient in a clinical study, the following plasma concentration–time relationship was observed during the terminal phase. The area under the curve associated with the distribution

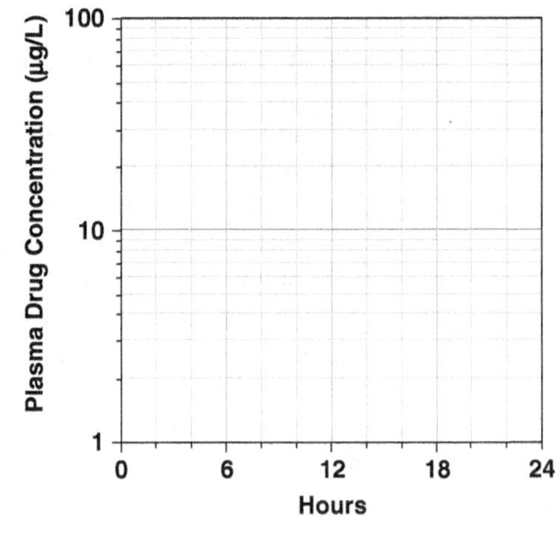

FIGURE 5-9

phase (first 2 hours) was small compared with the total area under the curve; therefore, a monoexponential model for the drug was deemed to be reasonable.

$$C = 25 \cdot e^{-0.05t} \text{ (} C \text{ in µg/L; } t \text{ in hours)}$$

Calculate the following values:

a. Volume of distribution
b. Elimination half-life
c. Total clearance
d. The plasma concentration 24 hours after a 4-mg dose.

7. The average clearance and volume of distribution of valproic acid, an antiepileptic drug, in the adult patient population are 0.5 L/hr and 9 L, respectively.
   a. Calculate the rate of elimination of valproic acid when the plasma concentration is 30 mg/L.
   b. Calculate the half-life of valproic acid.
   c. What is the amount of valproic acid in the body at distribution equilibrium when the plasma concentration is 60 mg/L?
   d. What is the expected plasma concentration 12 hours after an intravenous 700-mg dose of valproic acid (administered as the equivalent amount of the sodium salt)?
8. Fig. 5-10 shows a semilogarithmic plot of the plasma concentration–time profile of theophylline, used in the treatment of chronic obstructive airways disease, following a 500-mg intravenous bolus dose in a 70-kg patient. Notice that the decline is biexponential, with the break in the curve between 30 minutes and 1 hour. Theophylline is 40% bound in plasma and freely passes across membranes and distributes in all body water spaces. It is also extensively metabolized, with only 10% of the dose excreted in the urine unchanged.

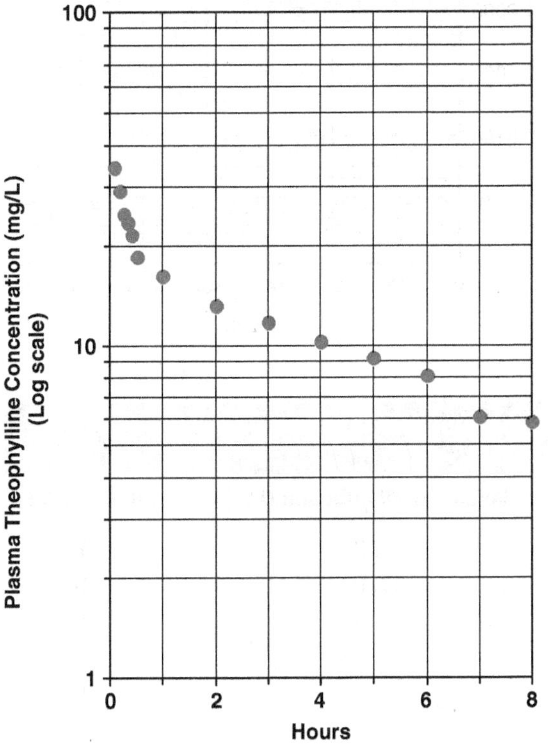

FIGURE 5-10 Semilogarithmic plot of the plasma concentration–time profile of theophylline following a 500-mg IV bolus dose in a 70-kg patient. (From Mitenko PA, Ogilvie RI. Pharmacokinetics of intravenous theophylline. *Clin Pharmacol Ther* 1973;14:509–513.)

a. The total area under the plasma concentration–time profile of theophylline is 125 mg-hr/L. Calculate the total clearance of theophylline.
b. Is it appropriate to call the initial decline phase up to about 30 minutes the distribution phase, knowing that the AUC of theophylline up to that time is 13.1 mg-hr/L?
c. The plasma concentration at the first sampling time of 5 minutes is 33 mg/L. What percentage of the dose has distributed out of the plasma by then? Also, what tissues are most likely to be involved, and why?
d. Calculate the renal clearance of theophylline.
e. From the graph, estimate the half-life of theophylline.
f. Estimate the volume of distribution of theophylline.
g. Determine the amount of theophylline remaining in the body 8 hours after a 500-mg intravenous dose.

9. As can be seen from Fig. 5-8 of this chapter, the half-lives of diazepam, nortriptyline, and warfarin are of a similar magnitude, around 30 hours.
   a. From the respective values of clearance and volume of distribution of these drugs obtained in Fig. 5-8 and listed in Table 5-2, plot on Fig. 5-11 the expected plasma concentration–time profiles of these drugs for 14 days (336 hours) following a 10-mg intravenous dose of each, assuming that the decline can be well characterized by a monoexponential equation.
   b. Comment on the statement "half-life depends on clearance and volume of distribution."

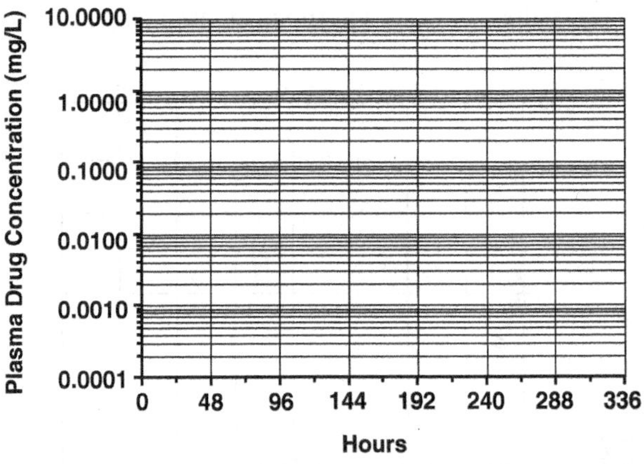

FIGURE 5-11

TABLE 5-2 | Estimated Pharmacokinetic Paramenters for Diazepam, Nortryptyline, and Warfarin from data in Fig. 5-8

Drug	Clearance (L/hr)	Volume of Distribution (L)	Half-life (hr)
Diazepam	1.6	80	35
Nortryptyline	30	1700	39
Warfarin	0.18	8	31

TABLE 5-3 | Plasma Concentrations of Cocaine Base After a Single IV Dose of 33 mg Cocaine Hydrochloride

Time (hr)	0.16	0.5	1.0	1.5	2	2.5	3.0
Concentration (μg/L)	170	122	74	45	28	17	10

10. The data given in Table 5-3 are the plasma concentrations of cocaine base as a function of time after i.v. administration of 33 mg cocaine hydrochloride to a subject. (Molecular weight of cocaine hydrochloride = 340 g/mol; molecular weight of cocaine = 303 g/mol.) (Adapted from Chow MJ, Ambre JJ, Ruo TI, et al. Kinetics of cocaine distribution, elimination, and chronotropic effects. *Clin Pharmacol Ther* 1985;38:318–324.)
    a. Prepare a semilogarithmic plot of plasma concentration versus time.
    b. Estimate the half-life.
    c. Estimate the total AUC of cocaine from the relationship AUC = $C(0)/k$, which is obtained by integrating the exponential equation, $C = C(0) \cdot e^{-kt}$
    d. Calculate the clearance of cocaine.
    e. Given that the body weight of the subject is 75 kg, calculate the volume of distribution of cocaine in L/kg.

CHAPTER 6

Physiologic and Physicochemical Determinants of Distribution and Elimination

OBJECTIVES

The reader will be able to:

- Describe the effects of a perfusion-rate limitation, a permeability-rate limitation, and the tissue-to-blood equilibrium distribution ratio on the time required for drug distribution to the tissues.
- Describe the relationship between volume of distribution of a drug and the size and affinity that it has for the tissues involved in its distribution.
- Describe the relationship between volume of distribution of a drug and its binding to constituents in plasma and tissues.
- Ascertain whether or not, for a given amount of drug in the body, the unbound plasma concentration is likely to be sensitive to variation in plasma protein binding when the volume of distribution is known.
- Calculate blood clearance when plasma clearance and plasma-to-blood concentration ratio are known.
- Calculate the extraction ratio of a drug across an eliminating organ given both blood clearance and blood flow associated with that organ.
- Describe what is meant by intrinsic hepatic clearance.
- Ascertain from the value of an organ's extraction ratio whether the clearance of a drug by that organ is likely to be sensitive to changes in perfusion rate, cellular activity, or plasma protein binding.
- Describe the role that biliary secretion can play in drug disposition.
- Describe where filtration, secretion, and reabsorption of drugs occur within the nephron.
- State the average values of hepatic blood flow, renal blood flow, and glomerular filtration rate in a typical 20-year-old patient.
- Given renal clearance and plasma protein binding data, determine whether a drug is predominately reabsorbed from or secreted into the renal tubule.
- Ascertain the relative contribution of the renal and hepatic routes to total elimination from total and renal clearance values.
- Define enterohepatic cycling of a drug and what is meant by enterohepatic cycling through a metabolite.

In Chapter 5, we explored the kinetics of drug disposition, that is, the change in the systemic exposure to a drug with time after its administration in an intravenous bolus dose. In this chapter, we examine the physiologic and physicochemical determinants of drug disposition.

WHY DOES DISTRIBUTION VARY SO WIDELY AMONG DRUGS?

In Chapter 5, we learned that the distribution of drugs varies widely. But why is this the case? Recall that **distribution** refers to the reversible transfer of drug from one location to another within the body. Definitive information on the distribution of a drug requires its measurement in various tissues. Such data have been obtained in animals, but for obvious reasons are lacking in humans, although there are some scattered data from autopsy studies and from imaging with positron emitting labeled drugs, which can be externally monitored. Much useful information on rate and extent of distribution in humans can be derived, however, from observations in blood or plasma alone. This section explores distribution and its applications in drug therapy. It begins with kinetic considerations and ends with equilibrium concepts.

Kinetics of Drug Distribution

Although it may have great viewer impact on TV and films to portray a person succumbing instantly to the deadly effects of an ingested drug or poison acting on the heart, brain, or respiratory center, reality is different. Even if systemic absorption and response at the target site were instantaneous—which they are not, as discussed in Chapters 7 and 8—tissue distribution also takes time; it occurs at various rates and to various extents, as illustrated by experimental data in Fig. 6-1. Several factors determine the distribution pattern of a drug with time. Included are delivery of drug to tissues by blood, ability to cross tissue membranes, binding to constituents within blood and tissues, and partitioning into fat. Tissue uptake from blood, commonly called **extravasation**, continues toward equilibrium of the diffusible form of the drug (unionized and not protein bound) between tissue and blood perfusing it. The kinetics of distribution to a tissue can be controlled, or rate-limited, by either blood **perfusion** (a delivery limitation) or tissue **permeability** (a membrane limitation), as discussed qualitatively in Chapter 4. We now consider these issues more quantitatively.

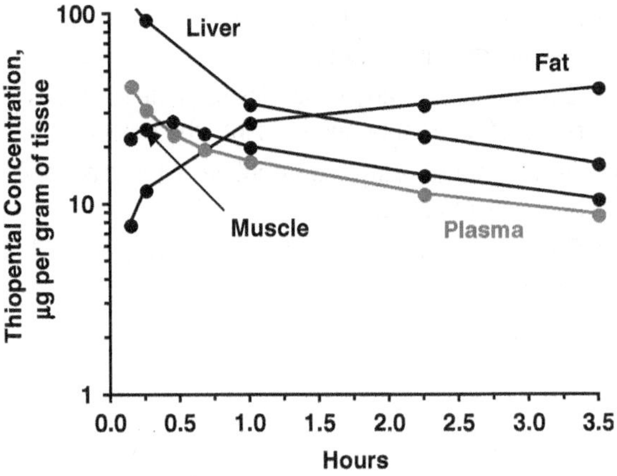

FIGURE 6-1 Semilogarithmic plot of the concentration (µg/g of tissue) of thiopental, a lipophilic drug in various tissues and plasma (*colored line*) following an IV bolus dose of 25 mg/kg to a dog. Note the early rise and fall of thiopental in a well-perfused tissue (liver), the slower rise in muscle, a poorly perfused tissue, and still slower rise in fat, a poorly perfused tissue with a high affinity for thiopental. After 3 hours, much of the drug remaining in the body is in adipose tissue. (Redrawn from Brodie BB, Bernstein E, Mark L. The role of body fat in limiting the duration of action of thiopental. *J Pharmacol Exp Ther* 1953;105:421–426 © Williams & Wilkins [1952].)

Perfusion-Rate Limitation

A **perfusion-rate limitation** prevails when the tissue membranes present essentially no barrier to distribution. As expected, this condition is likely to be met by small lipophilic drugs diffusing across most membranes of the body. As seen in Table 6-1, the perfusion rate of tissues varies enormously from approximately 10 mL/min/g for lungs down to a value on the order of only 0.025 mL/min/g for fat and resting skeletal muscle. To obtain the blood flow to a tissue, the perfusion rate must be multiplied by the mass of the tissue or organ of interest. All other factors, including organ mass, remaining equal, well-perfused tissues take up a drug much more rapidly than do poorly perfused tissues. Moreover, as the subsequent analysis shows, there is a direct correlation between tissue perfusion rate and the time required to distribute a drug to a tissue.

Fig. 6-2 (next page) shows blood perfusing a tissue in which distribution is perfusion rate–limited and no elimination occurs. The rate of presentation to the tissue, which in this scheme is maintained constant throughout, is the product of blood flow to it, Q, and arterial blood concentration, C_A, that is,

$$\text{Rate of presentation} = Q \cdot C_A \qquad \textbf{Eq. 6-1}$$

TABLE 6-1 | Blood Flow, Perfusion Rate, and Relative Sizes of Different Organs and Tissues Under Basal Conditions in a Standard 70-kg Human

Organ	Percent (%) of Body Weight	Blood Flow (mL/min)	Cardiac Output (%)	Perfusion Rate (mL/min/g of Tissue)
1. Adrenal glands	0.03	25	0.2	1.2
2. Blood	7	(5000)	(100)	–
3. Bone	16	250	5	0.02
4. Brain	2.0	700	14	0.5
5. Adipose	20[b]	200	4	0.03
6. Heart	0.4	200	4	0.6
7. Kidneys	0.5	1100	22	4
8. Liver	2.3	1350	27	0.8
Portal[a]	1.7 (gut)	(1050)	(21)	–
Arterial	–	(300)	(6)	–
9. Lungs	1.6	5000	100	10
10. Muscle (inactive)	43	750	15	0.025
11. Skin (cool weather)	11	300	6	0.04
12. Spleen	0.3	77	1.5	0.4
13. Thyroid gland	0.03	50	1	2.4
Total body	100	5000	100	0.071

[a]Some organs, e.g., stomach, intestines, spleen, and pancreas are not included separately, but together (total weight of 1.2 kg), as the blood perfusing them forms the hepatic portal system.
[b]Includes fat within organs.
Compiled and adapted from data in Guyton AC. *Textbook of Medical Physiology.* 7th ed. Philadelphia, PA: W.B. Saunders; 1986:230; Lentner C, ed. *Geigy Scientific Tables.* Vol. I. Edison, NJ: Ciba-Geigy, 1981; and Davies B, Morris T. Physiological parameters in laboratory animals and humans. *Pharm Res* 1993;10:1093–1095.

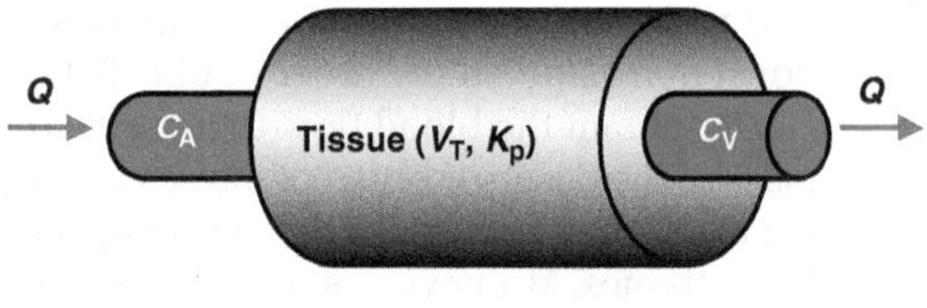

FIGURE 6-2 Drug is presented to a tissue at an arterial concentration of C_A and at a rate equal to the product of blood flow, Q_T, and C_A. The drug leaves the tissue at a venous concentration, C_V, and at a rate equal to $Q \cdot C_V$. The tissue concentration, C_T, increases when the rate of presentation exceeds the rate of leaving in the venous blood, and the converse. The amount of drug in the tissue is the product of V_T, the volume of the tissue, and the tissue drug concentration. K_p, the distribution ratio, is a measure of the affinity of tissue for drug.

The net rate of extravasation is the difference between the rate of presentation and the rate of leaving, $Q \cdot C_V$, where C_V is the emergent venous concentration. Therefore,

$$\text{Net rate of uptake} = Q \cdot (C_A - C_V) \qquad \text{Eq. 6-2}$$

Further, with no effective resistance to movement into the tissue, blood and tissue can be viewed kinetically as one compartment, with the concentration in emergent venous blood (C_V) in equilibrium with that in the tissue, C_T.

At any time, therefore,

$$\text{Amount of drug in tissue} = V_T \cdot C_T = V_T \cdot K_P \cdot C_V \qquad \text{Eq. 6-3}$$

where V_T is the tissue volume and K_P is the **tissue-to-blood equilibrium distribution ratio (C_T/C_V)**, a measure of the affinity of tissue for the drug. The higher the value of K_P, the greater is the tissue affinity. Furthermore, the fractional rate of exit, or **distribution rate constant, k_T**, is given by

$$k_T = \frac{\text{Rate of exit}}{\text{Amount in tissue}} = \frac{Q_T \cdot C_V}{V_T \cdot K_P \cdot C_V} \qquad \text{Eq. 6-4}$$

or

$$k_T = \frac{(Q_T / V_T)}{k_P} \qquad \text{Eq. 6-5}$$

where Q_T/V_T is the perfusion rate of the tissue. The parameter k_T, with units of reciprocal time, may be regarded as a measure of how rapidly drug would leave the tissue if the arterial concentration were suddenly to drop to zero. It is analogous to the elimination rate constant for loss of drug from the whole body, and, like elimination, the kinetics of tissue distribution can be characterized by a tissue **distribution half-life** for which

$$\text{Distribution half-life} = \frac{0.693}{k_T} = \frac{0.693 \cdot K_P}{(Q_T / V_T)} \qquad \text{Eq. 6-6}$$

Thus, drug leaves slowly from tissues that have a high affinity (K_P) for it and that are poorly perfused. The reason for this is that, when affinity is high there is much drug in the tissue, and with poor perfusion, it takes a long time to remove what is in the tissue. The distribution half-life applies not only to efflux from, but also to uptake into, tissues. That is, distribution is fastest into those tissues in which the tissue distribution half-life is shortest. Furthermore, it takes approximately one distribution half-life to reach 50% of the equilibrium value and, for practical purposes, 3.32 half-lives to reach the equilibrium value. For example, with an average perfusion rate for the whole body

TABLE 6-2 | Influence of Changes in Perfusion Rates and Tissue Affinity on the Time to Achieve Distribution Equilibrium

Tissue/Drug	Perfusion Rate (mL/min/g of Tissue)[a]	K_p	Tissue Distribution Half-Life (min)[b]	Time to Achieve Distribution Equilibrium (min)[c]
Influence of Perfusion Rate on Drug A				
Kidney	4	1	0.173	0.57
Brain	0.5	1	1.386	4.60
Adipose	0.03	1	23.10	76.7
Influence of Affinity for Adipose				
Drug A	0.03	1	23.10	76.7
Drug B	0.03	2	46.20	153
Drug C	0.03	10	231.0	767

[a]Although usually expressed and measured in these units, for calculating the times for drug distribution, the density of the tissues is assumed to be 1, that is, 1 g/mL of tissue.
[b]Calculated using Equation 6-6.
[c]3.32 × tissue distribution half-life.

of 5 L/min/70 kg (see Table 6-1) and for a drug with a tissue-to-blood equilibrium ratio of 1, the average tissue distribution half-life is 10 minutes and, therefore, distribution within the body would be complete well within 1 hour (6 half-lives). However, because both perfusion and K_P vary among tissues, so does the time for achievement of distribution equilibrium among them.

To appreciate the foregoing, consider the data provided in Table 6-2, in which are listed the perfusion rates (from Table 6-1), K_P values, and corresponding tissue distribution half-lives for various selected tissues, calculated using Equation 6-6. First, consider the data for drug A in which K_P values in kidneys, brain, and fat are the same and equal to 1. Given that the perfusion rates to these tissues are 4, 0.5, and 0.03 mL/min/g of tissue, respectively, it follows that the corresponding half-lives for distribution are 0.17, 1.4, and 23 minutes. Thus, by 0.57 minutes (3.32 half-lives), drug in the kidneys has reached equilibrium with that in blood, whereas it takes closer to 5 and 77 minutes for equilibrium to be reached in brain and fat, respectively, which are tissues of lower perfusion. Next, consider events in fat for drugs with different K_P values, namely 1, 2, and 10. Here, the corresponding half-lives are 23, 46, and 231 minutes. Now, not only is the time taken for drug in tissue to reach equilibrium different, but so are the equilibrium tissue concentrations for a given plasma drug concentration.

These simple examples illustrate two basic principles: Both the approach toward equilibrium during drug input and the loss of drug from a tissue on stopping drug input take longer, the poorer the perfusion and the greater the partitioning of drug into a tissue. The latter is contrary to what one might intuitively anticipate. However, the greater the tendency to concentrate in a tissue, the longer it takes to deliver to that tissue the amount needed to achieve distribution equilibrium, and the longer it takes to redistribute drug out of that tissue. Stated differently, an increased affinity of drug for a tissue accentuates an existing limitation imposed by perfusion.

Permeability Limitation

As discussed in Chapter 4, a **permeability-rate limitation** arises particularly for polar drugs diffusing across tightly knit lipoidal membranes, such as the brain where

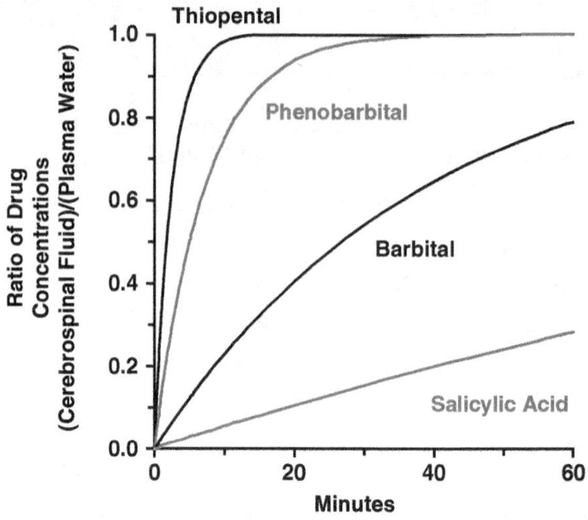

FIGURE 6-3 The approach to equilibrium of drug in the cerebrospinal fluid (essentially devoid of protein) with that unbound in plasma is often permeability-rate limited. The rise in the ratio of drug concentrations (cerebrospinal fluid/unbound drug in plasma) to equilibrium (when the ratio = 1) is shown for various drugs in the dog. The plasma concentration was kept relatively constant throughout the study. Notice that when a permeability rate limitation occurs, the time to achieve equilibration is longer than that when uptake is perfusion-rate limited, as occurs with the lipophilic thiopental. (Redrawn from the data of Brodie BB, Kurz H, Schanker LS. The importance of dissociation constant and lipid solubility in influencing the passage of drugs into the cerebrospinal fluid. *J Pharmacol Exp Ther* 1960;130:20–25. Copyright 1960, The Williams & Wilkins Co., Baltimore).

the barrier is at the vascular level. Under these circumstances, there are large differences in the permeability—hence ease of entry—among compounds for the same tissue. A permeability-rate limitation simply decreases the speed of entry and hence increases the time to reach distribution equilibrium *over that of perfusion alone.* This is illustrated in Fig. 6-3, which shows the time course for approach to equilibrium of various compounds between the cerebrospinal fluid of brain and that unbound in plasma. The anesthetic thiopental is very lipophilic, and its entry into brain is essentially perfusion-rate limited. The remaining compounds are more polar, and uptake is slower. In addition to lipophilicity, degree of ionization is a determinant in that only unionized drug penetrates the brain. For example, the partition coefficients of the anti-inflammatory agent salicylic acid (pK_a, 3) and pentobarbital (pK_a, 7.8), a sedative hypnotic, are similar; yet the time required to reach distribution equilibrium is far shorter for pentobarbital than for salicylic acid because, being the weaker acid, a greater percentage of pentobarbital is un-ionized within the plasma and tissue pH range, 7.2–7.4.

At equilibrium, the unbound concentration in tissue would be expected to be the same as that in plasma. Sometimes, however, this equality is not observed. Reasons for lack of equality, such as pH gradients across cell membranes and active transport, have been discussed in Chapter 4. Another reason for its occurrence in an eliminating organ is maintenance of sink conditions by cellular metabolism.

Extent of Distribution

Multiple equilibria occur within plasma in which drugs can bind to various proteins, examples of which are listed in Table 6-3. In plasma, acidic drugs commonly bind to albumin, the most abundant plasma protein. Basic drugs often bind to α_1-acid glycoprotein and neutral compounds to lipoproteins. Some hormones bind preferentially to specific proteins, such as cortisol to transcortin, thyroxine to thyroid-binding globulin, and testosterone to one of the sex-binding globulins. Distribution within each tissue also involves multiple equilibria. Within tissues, drugs can bind to a wide variety of substances, such as neutral and acidic phospholipids, as well as partition into fat.

TABLE 6-3 | Representative Proteins to Which Drugs Bind in Plasma

Protein	Molecular Weight (g/mol)	Normal Concentrations g/L	Normal Concentrations μM
Albumin	67,000	35–50	500–700
α_1-Acid glycoprotein	42,000	0.4–1.0	9–23
Lipoproteins	200,000–2,400,000	Variable	–
Cortisol binding globulin (transcortin)	53,000	0.03–0.07	0.6–1.4
Sex-binding globulin	90,000	0.0036	0.04

Apparent Volume of Distribution

The concentration in plasma achieved after distribution of drug throughout the body is complete is a result of the dose administered and the extent of tissue distribution, reflected by the volume of distribution. Recall from Equation 5-22 in the last chapter, and repeated here, that

$$V = \frac{\text{Amount in body at equilibrium}}{\text{Plasma drug concentration}} = \frac{A}{C}$$

This parameter is useful in relating amount in body to plasma concentration, and the converse. Recall, also, that V varies widely, with illustrative values ranging from 3 to 7000 L in an average 70-kg adult, the latter being a value far in excess of total body size. On examination, most acids tend to have small volumes of distribution (<50 L), and basic compounds much larger ones (>100 L). For example, reference to Fig. 5-8 (chapter 5) shows that the values of V for acidic drugs, such as the analgesic aspirin, the diuretic furosemide, and the oral anticoagulant warfarin, all cluster around 10 L/70 kg. In contrast, for basic drugs such as the antihypertensive β-blocker propranolol, the analgesic morphine, and the antidepressant nortriptyline, V exceeds 100 L and can be much higher, e.g., 7000 L, as seen for the antiarrhythmic drug amiodarone.

Knowing plasma volume, V_P, and volume of distribution, V, the fraction of drug in body that is in and outside of plasma can be estimated. The amount in plasma is $V_P \cdot C$; the amount in the body is $V \cdot C$. Therefore,

$$\text{Fraction of drug in body in plasma} = \frac{V_P}{V} \qquad \text{Eq. 6-7}$$

It is evident that the larger the volume of distribution, the smaller is the percentage in plasma. For example, for a drug with a volume of distribution of 100 L, only 3% resides in plasma.

The remaining fraction, given by

$$\text{Fraction of drug in body outside plasma} = \frac{(V - V_P)}{V} \qquad \text{Eq. 6-8}$$

includes drug in blood cells. For the example considered above, 97% is outside plasma. Although this fraction can be readily determined from plasma data, the actual tissue distribution of drug outside plasma cannot.

The reason why the volume of distribution is an apparent volume and why its value differs among drugs may be appreciated by considering the simple model shown

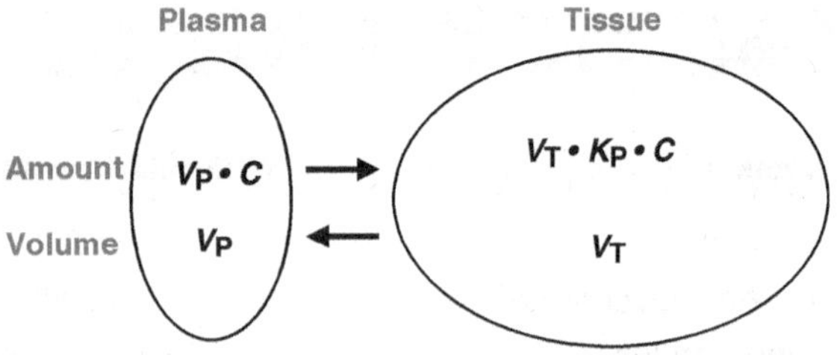

FIGURE 6-4 The effect of tissue binding on volume of distribution is illustrated by a drug that distributes between plasma and a tissue. The physiologic volumes are V_P and V_T, respectively. At equilibrium, the amount of drug in each location depends on the equilibrium distribution (partition) ratio, K_P, the plasma and tissue volumes, and the plasma concentration.

in Fig. 6-4. In this model, drug in the body is entirely accounted for in plasma, of volume V_P, and one tissue compartment, of volume V_T. At distribution equilibrium, the amount of drug in each location can be expressed in terms of their respective volumes and concentrations (C, C_T)

$$\underset{\text{Amount in body}}{A} = \underset{\text{Amount in plasma}}{V_P \cdot C} + \underset{\text{Amount in tissue}}{V_T \cdot C_T} \qquad \text{Eq. 6-9}$$

And, since $A = V \cdot C$ (Equation 5-22), it follows, on dividing the equation above by C, that

$$V = V_P + V_T \cdot K_P \qquad \text{Eq. 6-10}$$

Since $K_p = C_T/C$, the product $V_T \cdot K_P$ is the apparent volume of a tissue viewed from measurement of drug in plasma. Thus, by expanding the model to embrace all tissues of the body, it is seen that the volume of distribution of a drug is the volume of plasma plus the sum of the apparent volumes of distribution of each tissue. For some tissues, the value of K_P is large, which explains why the volume of distribution of some drugs, such as basic compounds, can be much greater than total body size. Also, fat, for example, occupies approximately 20% of body volume. If the K_P value of a drug in fat is 10, then this tissue alone has an apparent volume of distribution of 140 L (0.2 × 70 × 10), twice that of body volume. Remember, that even when perfusion rate-limits distribution, it takes many hours longer for distribution equilibrium to be achieved when the drug has a high affinity for fat.

The volume of distribution of a specific drug can also vary widely among patients. The reasons for such differences are now explored.

Plasma Protein Binding

The principal concern with plasma protein binding of a drug is related to its variability within and among patients in various therapeutic settings. The degree of binding is frequently expressed as the bound-to-total concentration ratio. This ratio has limiting values of 0 and 1.0. Drugs with values greater than 0.90 are said to be highly bound.

As stated previously, unbound, rather than bound, concentration is more important in therapeutics. Consequently, the fraction unbound is more useful in pharmacokinetics than the fraction bound. The **fraction in plasma unbound,** fu, is

$$fu = \frac{Cu}{C} \qquad \text{Eq. 6-11}$$

Binding is a function of the affinity between protein and drug. Because the number of binding sites on a protein is limited, binding also depends on the molar concentrations of both drug and protein. The greater the protein concentration for a given drug concentration, the greater the fraction bound and the converse. In practice, only a small

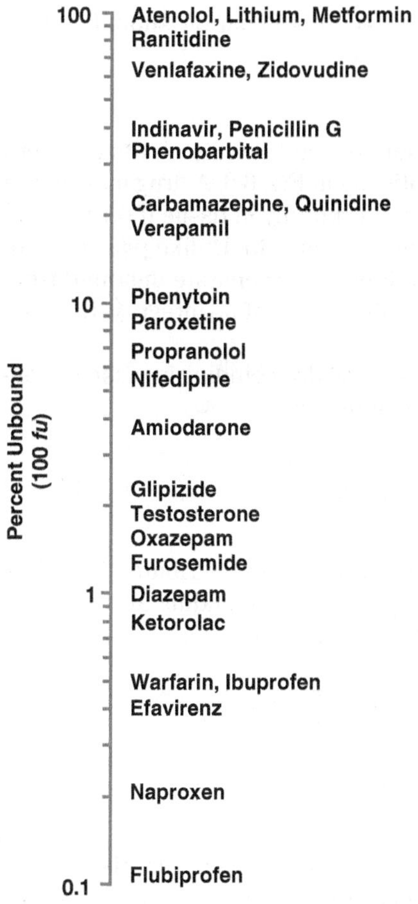

FIGURE 6-5 The fraction of drug in plasma unbound (expressed here in percent) varies widely among drugs.

percentage of the available sites on binding proteins is occupied at the therapeutic concentrations of most drugs; *fu* is then relatively constant at a given protein concentration and independent of drug concentration. Then, total plasma concentration is a good measure of changes in unbound drug concentration. Occasionally, therapeutic concentrations are sufficiently high that most of the available binding sites are occupied, in which case *fu* is concentration-dependent. Approximate values of *fu* usually associated with therapy for representative drugs are shown in Fig. 6-5.

For the remainder of the book, it is helpful to remember that pharmacologic activity relates to the unbound concentration. Plasma protein binding, then, is often only of interest because the total plasma concentration is commonly measured and binding sometimes varies, such as in renal and hepatic disease and with drug concentration. The total concentration is commonly measured because of technical problems in readily measuring the unbound concentration, such as physical problems in quantitatively separating small molecular weight unbound drug from very large protein-bound drug, and because of assay sensitivity problems, especially when *fu* is very small. The total plasma concentration depends on both the extent of protein binding and the unbound concentration, that is,

$$C = \frac{Cu}{fu} \qquad \text{Eq. 6-12}$$

When conceptualizing dependency and functionality, this equation should not be rearranged.

Tissue Binding

The fraction of drug in the body located in plasma depends on its binding to both plasma and tissue components, as shown schematically in Fig. 6-6. A drug may have a high affinity for plasma proteins, but may be located primarily in tissue if tissue components have a higher affinity for drug than plasma proteins do. Unlike plasma binding, tissue binding of a drug cannot be measured directly. To separate unbound from bound drug, the tissue must be disrupted, resulting in the loss of its integrity. Even so, tissue binding is important in drug distribution.

Tissue binding may be inferred from measurement of drug binding in plasma. Consider, for example, the following mass balance relationship:

$$\underset{\text{Amount in body}}{V \cdot C} = \underset{\text{Amount in plasma}}{V_P \cdot C} + \underset{\text{Amount in tissue}}{V_T \cdot C_T} \qquad \text{Eq. 6-13}$$

in which V_T is the volume outside plasma into which the drug distributes (which is close to the total volume of tissue water), and C_T is the corresponding average total tissue concentration that accounts for mass of drug in the tissues.
Dividing by C,

$$\underset{\text{Apparent volume of distribution}}{V} = \underset{\text{Volume of plasma}}{V_P} + \underset{\text{Apparent volume of tissue}}{V_T \cdot \left(C_T/C\right)} \qquad \text{Eq. 6-14}$$

Recall that $fu = Cu/C$. Similarly, for the tissue, $fu_T = Cu_T/C_T$. Given that distribution equilibrium is achieved when the unbound concentrations in plasma, Cu, and in tissue, Cu_T, are equal, that is, that there is no active transport into or out of the tissue, it follows that

$$\frac{C_T}{C} = \frac{fu}{fu_T} \qquad \text{Eq. 6-15}$$

which, on substituting into Equation 6-14, yields

$$V = V_P + V_T \cdot \frac{fu}{fu_T} \qquad \text{Eq. 6-16}$$

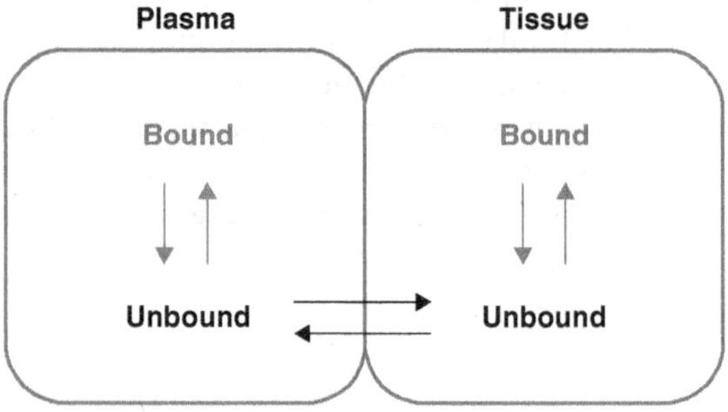

FIGURE 6-6 At equilibrium, the distribution of a drug within the body depends on binding to both plasma proteins and tissue components. In the model, only unbound drug is capable of entering and leaving the plasma and tissue compartments.

From this relationship, it is seen that V increases when either fu increases or fu_T decreases, and the converse.

By comparing Equations 6-10 and 6-16, it is seen that $K_P \approx fu/fu_T$. That is, K_P is a measure of the relative binding of a drug between plasma and tissue. However, although equivalent, the advantage of Equation 6-16 over Equation 6-10 is that it allows for the interpretation of drug distribution among drugs, as well as when binding is altered for a specific compound. To appreciate this interpretation, first consider the statement, made earlier, that the volumes of distribution of basic drugs are much larger than those of acidic ones. The difference cannot be ascribed to differences in plasma binding. Examination of the data in Fig. 6-5 shows that there is no clear pattern in the fraction unbound in plasma between these two classes of compounds. For example, fu is 0.02–0.04 for furosemide and amiodarone, an acidic and a basic drug, respectively. Yet, the former has a volume of distribution of 10 L, and the latter 7000 L. Therefore, the difference between acidic and basic drugs must lie in a much higher tissue binding of bases (lower fu_T). The major group of binding constituents for basic drugs in tissues, to which acids do not bind, are acidic phospholipids, in addition to adipose. Next, consider the data for propranolol in Fig. 6-7, which shows large differences in V among subjects. The linear relationship between V and fu not only indicates, from Equation 6-15, that V_T/fu_T is relatively constant (and, as the body water content does not vary much among individuals, hence tissue binding is constant), but also that differences in binding of propranolol in plasma among subjects account for most of the variation observed in its volume of distribution.

The relationship expressed in Equation 6-15 explains why, because of plasma and tissue binding, V rarely corresponds to a defined physiologic space, such as plasma volume (3 L), extracellular water (16 L), or total body water (42 L). Even if V corresponds to the value of a physiologic space, one cannot conclude unambiguously that the drug distributes only into that volume. Binding of drugs in both plasma and specific tissues complicates the situation and often prevents any conclusion from being made about the actual volume into which the drug distributes. An exception is when drug is restricted to plasma; the volumes of distribution, apparent and real, are then the same, about 3 L in an adult.

For drugs of high molecular weight, particularly antibody drugs, extravascular distribution is very slow. For such drugs, the volume of distribution tends to be very low, sometimes approaching that of plasma, 3 L. For example, for most antibody drugs, V ranges between 3 and 8 L. However, for small molecular weight drugs, an

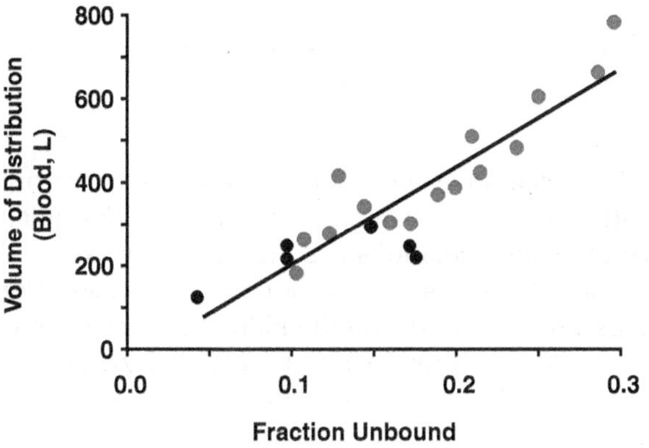

FIGURE 6-7 The volume of distribution of (+)-propranolol varies with the fraction unbound in plasma. The observation was made in six control subjects (*black circle*) and in 15 patients with chronic hepatic disease (*red circle*) after an IV 40 mg bolus dose of (+)-propranolol. (Data redrawn from Branch RA, Jones J, Read AE. A study of factors influencing drug disposition in chronic liver disease, using the model drug (+)-propranolol. *Br J Clin Pharmacol* 1976;3:243–249.)

apparent volume of 3 L cannot be an equilibrium value, because plasma proteins themselves equilibrate slowly between plasma and other extracellular fluids. The apparent volume of plasma proteins, about 7.5 L for albumin, is perhaps a better estimate of the minimum value for drugs strongly and predominantly bound to this protein. For reasons just discussed, this lower limit tends to be seen more frequently with acidic, predominantly ionized at pH 7.4, nonpolar drugs than with neutral, polar, or basic ones.

For very polar, small (MW < 1000 g/mol) drugs that are not bound in either tissues or plasma, the volume of distribution varies between the extracellular fluid volume (16 L) and the total body water (42 L), depending on the degree to which the drug gains access to intracellular fluids. Examples of compounds that distribute in total body water, and that do not appreciably bind within plasma or in tissues, are caffeine and alcohol, both small neutral molecules that pass freely through membranes. The volume of distribution of these two compounds is about 40 L.

Amount in Body and Unbound Concentration

For many drugs, volume of distribution is greater than 50 L, implying that only a small fraction of drug in body resides in plasma. Therefore, ignoring the first term, V_P (3 L), in Equation 6-16 and noting that $fu \cdot C = Cu$, it follows that

$$\text{Amount in body} = V \cdot C \approx \frac{V_T}{fu_T} \cdot Cu \qquad \text{Eq. 6-17}$$

This equation indicates that the unbound concentration, Cu, which drives response, is independent of plasma protein binding for a given amount of drug in the body and that amount in the body is better reflected by Cu than C when plasma protein binding is altered.

Sometimes, a larger than usual dose, often termed a loading dose, is given to rapidly achieve a therapeutic response, putatively by rapidly producing a desired unbound concentration (see Chapter 12). The question arises whether or not the loading dose needs to be adjusted with variations in both plasma and tissue binding. Based on the foregoing consideration, for drugs with a volume of distribution greater than 50 L, it should be apparent that no adjustment in loading dose for altered plasma protein binding is needed. The total plasma concentration does, of course, change with altered plasma binding, but this is of no therapeutic consequence with respect to loading dose requirements. If, however, tissue binding (fu_T) were to change, so would the initial value(s) of Cu (and C), necessitating a decision to change the loading dose.

WHY DOES CLEARANCE VARY SO WIDELY AMONG DRUGS?

Processes of Elimination

Before answering the question as to why clearance varies so widely, a few words are in order about processes of elimination and about clearance in general. For small molecules, elimination occurs by excretion and metabolism. Some drugs are excreted via the bile. Others, particularly volatile substances, are excreted in the breath. For most drugs, however, excretion occurs predominantly via the kidneys. Indeed, some drugs are eliminated almost entirely by urinary excretion, but these are relatively few. Rather, metabolism is the major mechanism for elimination of drugs from the body,

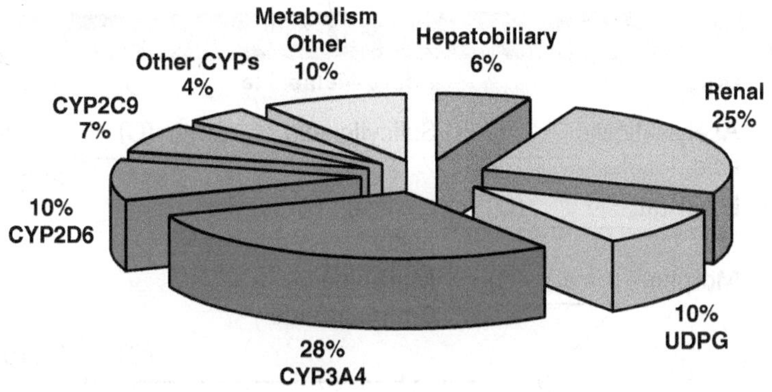

FIGURE 6-8 Relative importance of route and mechanism of elimination of the top 200 prescribed drugs. The segments of the pie in color refer to phase I metabolic reactions. The remaining segments refer to either phase II conjugative reactions or excretory processes within the liver and kidney. (From Williams JA, Hyland R, Jones BC, et al. Drug-drug interactions for the UDP-glucuronosyltransferase substrates: a pharmacokinetic explanation for typically observed low exposure [AUCi/AUC] ratios. *Drug Metab Dispos* 2004;32:1201–1208.)

as shown in Fig. 6-8 for the top 200 prescribed drugs. For most of these, metabolism occurs predominately in the liver; for some, the intestinal wall is an additional site of metabolism, which has implications for oral administration (see Chapter 8). For a few drugs, metabolism is extensive in one or more other tissues, such as the kidneys, lungs, and blood. These remarks should be contrasted with the processes responsible for the elimination of polypeptide drugs and therapeutic proteins. These undergo degradation in the body to their constituent amino acids, which are then reutilized by the body.

The most common routes of drug metabolism are oxidation, reduction, hydrolysis, and conjugation. Frequently, a drug simultaneously undergoes metabolism by several competing (primary) pathways. The fraction going to each metabolite depends on the relative rates of each of the parallel pathways. Metabolites may undergo further (secondary) metabolism. For example, oxidation, reduction, and hydrolysis are often followed by conjugation. These reactions occur in series or are said to be **sequential reactions**. Because oxidation, reduction, and hydrolysis often occur first, they are commonly referred to as **phase I reactions**, and conjugations as **phase II reactions**. Some drugs, however, undergo only phase II reactions, and for others conjugation occurs in parallel with Phase I reactions.

Generally, the liver is the major—sometimes only—site of drug metabolism. Occasionally, however, a drug is extensively metabolized in one or more other tissues, such as the kidneys, lungs, blood, and gastrointestinal wall.

Table 6-4 (next page) illustrates patterns of biotransformation (metabolism) of representative drugs. The pathways of metabolism are classified by chemical alteration. Several of the transformations occur in the endoplasmic reticulum of cells of the liver and certain other tissues. On homogenizing these tissues, the endoplasmic reticulum is disrupted with the formation of small vesicles called **microsomes**. For this reason, metabolizing enzymes of the endoplasmic reticulum are called **microsomal enzymes**. Drug metabolism, therefore, may be classified as microsomal and nonmicrosomal.

The major enzymes responsible for the oxidation and reduction of many drugs belong to the superfamily of cytochrome P450 enzymes. The drug metabolizing enzymes of this vast superfamily are divided in humans into three major distinct families,

TABLE 6-4 | Patterns of Biotransformation[a] of Representative Drugs[b]

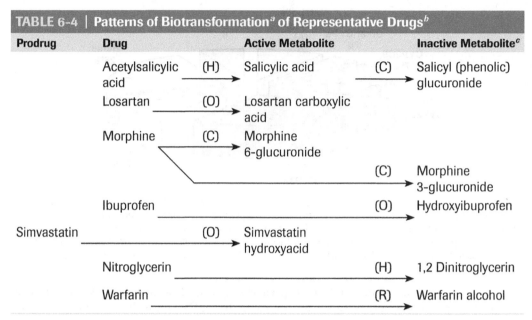

Prodrug	Drug		Active Metabolite		Inactive Metabolite[c]
	Acetylsalicylic acid	(H) →	Salicylic acid	(C) →	Salicyl (phenolic) glucuronide
	Losartan	(O) →	Losartan carboxylic acid		
	Morphine	(C) →	Morphine 6-glucuronide		
	Morphine			(C) →	Morphine 3-glucuronide
	Ibuprofen			(O) →	Hydroxyibuprofen
Simvastatin		(O) →	Simvastatin hydroxyacid		
	Nitroglycerin			(H) →	1,2 Dinitroglycerin
	Warfarin			(R) →	Warfarin alcohol

[a]Classification: C, conjugation; H, hydrolysis; O, oxidation; R, reduction.
[b]For some drugs, only representative pathways are indicated.
[c]Inactive at concentrations obtained following the administration of a therapeutic dose of the parent drug.

designated CY(cytochrome)P(450) 1, 2 and 3, each further divided into subfamilies, designation by capital letters A, B, and so on. Arabic numerals are used to refer to individual enzymes (gene products) within each subfamily. These enzymes display a relatively high degree of structural specificity in that a drug is often a good substrate for one enzyme but not another. Fig. 6-9 displays the major P450 enzymes by abundance and by relevance to drug metabolism. The most abundant, CYP3A4, metabolizes many drugs of relatively diverse structure and size, and, unlike most of the other P450 enzymes, is found in the intestinal wall as well as in the liver. The abundance of a particular cytochrome in the liver does not necessarily reflect its importance to drug metabolism. For example, although making up only approximately 2% of the total CYP content, CYP2D6 is responsible for the metabolism of approximately 25% of the metabolism of prescribed drugs, and particularly basic compounds, many of which act on the central nervous system. Many acidic drugs are metabolized preferentially by CYP2C9 and CYP2C19. There are other drug metabolizing enzymes, in addition to the CYP450s, including monooxygenases, aldehyde oxidases, and various reductases.

The consequences of drug metabolism are manifold. Biotransformation provides a mechanism for ridding the body of undesirable foreign compounds and drugs; it also provides a means of producing active compounds. Often, both the drug and its metabolite(s) are active. The duration and intensity of the responses relate to the time courses of all active substances in the body.

Clearance in General

Of the concepts in pharmacokinetics, **clearance** has the greatest potential for clinical applications. It is also the most useful parameter for the evaluation of an elimination mechanism.

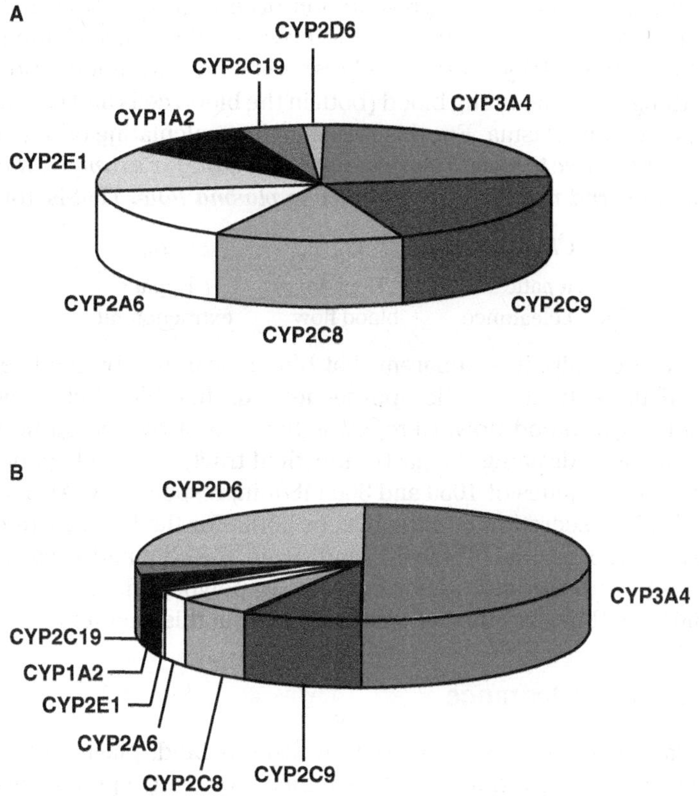

FIGURE 6-9 **A.** Relative abundance of the major hepatic P450 cytochromes in human liver. **B.** Relative contribution of the major hepatic P450 cytochromes in the P450-mediated clearance of 403 marketed drugs in the United States and Europe. (Redrawn from Clarke SE, Jones BC. Hepatic cytochromes P450 and their role in metabolism-based drug-drug interactions. In: Rodriguez AD, ed. *Drug-Drug Interactions.* New York, NY: Marcel Dekker, 2002:55–88.)

Recall from Chapter 5 that clearance is defined as the proportionality factor that relates rate of drug elimination to the plasma (drug) concentration, that is,

$$\text{Rate of elimination} = CL \cdot C$$

Alternatively, recall also that clearance may be viewed from the loss of drug across an organ of elimination, yielding the relationship (Equation 5-5 in Chapter 5)

$$CL = Q \cdot E$$

where Q is the flow rate to the organ, and E is the extraction ratio. This latter physiologic approach has a number of advantages, particularly in predicting and in evaluating the effects of changes in blood flow, plasma protein binding, enzyme activity, and secretory activity on the elimination of a drug, as will be seen.

Before proceeding, however, a point of distinction needs to be made between these two relationships for clearance. In the first, clearance is simply a proportionality term. In the second, it is derived from mass balance considerations, in the context of rates of presentation and exit from an eliminating organ. In the reservoir model used to introduce this concept, the fluid perfusing the eliminating organ (the extractor) is water, containing drug (Fig. 5-3). In vivo, the fluid presented to the liver and kidneys is whole blood, and the rate of presentation of drug to the kidneys, for example, is $Q_R \cdot C_A$, where Q_R and C_A are renal blood flow and the concentration in the arterial blood perfusing the kidneys, respectively. So when the extraction ratio, E, approaches one, everything in the incoming blood (both in the blood cells and plasma) is cleared of drug, not just that in plasma. For this reason, when calculating organ extraction ratio, *it is important to relate blood clearance of the organ, for example, the liver,* ($CL_{b,H}$), *to its blood flow and not plasma clearance to plasma flow.* That is, for the liver

$$\underset{\text{Hepatic blood clearance}}{CL_{b,H}} = \underset{\text{Hepatic blood flow}}{Q_H} \cdot \underset{\text{Hepatic extraction ratio}}{E_H} \qquad \text{Eq. 6-18}$$

From this relationship, it is apparent that blood clearance by the liver cannot be of any value. If the extraction ratio approaches 1.0, then blood clearance approaches a maximum, organ blood flow. Here, Q_H is the sum of two blood flows, the hepatic portal venous flow, draining the gastrointestinal tract, and the hepatic arterial blood flow, with average values of 1050 and 300 mL/min, respectively. Also, elimination can be by metabolism, secretion into the bile, or both. For the kidneys, the average blood flow in an adult is 1.1 L/min (Table 6-1) and, again, the elimination can be by excretion or metabolism, with the latter being common to polypeptide and protein drugs up to about 30,000 g/mol in size (further discussed later in this chapter).

Plasma Versus Blood Clearance

Because plasma is the most commonly measured fluid, plasma clearance is much more frequently reported than blood clearance. For many applications in pharmacokinetics, all that is needed is a proportionality term, in which case it matters little which clearance value for a drug is used. As seen above, the exception is if one wishes to estimate extraction ratio. Then, one needs to convert plasma clearance to blood clearance. This conversion is readily accomplished by experimentally determining the **plasma-to-blood concentration ratio (C/C_b)**, most often by preparing a known concentration in whole blood, centrifuging, and determining the resulting concentration in the plasma. This ratio generally ranges from 0.3 to 2, although it can be very much lower for drugs that associate extensively with blood cells, such as tacrolimus (0.05), an immunosuppressant drug used to prevent organ transplant rejection. Because, by definition, the product of clearance and concentration is equal to the rate of elimination, which is independent of what fluid is measured, it follows that:

$$\text{Rate of elimination} = CL \cdot C = CL_b \cdot C_b \qquad \text{Eq. 6-19}$$

so that blood clearance, CL_b, is

$$CL_b = CL \cdot \left(\frac{C}{C_b} \right) \qquad \text{Eq. 6-20}$$

For example, if the plasma clearance of a drug, by default simply called clearance, is 1.3 L/min, and the drug is extensively eliminated by hepatic metabolism, there is a potential danger in concluding that it has a high extraction ratio. However, knowing that the plasma-to-blood concentration ratio (from measurement of drug concentrations in plasma and whole blood) is 0.1 indicates that blood clearance is only 0.13 L/min, much lower than hepatic blood flow, 1.35 L/min. Hence, this drug is one of low extraction ratio, and clinically, the implications are very different, as discussed below.

Clearances of drugs by the liver and the kidneys are now examined. Each organ has special anatomic and physiologic features that require its separate consideration.

Hepatic Clearance

The functional unit of the liver is the acinus. It comprises hepatocytes (that metabolize some drugs and secrete others into the bile canniliculi), and associated hepatic arterioles and portal venules, which merge into the sinusoid just before reaching the hepatocytes. As with other organs of elimination, the removal of drug by the liver may be considered from mass balance relationships, as summarized in Equation 6-18.

Perfusion, Protein Binding, and Hepatocellular Activity

The clearances of drugs vary widely among compounds and between and within subjects owing to differences in organ perfusion, plasma protein binding, and inherent elimination characteristics within hepatocytes. Changes in perfusion can occur in disease and during exercise. One drug can compete for the binding sites of another within plasma, thereby increasing the fraction unbound of the affected drug. The cellular activity, controlling the elimination processes, is sometimes affected by disease and by other drugs taken by a patient. Although the following principles, relating changes in clearance and extraction ratio, are exemplified here with hepatic extraction, they apply in general to all organs of elimination.

At least six processes, as shown in Fig. 6-10, may affect the ability of the liver to extract and eliminate drug from the blood. In addition to perfusion (not shown), there is binding within the perfusing blood, to blood cells and proteins, and permeation or transport of unbound drug into the hepatocyte, where subsequent elimination occurs, via metabolism or secretion into the bile, or both (processes a to e). The scheme in Fig. 6-10 appears to be such a complex interplay of processes as to preclude any ready conclusion about how any one of these factors may influence clearance. Fortunately, the task becomes relatively simple by dividing drugs into whether they are of high, low, or intermediate extraction ratio within the liver, as has been done for representative drugs in Table 6-5. However, before addressing the specific issues of perfusion and plasma protein binding, we need to bring forward the concept of **intrinsic clearance**.

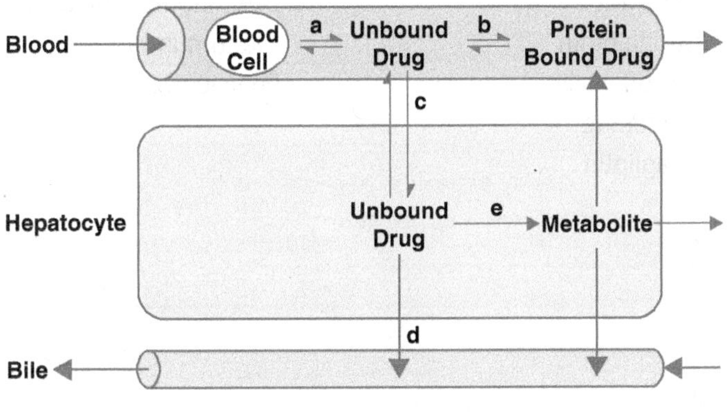

FIGURE 6-10 Drug in blood is bound to blood cells (process *a*) and to plasma proteins (process *b*); however, it is the unbound drug that permeates (process *c*) into the hepatocyte. Within the hepatocyte, unbound drug is subjected to secretion into bile (process *d*) or to metabolism (process *e*). Any one of these five processes, or perfusion, can be the slowest, or rate-limiting, step in the overall process of drug elimination within the liver. The formed metabolite leaves the hepatocyte via blood or bile or is subjected to further metabolism (not shown).

INTRINSIC CLEARANCE

Although clearance is measured from observations in plasma or blood, elimination occurs only because a drug is a substrate for one or more of the eliminating mechanisms *within the cell*. In all cases, the externally observed rate of elimination is therefore a measure of, and indeed equal to, the rate of elimination occurring within the cell. This rate is dependent on the intracellular unbound concentration, Cu_H, to which the metabolic enzymes and excretory transporters are exposed. Because, by definition, clearance is simply the proportionality constant between rate of elimination and concentration, it therefore follows that

$$\text{Rate of elimination} = CL \cdot C = CL_{int} \cdot Cu_H \quad \text{Eq. 6-21}$$

where CL_{int} is the **intrinsic clearance** of the drug, so called because it is a measure of the **intrinsic hepatocellular** eliminating activity, separated from other external factors, such as blood flow and plasma protein binding. Many drugs are substrates for more than one enzyme or eliminating transporter, so that analogous to the partitioning of hepatic clearance into hepatic metabolic and excretory (biliary) clearances, hepatic intrinsic clearance is equal to the sum of the intrinsic metabolic and excretory clearances associated with each of the primary elimination processes.

TABLE 6-5 | Hepatic and Renal Extraction Ratios of Representative Drugs

Low (<0.3)	Intermediate (0.3–0.7)	High (>0.7)
Hepatic Extraction[a]		
Carbamazepine	Aspirin	Alprenolol
Diazepam	Codeine	Cocaine
Ibuprofen	Cyclosporine	Meperidine
Nitrazepam	Ondansetrone	Morphine
Paroxetine	Nifedipine	Nicotine
Itraconazole	Nortriptyline	Nitroglycerin
Valproic acid		Propoxyphene
Warfarin		Verapamil
Renal Extraction[a]		
Amoxicillin	Acyclovir	*p*-Aminohippuric acid[b]
Atenolol	Cephalothin	Metformin
Cefazolin	Ciprofloxacin	Peniciclovir
Digoxin	Ranitidine	
Fexofenadine	Sitagliptin	
Furosemide		
Gentamicin		
Methotrexate		
Pamidronate		

[a]At least 30% of drug eliminated by pathway.
[b]Used as a diagnostic to measure renal plasma flow.

High Extraction Ratio

When the hepatic extraction ratio of a drug approaches 1.0 ($E_H > 0.7$), its hepatic blood clearance approaches hepatic blood flow. The drug must have had sufficient time while passing through the liver to partition out of the blood cells, dissociate from the plasma proteins, pass across the hepatic membranes, and be either metabolized by an enzyme or transported into the bile, or both. To maintain the sink conditions necessary to promote the continuous entry of more drug into the cell to be eliminated, as depicted in Fig. 6-11A, drug must obviously be a very good substrate for the elimination processes within the hepatic cells. In this condition, with hepatic blood clearance approaching its maximum value, hepatic blood flow, hepatic elimination becomes rate-limited by perfusion and not by the speed of any of the other processes depicted in Fig. 6-10. Clearance is then sensitive to changes in blood flow but relatively insensitive to changes in, for example, plasma protein binding or cellular eliminating activity (i.e., intrinsic clearance). Furthermore, for a given systemic concentration, changes in blood flow produce corresponding changes in rate of elimination, but the extraction ratio is virtually unaffected.

Low Extraction Ratio

In contrast to high extraction, elimination of a drug with a low hepatic extraction ratio ($E_H < 0.3$) must be rate-limited somewhere else in the overall scheme other than perfusion (Fig. 6-10). The most common reason is that the drug is a poor substrate for the elimination process(s), usually metabolism. Occasionally, for polar drugs, of insufficient lipophilicity to readily permeate the cell, elimination may be rate-limited by membrane permeability, in which case uptake and efflux transporters can play a substantial part in influencing the concentration of drug within the hepatocyte, and hence its clearance. Whatever the cause of the limitation, drug concentration in arterial and venous blood, entering and leaving the liver, are virtually identical when the extraction ratio is low (Fig. 6-11B). This virtual identity also applies to unbound concentration within blood, the driving force for entering the hepatocyte or for elimination within it. Accordingly, changes in blood flow are expected to produce little or no change in the

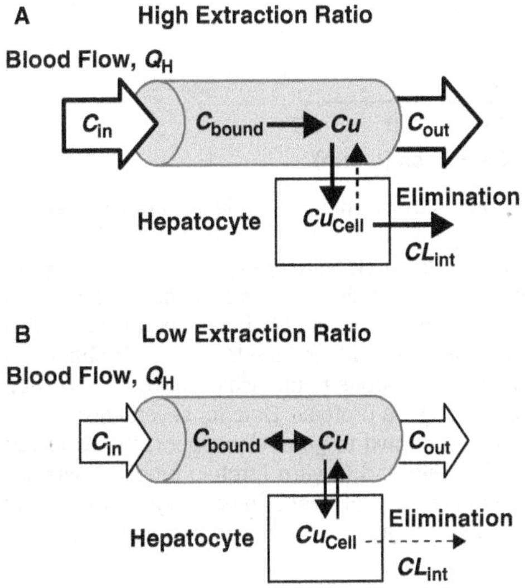

FIGURE 6-11 Exchange of drug between plasma and hepatocyte and its removal from this cell involves unbound drug (Cu). When the extraction ratio is high ($E_H > 0.7$), Case A, essentially all the drug is removed from blood on entering the liver (entering concentration, C_{in}), whether bound to blood cells or to plasma proteins. Clearance is then rate-limited by perfusion. In contrast, when the extraction ratio is low ($E_H < 0.3$), Case B, little drug is removed (exiting concentration, C_{out}), approaching C_{in}, and any one of the many processes (other than perfusion) can rate limit drug elimination. Generally, it is because the drug is a poor substrate for the hepatic enzymes or biliary transporters (low intrinsic clearance). Occasionally, it is cell membrane permeability. Clearance is then governed by hepatocellular activity and fraction unbound in plasma. Arrows denote mass flow of drug; the thicker the arrow, the greater the speed of mass transfer occurring via the associated process.

rate of elimination and therefore, by definition, in clearance. From Equation 6-18, however, it follows that E_H varies inversely with blood flow when clearance is constant.

When E_H is low, clearance is expected to be influenced by changes in plasma protein binding or intracellular hepatic activity. Concerning plasma protein binding, it should be clear from the above that any change in binding for a given total plasma concentration entering the liver would be reflected in a corresponding change in the unbound concentration perfusing the liver, and hence in the rate of elimination and so, by definition, in clearance. The influence of changing the activity of the elimination process within the liver cell may perhaps be most easily visualized by examining Fig. 6-12, which shows anticipated changes in extraction ratio as a function of hepatic intrinsic clearance. When E_H is low because the limitation is hepatic intrinsic clearance, any change in this activity is directly reflected by a change in the extraction ratio, and hence clearance. In contrast, when eliminating activity is very high, E_H and clearance both approach their limiting values, of one and blood flow, respectively. Then, both parameters are relatively insensitive to even large changes in intrinsic clearance.

Finally, some drugs have intermediate extraction ratios, such as codeine and nortriptyline (Table 6-5). The clearance of these compounds is sensitive to all the above-mentioned factors, but not to the same extent as expected at the extremes of extraction ratio. The concept of high and low hepatic extraction ratio becomes important for considering the effect of changes in blood flow on oral bioavailability, a topic covered in Chapter 8.

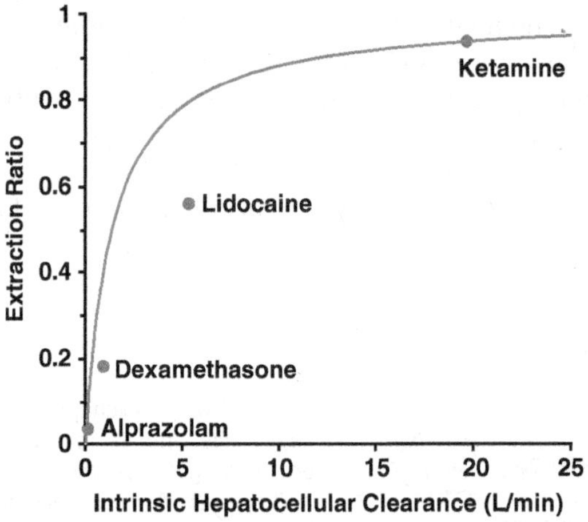

FIGURE 6-12 Relationship between hepatic extraction ratio and intrinsic hepatocellular clearance, the parameter that relates rate of hepatic elimination to the unbound concentration in the hepatocyte (see Fig. 6-10). When intrinsic hepatocellular clearance is low, extraction ratio (and blood clearance) increase in almost direct proportion to intrinsic hepatocellular activity. However, as intrinsic hepatocellular clearance increases, extraction ratio approaches the limiting value of 1 (and blood clearance to the limiting value of hepatic blood flow). In this upper limiting region, large changes in intrinsic hepatocellular clearance produce little to negligible change in extraction ratio (or blood clearance). The solid line is the expected continuous relationship between extraction ratio and hepatic intrinsic clearance for drugs that are not bound to plasma proteins. Data for several drugs with weak binding and predominantly cleared by hepatic metabolism are shown to generally support the expected relationship. (Experimental data are based on a combination of in vivo and in vitro [protein binding, plasma-to-blood ratio] data provided in Obach RS. Prediction of human clearance of twenty-nine drugs from hepatic microsomal intrinsic clearance data: an examination of in vitro half-life approach and nonspecific binding to microsomes. *Drug Met Disp* 1999;27:1350–1359).

Biliary Excretion and Enterohepatic Cycling

Biliary secretion is restricted to small molecular weight drugs; protein drugs are too large to enter the hepatocyte and are not substrates for the biliary transport processes. Drugs in bile enter the small intestine via the common bile duct after storage in the gallbladder. In the small intestine, they may be reabsorbed to complete an **enterohepatic cycle**. Recall from Chapter 2 that enterohepatic cycling is a component of distribution, not elimination. Drug excreted in the bile that is not reabsorbed in the intestines must be either excreted in the feces or degraded there. Thus, for some drugs biliary excretion can become the major route of elimination even when given intravenously.

A few generalizations can be made regarding the characteristics of a drug needed to ensure high biliary clearance. First, the drug must be actively secreted by transporters, as occurs extensively for the relatively hydrophilic statin, pravastatin; separate secretory mechanisms exist for acids, bases, and un-ionized compounds. Second, it must be polar (to prevent or slow reabsorption in the biliary tract), and, last, its molecular weight must exceed about 350 g/mol. These arguments do not aid in predicting the nature and specificity of the secretory mechanisms, but they do aid in predicting the likelihood of a high biliary clearance. For example, glucuronide conjugates of drugs are polar, ionized, pK_a about 3, and have molecular weights exceeding 350 g/mol. They are often highly cleared into bile and in many cases are hydrolyzed in the small intestine back to the parent drug which may be reabsorbed, thereby undergoing enterohepatic cycling of drug via a metabolite.

An example of a drug undergoing enterohepatic recycling through a glucuronide metabolite is mycophenolate mofetil, an immunosuppressive agent used in transplant medicine (Fig. 6-13). The administered compound itself is inactive but forms an active metabolite, mycophenolic acid, during its first pass through the gut wall and liver. The absorbed mycophenolic acid is further metabolized to a glucuronide that is secreted into the bile and stored in the gall bladder. When food is ingested, the glucuronide moves into the small intestine, via the common bile duct. There it is hydrolyzed back to the active metabolite, which is reabsorbed into the body and again converted to the glucuronide. The net result is that the plasma concentrations of both the active metabolite and its glucuronide increase soon after eating.

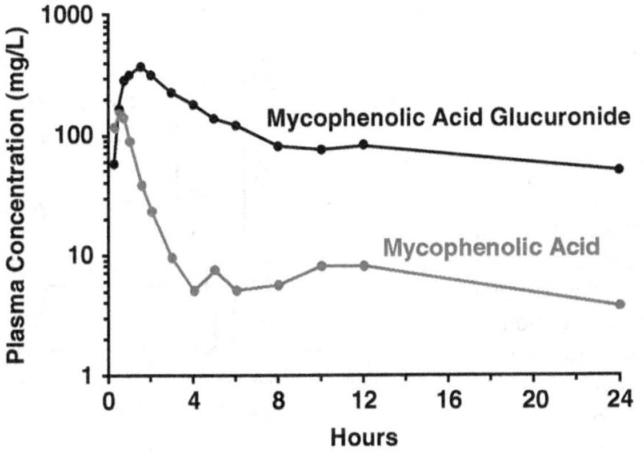

FIGURE 6-13 Mean observed plasma concentration–time profiles of mycophenolic acid and its glucuronide metabolite after administration of 500 mg of mycophenolate mofetil, to 42 subjects. The administered compound undergoes extensive first-pass metabolism to the active metabolite, mycophenolic acid, which, in turn, is rapidly conjugated in the liver to its glucuronide. The glucuronide is secreted into the bile, stored in the gall bladder, and emptied into the small intestine with the bile. The effect of rapid emptying of the gall bladder is apparent after the evening meal at about 10 hours. (Redrawn from Jiao Z, Ding J, Shen J, et al. Population pharmacokinetic modeling for enterohepatic circulation of mycophenolic acid in healthy Chinese and the influence of polymorphisms in UGT1A9. *Br J Clin Pharmacol* 2008;65(6):893–907.)

In addition, the active metabolite, in general, stays in the body much longer than it would have had it not undergone enterohepatic recycling through its glucuronide metabolite.

Hepatic Handling of Protein Drugs

For small molecular weight protein drugs (less than 60,000 g/mol), the liver can be a major site of elimination. Some, for example, somatropin (22,124 g/mol), a recombinant growth hormone, are transported into the liver, where proteases break them down. For most other small protein drugs, elimination is primarily by the kidneys, as discussed later. Some larger proteins, such as asparaginase (175,000 g/mol), an oncolytic agent, and alteplase (59,042 g/mol), a thrombolytic drug, are primarily eliminated by the liver. Monoclonal antibodies, on the other hand, are not handled by this organ.

In general, metabolites are not of interest for protein drugs, because they are usually fully metabolized back to their basic amino acids, which are the building blocks for all proteins made by the body.

Renal Clearance

Drugs vary widely in their renal clearance (see Table 6-5). Although the general principles governing renal clearance are the same as for the liver, the mechanisms involved and the relative importance of each differ.

The Nephron: Anatomy and Function

The basic anatomic and functional unit of the kidney is the nephron (Fig. 6-14). The basic components are the glomerulus, tubule (consisting of the proximal tubule, loop of Henle, and distal tubule), and collecting tubule. The glomerulus receives blood first and filters about 102 (in women) to 120 mL (in males) of plasma water each minute in a typical 20-year-old patient or 68 (in women) to 80 (in males) mL/min in a 60 year-old patient. The filtrate passes down the tubule. Most of the water is reabsorbed; only 1–2 mL/min, a value highly dependent on water intake, leaves the kidneys as urine. On

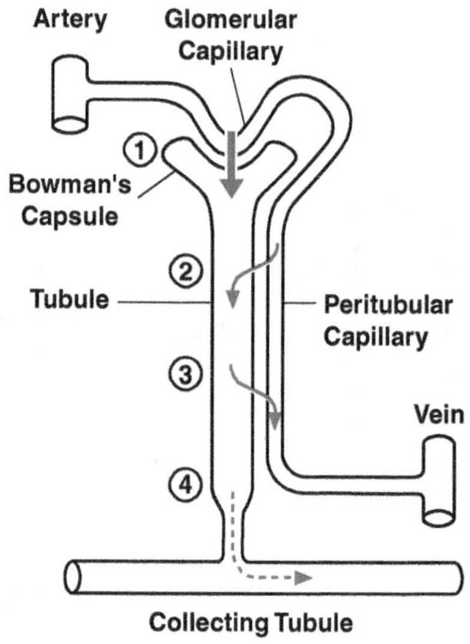

FIGURE 6-14 Schematic representation of the functional unit of the kidney, the nephron. Drug enters the kidney via the renal artery and leaves partly in the exiting renal vein and partly in urine. Urinary excretion (*4*) is the net effect of glomerular filtration of unbound drug (*1*) and tubular secretion (*2*), processes adding drug into the proximal part of the lumen of the tubule, and tubular reabsorption of drug from the distal lumen back into the perfusing blood (*3*).

leaving the glomerulus, the same blood perfuses both proximal and distal portions of the tubule through a series of interconnecting vascular channels.

Appearance of drug in the urine is the net result of filtration, secretion, and reabsorption. The first two processes add drug to the proximal part of the lumen of the nephron; the last process involves the movement of drug from the lumen back into the bloodstream. The excretion rate is, therefore,

$$\text{Rate of excretion} = (1 - F_R)\,[\text{Rate of filtration} + \text{Rate of secretion}] \qquad \textbf{Eq. 6-22}$$

where F_R is the fraction reabsorbed from the lumen. A schematic representation of these processes and their approximate location in the nephron are given in Fig. 6-14. Let us examine each process in turn.

Glomerular Filtration

Approximately 20%–25% of cardiac output, or 1.1 L of blood per minute, goes to the kidneys. Of this volume, about 10% is filtered at the glomerulus by the hydraulic pressure exerted by the heart. Small- to medium-sized molecules (MW < 2000 g/mol) pass through the sieve with ease. Even for small proteins such as insulin (5058 g/mol) and myoglobulin (17,670 g/mol), the ultrafiltrate concentration in the lumen immediately below the glomerulus is close to that in plasma. Only when the molecular weight of the protein exceeds about 30,000 g/mol does filtration fall off sharply, depending on charge and shape as well. Indeed, virtually no albumin (MW, 69,000 g/mol, and anionic at plasma pH) is normally found in the ultrafiltrate. Accordingly, as the binding of most drugs in plasma is to albumin or other proteins of similar or higher molecular weight, as a general rule, only unbound drug in plasma water (concentration Cu) is filtered.

The rate at which plasma water is filtered is conventionally called the **glomerular filtration rate, GFR**. Therefore,

$$\text{Rate of filtration} = \text{GFR} \cdot Cu \qquad \textbf{Eq. 6-23}$$

Recall that fu is the ratio of the unbound to total plasma drug concentration; therefore,

$$\text{Rate of filtration} = fu \cdot \text{GFR} \cdot C \qquad \textbf{Eq. 6-24}$$

If a drug is only filtered and all filtered drug is excreted into the urine, then the rate of excretion is the rate of filtration. Since renal clearance, CL_R, by definition, is

$$CL_R = \frac{\text{Rate of excretion}}{\text{Plasma concentration}} \qquad \textbf{Eq. 6-25}$$

it follows that for such a drug its renal clearance (by filtration) is $fu \cdot$ GFR. The extraction ratio of such a drug is low. For example, even if the drug is totally unbound in blood ($Cu = C_b$), the extraction ratio in a young male 70 kg adult (GFR =120 mL/min; renal blood flow 1100 mL/min) is still only 0.11. This follows because

$$\text{Extraction ratio} = \frac{\text{Rate of excretion}}{\text{Rate of presentation}} = \frac{\text{GFR} \cdot Cu}{Q_R \cdot C_b} = \frac{120\ \text{mL/min}}{1{,}100\ \text{mL/min}} = 0.11$$

Creatinine, an endogenously produced compound, is neither bound to plasma proteins nor secreted, and the entire filtered load is excreted into the urine. Accordingly, its renal clearance is a measure of GFR. Under normal conditions, GFR is relatively stable and insensitive to changes in renal blood flow.

ACTIVE SECRETION

Filtration always occurs, but, as shown above, renal extraction of a drug by this mechanism alone is low, especially if drug is highly bound in plasma. Secretion, active transport from blood to lumen of nephron, facilitates extraction. Mechanisms exist for secreting acids (anions) and bases (cations). The secretory processes are located predominantly in the proximal tubule. As expected, substances transported by the same system can compete with each other and in doing so may affect their renal clearances.

Secretion is inferred when rate of excretion ($CL_R \cdot C$) exceeds the rate of filtration ($fu \cdot \text{GFR} \cdot C$). Stated differently, secretion is apparent when $CL_R > fu \cdot \text{GFR}$. Some reabsorption may still occur, but it must be less than secretion. Some drugs are such excellent substrates for the secretory system that they are virtually completely removed from blood within the time they are in contact with the active transport site, even when they are bound to plasma proteins or located in blood cells. In such cases, evidently dissociation of the drug–protein complex and movement of drug out of the blood cells are both rapid enough not to limit the secretory process. Para-aminohippuric acid (PAH) is handled in this manner and is not reabsorbed. Accordingly, the renal extraction ratio of PAH is close to 1.0. This compound is restricted in blood to plasma; hence, its renal plasma clearance is a measure of renal plasma flow, the clinical use of the compound. Obviously, under these circumstances, clearance is perfusion-rate limited and insensitive to changes in plasma protein binding.

ACTIVE REABSORPTION

Tubular reabsorption is the third factor controlling the renal handling of drugs; it is primarily seen with small molecular weight compounds. One does not always know whether reabsorption is passive or active, but that it occurs can be confidently concluded when renal clearance is less than the calculated clearance by filtration ($CL_R < fu \cdot \text{GFR}$). Many endogenous compounds, including B vitamins, vitamin C, electrolytes, glucose, and amino acids are actively reabsorbed in the renal tubule. One can develop therapeutic maneuvers around these transport systems. As an example, consider the use of canagliflozin (Invokana), a new drug for treating type 2 diabetes. By blocking the sodium glucose transporter (SGLT2) in the proximal tubule of the nephron, which accounts for 90% of glucose active reabsorption, about 50–80 g of glucose is excreted into the urine per day, helping to lower the systemic exposure to this substance. The drug has additional advantages in that it lowers blood pressure (due to an osmotic effect of glucose in the renal tubule) and decreases body weight, probably accounted for by the daily 200–320 kcal contained in the excreted glucose.

PASSIVE REABSORPTION

For the majority of drugs, reabsorption appears to be passive. The extent of reabsorption varies among drugs from being almost absent to being virtually complete. The driving force for reabsorption of drug is the concentration gradient generated by the extensive reabsorption of filtered water, from 120 mL/min at the glomerulus to only 1–2 mL/min as formed urine, which tends to concentrate drug in the lumen of the nephron by roughly a factor of 100, if no reabsorption occurs. Extensive reabsorption is commonly seen for lipophilic drugs, which readily pass across the luminal membrane back into the blood perfusing the nephron. Accordingly, their renal clearances are very low. Indeed, when the urine drug concentration equals the unbound concentration in plasma, that is, when equilibrium is achieved, the rate of excretion becomes Urine Flow · *Cu*, and the renal clearance (rate of excretion/*C*) becomes Urine Flow · *fu*, an extremely low value.

Renal Handling of Protein Drugs

As mentioned, insulin is readily filtered at the glomerulus. However, negligible amounts are found excreted in urine. This occurs because this protein and many other filtered protein drugs are virtually completely metabolized back to constituent amino acids, by enzymes either located in the brush border of the lumen or after uptake within the luminal cells of the nephron. Although well-studied examples are limited, it appears that for many polypeptide and protein drugs with molecular weights less than about 30,000 g/mol, the kidney is a, if not *the*, major organ of elimination, as is the case for anakinra (see text discussing Fig. 5-7 in Chapter 5). Monoclonal antibodies and other large (>about 60,000 g/mol) proteins, because of their size, are not filtered at the glomerulus. They are therefore not eliminated by the kidneys.

Clearance by Other Organs

Up to this point, we have assumed that metabolism occurs in either the liver or the kidneys, but for a few small molecules a large percentage of their elimination may occur in other organs. Nitroglycerin is an example; its metabolism is extensive in both red blood cells and the walls lining the vasculature. Many ester drugs, particularly ester prodrugs, such as valganciclovir, are metabolized extensively in the gut lumen and gut wall before being systemically absorbed as the active ganciclovir. The liver, although replete with esterases, may then contribute little to the metabolism of the administered prodrug as most of it has been already hydrolyzed before entering the liver.

TARGET-MEDIATED DISPOSITION

For most drugs, the amount bound on the target is only a minute fraction of that in the body. Most is found elsewhere, in plasma and tissues, such that the engagement with the target does not affect the overall pharmacokinetics of the drug. There are, however, a number of exceptions in which their pharmacokinetic and pharmacodynamic behaviors are intimately linked because a major fraction of drug in the body is bound to the target site, at least at low doses, resulting in a phenomenon known as **target-mediated disposition**. Imirestat, an experimental aldose reductase inhibitor, and bosentan, a drug used in the treatment of certain types of pulmonary arterial hypertension, are examples of small molecular weight drugs showing this behavior. Target-mediated disposition is much more commonly encountered with monoclonal antibody drugs. Unlike with small molecules, the antibody-target complex is internalized and eliminated by the cell, resulting in a more rapid elimination than would be the case if not complexed. Clinically, these protein drugs are highly selective and often administered at doses far in excess of that required to saturate the target. Although not fully elucidated, at these high saturating doses, the majority of monoclonal antibodies are broken down by generalized intracellular catabolism occurring throughout much of the body. This process is a very slow one, so that the half-life of these agents at these doses is typically weeks or months, facilitating infrequent dosing.

In this chapter, we have examined the physiologic and physicochemical determinants of the kinetics of a drug after an intravenous bolus dose. We turn our attention in the next chapter to the much more common situation, namely, events following extravascular administration—in particular, oral administration.

SUMMARY

Kinetics of Distribution

- Small lipophilic molecules are generally perfusion-rate limited in their tissue distribution.
- Cell membrane permeability is rate-limiting for larger and more polar compounds.
- Tissue affinity is an additional factor influencing distribution kinetics.

Extent of Distribution

- Volume of distribution depends on binding in plasma and tissues, the accessibility of cells, and partitioning into fat.
- Volume of distribution and fraction in plasma unbound are the major measures of drug distribution in pharmacokinetics.

Elimination

- Clearance relates plasma concentration to rate of drug elimination.
- Organ blood clearance is the product of organ blood flow and extraction ratio.
- For drugs of high extraction ratio, blood clearance is limited by and dependent on organ blood flow and insensitive to changes in either plasma protein binding or intrinsic hepatocellular activity.
- For drugs of low extraction ratio, clearance is dependent on fraction in plasma unbound and intrinsic hepatocellular activity, and insensitive to changes in organ blood flow.
- Total clearance is the sum of hepatic and renal clearances.
- Biliary clearance is generally greater for polar molecules that are substrates of both hepatic uptake transporters and efflux biliary transporters.
- Renal excretion is the net effect of filtration, secretion, and tubular reabsorption.
- For drugs that are filtered, but neither secreted nor reabsorbed in the renal tubules, renal clearance depends only on GFR and fraction unbound in plasma.
- Tubular secretion is an active process, exhibiting the potential for saturation and competition.
- Tubular reabsorption is generally by passive diffusion.
- By relating filtration clearance to renal clearance, information can be gained as to whether there is net secretion or net reabsorption of a compound.
- For some compounds, especially protein drugs, the kidney is also a metabolic organ. Sometimes, it is the major metabolic organ.
- Some small molecular weight drugs and many monoclonal antibodies exhibit target-mediated disposition at low doses.

KEY TERM REVIEW

Blood clearance
Clearance
Distribution half-life
Distribution rate constant
Elimination half-life
Elimination rate constant
Extraction ratio
Fraction in plasma unbound
Fractional rate of elimination
Glomerular filtration rate
Half-life
Hepatic clearance

Intrinsic clearance
Intrinsic hepatocellular activity
Microsomal enzymes
Perfusion rate limitation
Permeability-rate limitation
Phase I and II reactions
Plasma-to-blood concentration ratio
Renal clearance
Sequential reactions
Target-mediated disposition
Tissue binding
Volume of distribution

KEY RELATIONSHIPS

$$\text{Distribution half-life} = \frac{0.693}{k_T} = \frac{0.693 \cdot K_P}{(Q_T/V_T)}$$

$$\text{Fraction of drug in body in plasma} = \frac{V_P}{V}$$

$$V = V_P + V_T \cdot K_P$$

$$fu = \frac{Cu}{C}$$

$$V = V_P + V_T \cdot \frac{fu}{fu_T}$$

$CL_{b,H}$	=	Q_H	·	E_H
Hepatic blood clearance		Hepatic blood flow		Hepatic extraction ratio

$$CL_b = CL \cdot \left(\frac{C}{C_b}\right)$$

$$\text{Rate of filtration} = \text{GFR} \cdot Cu$$

$$CL_R = \frac{\text{Rate of excretion}}{\text{Plasma concentration}}$$

STUDY PROBLEMS

1. Which of the following statements apply(ies) to the distribution of drugs in the body?
   I. When distribution to a given tissue is perfusion-rate limited, the time to approach distribution equilibrium is shorter for a drug with a high affinity for that tissue than for one with a low affinity.
   II. For a drug whose distribution to tissues throughout the body is perfusion-rate limited, distribution equilibrium will always be achieved more quickly and in the same order as that of the tissue perfusion rate (blood flow/mL of tissue).
   III. The greater the fraction unbound in tissues (fu_T), the larger is the volume of distribution of a drug.
   A. I only
   B. II only
   C. III only
   D. I and II
   E. I and III
   F. II and III
   G. All
   H. None

2. Which of the following statements is (are) correct?
   I. Because the volume of distribution of a drug is 15 L in a 70 kg patient in whom the fraction unbound in plasma is 0.1, it must distribute intracellularly.
   II. The volume of distribution of a drug in a patient is 850 L; therefore, the tissue to plasma concentration ratio must exceed 10 in at least one tissue or organ.
   III. The expected volume of distribution of a large polar drug, which does not bind to plasma or tissue proteins and cannot enter cells, is 42 L in a 70-kg patient.
   A. I only **E.** I and III
   B. II only **F.** II and III
   C. III only **G.** All
   D. I and II **H.** None
3. Which of the following statements correctly summarize(s) features of the hepatic extraction of drugs?
   I. The intrinsic clearance of a drug for both low and high extraction ratio drugs is estimated from the ratio of hepatic blood clearance and fraction unbound in whole blood.
   II. The hepatic clearance of low extraction ratio drugs tends to be sensitive to changes in hepatic blood flow and plasma protein binding.
   III. The hepatic blood clearance of high hepatic extraction ratio drugs tends to be relatively insensitive to changes in plasma protein binding and hepatocellular activity (intrinsic clearance).
   A. I only **E.** I and III
   B. II only **F.** II and III
   C. III only **G.** All
   D. I and II **H.** None
4. Creatinine clearance is an estimate of which one of the following?
   a. Hepatic function
   b. Active tubular secretion
   c. Rate at which water is filtered in the glomerulus
   d. Effective renal plasma flow
   e. Muscle metabolism
5. Which *one* of the following statements is correct?
   a. The renal clearance of a drug that is glomerularly filtered and neither reabsorbed nor secreted in the kidneys is equal to GFR · *Cu*.
   b. The renal clearance of a small, lipophilic, nonionizable drug is expected to approach a value of Urine Flow · *Cu*.
   c. Renal clearance is less than *fu* · GFR when reabsorption is greater than secretion in the renal tubule.
   d. Small nonprotein and small protein (<20,000 g/mol) drugs are filtered at the glomerulus at a rate equal to GFR · *C*.
6. Appropriately complete the following table by placing ↑, ↓, or ↔ arrows to signify increase, decrease, or little or no change, respectively, in the blank spaces to indicate the expectation for drugs that are primarily cleared by the liver and for which a modest change in the parameter occurs. For Case 6, indicate whether the drug is of low or high extraction ratio.

Case	Hepatic Extraction Ratio	Hepatic Blood Flow	Unbound Fraction in Blood	Intrinsic Clearance	Total (Plasma) Clearance
1.	High	↑	↔	↔	
2.	Low	↔	↓	↔	
3.	High	↔	↔	↑	
4.	Low	↔		↔	↑
5.	High	↔	↓	↔	
6.		↓	↔	↔	↔

↑, increase; ↔, little or no change; ↓, decrease.

7. Which of the following generalizations made about the body's ability to handle protein drugs is (are) reasonable?
   I. Small molecular weight protein drugs (MW < 20,000 g/mol) tend to be filtered and metabolized in the kidney, with little excreted unchanged.
   II. Monoclonal antibody drugs are eliminated throughout the body with only a minor contribution by the liver, and none by the kidneys.
   III. Protein drugs of all kinds cannot be given orally for systemic activity because they are degraded in the intestine to their constitutive amino acids.
   A. I only **E.** I and III
   B. II only **F.** II and III
   C. III only **G.** All
   D. I and II **H.** None
8. The immunosuppressive drug tacrolimus has the following characteristics: plasma clearance = 4.2 L/hr; fraction in plasma unbound = 0.01; plasma-to-blood concentration ratio = 0.05; and essentially all of the drug is eliminated by CYP3A4-catalyzed hepatic metabolism, with a negligible fraction excreted unchanged in urine.
   a. Comment on whether tacrolimus has a high or low hepatic extraction ratio.
   b. Why is the plasma-to-blood concentration ratio so low?
   c. What are the expected changes in the clearance and half-life of tacrolimus after induction of CYP3A4, which results in an increase in the intrinsic hepatocellular metabolic clearance of the drug?
9. Table 6-6 (next page) contains the equilibrium distribution ratios of a drug for various tissues and the corresponding perfusion rates.
   a. Calculate the time required for the amounts in each of the tissues listed to reach 50% of the equilibrium value for this drug, which is perfusion-rate limited in its distribution, when the arterial concentration is kept constant with time. Rank the times and list the corresponding tissues.
   b. What would be the expectation for temporal events in the heart if distribution to this organ were permeability-rate limited?
10. The following information regarding theophylline is either provided in Problem 8 of Chapter 5, or was calculated from the data provided. Clearance is 4 L/hr, volume of distribution is 29 L, half-life is 5 hours. The drug is 40% bound in plasma and freely

TABLE 6-6 | Equilibrium Distribution Ratio and Perfusion Rate of Selected Tissues

Tissue	Equilibrium Distribution Ratio (K_p)	Perfusion Rate (mL/min/g Tissue)[a]
Heart	3	0.6
Kidneys	40	4
Liver	15	0.8
Lungs	1	10
Skin	12	0.024

[a]1 g of each tissue occupies approximately 1 mL.

passes across cell membranes and distributes in all body water spaces. It is also extensively metabolized, with only 10% of the dose excreted in the urine unchanged following an intravenous dose.

a. Comment, with justification, on whether theophylline has a low or high hepatic extraction ratio.

b. Comment on whether a definite statement can be made as whether there is net renal secretion or net renal tubular reabsorption.

c. Knowing the volume of distribution and fraction unbound in plasma, calculate:

(1) a. The fraction of theophylline in the body unbound at distribution equilibrium.

b. The unbound concentration when there is 500 mg theophylline in the body at distribution equilibrium.

(2) a. The volume of distribution of theophylline in an individual receiving a 500-mg dose in whom the fraction unbound in plasma is 0.30.

b. The unbound concentration in that individual when there is 500 mg theophylline in the body. Comment on the sensitivity of unbound concentration to changes in fraction unbound in plasma.

CHAPTER 7

Quantifying Events Following an Extravascular Dose

OBJECTIVES

The reader will be able to:

- Describe the characteristics of, and the differences between, first-order and zero-order absorption processes.
- Estimate the bioavailability of a drug, when provided with plasma concentration–time profiles following both extravascular and intravascular administrations.
- Define the following drug products: immediate-release, modified-release, extended-release, and delayed-release.
- Estimate the relative bioavailability of a drug in different dosage forms given by the same route of administration, when provided with appropriate plasma concentration–time data.
- Determine whether absorption or disposition rate limits drug elimination, given plasma concentration–time data following different dosage forms by the same route of administration.
- Anticipate the effect of altering the kinetics of absorption, extent of absorption, clearance, or volume of distribution on the systemic exposure–time profile following extravascular administration.
- Given the concentration–time profile after a single oral dose, state what additional information might be needed to determine whether the terminal decline in the plasma concentration is rate limited by absorption.
- Define bioequivalence, and briefly describe how it is assessed.

Drugs are more frequently administered extravascularly (common routes are listed in Table 7-1 on next page) than intravascularly, and the majority are intended to act systemically rather than locally. For these drugs, systemic absorption, the focus of this and the next chapter, is a prerequisite for activity. Delays or losses of drug during systemic input may contribute to variability in drug response and occasionally may result in failure of drug therapy. It is primarily in this context, as a source of variability in systemic response and as a means of controlling the plasma concentration–time profile, that systemic absorption is considered here and throughout the remainder of the book. Keep in mind, however, that even for those drugs that are used locally (e.g., mydriatics, local anesthetics, nasal decongestants, topical agents, and aerosol bronchodilators), systemic absorption may influence time of onset, intensity, and duration of adverse systemic effects.

TABLE 7-1 | Extravascular Routes of Administration for Systemic Drug Delivery[a]

Via alimentary canal	
Buccal	Rectal
Oral	Sublingual
Other routes	
Inhalation	Subcutaneous
Intramuscular	Transdermal
Intranasal	

[a]Routes such as intradermal, intra-articular, intrathecal, intravaginal, ocular, subdural, and so on, are usually used to produce a local effect.

Although other routes of administration are considered, this chapter deals primarily with assessment of the kinetics and extent of systemic drug absorption from the gastrointestinal tract. This is not only because the oral mode of administration is the most prevalent for systemically acting drugs, but because it also illustrates aspects of variability encountered with extravascular routes of administration in general.

A number of oral dosage forms are commercially available. Some are liquids (e.g., syrups, elixirs, suspensions, and emulsions), whereas the more common ones are solids (tablets and capsules). Tablets and capsules are generally formulated to release drug immediately after their administration to hasten systemic absorption. These are called **immediate-release products.** Other products, **modified-release dosage forms,** have been developed to release drug in a controlled manner. Modified-release products fall into two categories. One is **extended-release,** a dosage form that allows a reduction in dosing frequency or diminishes the fluctuation of drug levels on repeated administration compared with that observed with immediate-release dosage forms. Controlled-release and sustained-release products fall into this category. The second category is that of **delayed-release.** This kind of dosage form releases drug, in part or in total, at a time other than promptly after administration. Enteric-coated dosage forms are the most common delayed-release products, and are designed to prevent release of drug in the stomach, where the drug may decompose in the acidic environment there or cause gastric irritation, and then to release drug for immediate absorption once in the small intestine. Modified-release products are also administered by nonoral extravascular routes. For example, repository (depot) dosage forms are given intramuscularly and subcutaneously in the form of emulsions, solutions in oil, suspensions, and tablet implants.

KINETICS OF ABSORPTION

The oral absorption of drugs often approximates first-order kinetics, especially when given in solution. The same holds true for the systemic absorption of drugs from many other extravascular sites, including subcutaneous tissue and muscle. Under these circumstances, absorption is characterized by an **absorption rate constant**, k_a. The corresponding **absorption half-life** is related to the absorption rate constant in the same way that elimination half-life is related to elimination rate constant, that is,

$$\text{Absorption half-life} = \frac{0.693}{k_a} \qquad \textbf{Eq. 7-1}$$

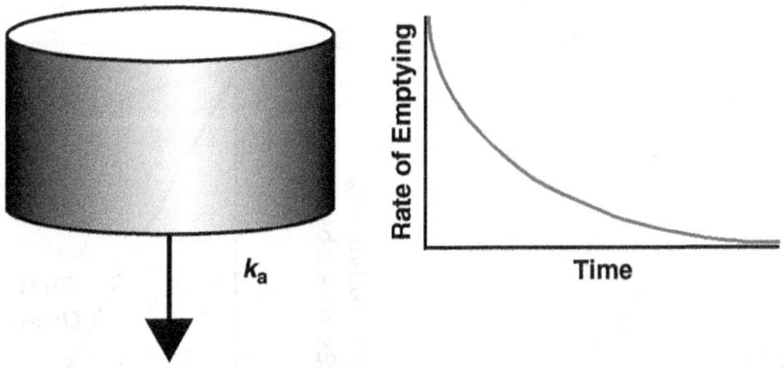

FIGURE 7-1 First-order systemic absorption is analogous to the emptying of water from a hole in the bottom of a cylindrical bucket, which represents the absorption site. The level of water, or amount remaining to be absorbed, in the bucket decreases with time, as does the rate of emptying. The slowing of the rate of decline of the water level or rate of emptying is due to the decrease in water pressure, which depends on the water level (or amount of water) in the bucket. The rate of emptying (g/min), which declines exponentially with time, is proportional to the amount (g) of water in the bucket and the size of the hole. The rate of emptying relative to the amount in the bucket is the fractional rate of emptying, which does not vary with time. In absorption terms, this constant is called the **absorption rate constant, k_a**.

The half-lives for the absorption of drugs administered orally in solution or in a rapidly dissolving (immediate-release) dosage form usually range from 10 minutes to 1 hour. They tend to be longer when administered as a solid dosage form, especially if dissolution or release from the dosage form is slow.

When absorption occurs by a **first-order** process,

$$\underset{\text{Absorption}}{\text{Rate of}} = \underset{\substack{\text{Absorption}\\ \text{rate constant}}}{k_a} \cdot \underset{\substack{\text{Amount}\\ \text{remaining}\\ \text{to be absorbed}}}{A_a} \qquad \text{Eq. 7-2}$$

that is, the rate is proportional to the **amount remaining to be absorbed, A_a**. First-order absorption is schematically depicted in Fig. 7-1 by the emptying of water from a cylindrical bucket. The rate of emptying depends on the amount of water (and its height) in the bucket and the size of the hole at the bottom. With time, the level of water decreases, reducing the rate at which water leaves the bucket. Indeed, the rate of emptying is directly proportional to the level or amount of water in the cylindrical bucket.

Sometimes, a drug is absorbed at essentially a constant rate driven, for example, by the maintenance of a saturated solution by the presence of excess dissolving solid. The absorption kinetics is then called **zero order.** Differences between first-order and zero-order kinetics are illustrated in Fig. 7-2 (next page). For zero-order absorption, a plot of amount remaining to be absorbed against time yields a straight line, the slope of which is the rate of absorption (Fig. 7-2A). Recall from Chapter 5 that the fractional rate of decline is constant for a first-order process; the amount declines linearly with time when plotted semilogarithmically. In contrast, for a zero-order absorption process, the fractional rate increases with time, because the rate is constant, whereas the amount remaining to be absorbed decreases linearly with time. This is reflected in an ever-increasing negative gradient with time in a semilogarithmic plot of the amount remaining to be absorbed (Fig. 7-2B). For the remainder of this chapter, and for much of the book, systemic absorption is modeled as a first-order process.

EXPOSURE–TIME AND EXPOSURE–DOSE RELATIONSHIPS

The systemic exposure to a drug after a single extravascular dose depends on both systemic absorption and disposition. Consider first how exposure with time after an extravascular dose compares with that seen after an intravenous dose.

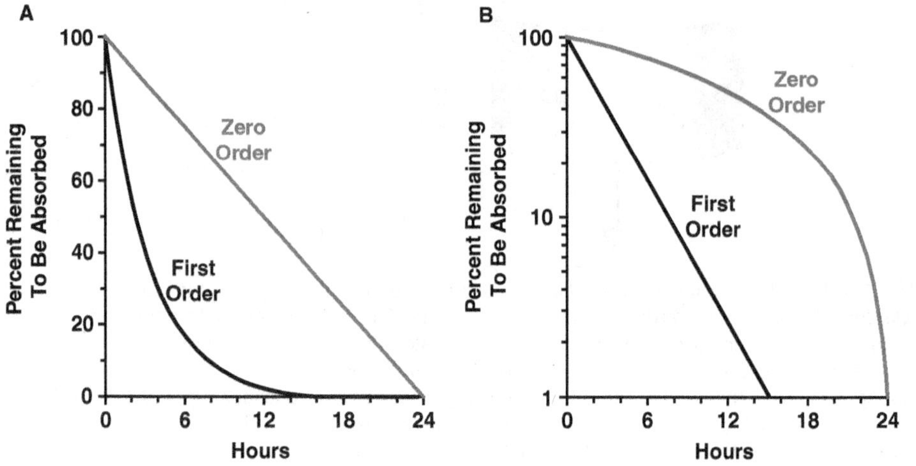

FIGURE 7-2 A comparison of zero-order and first-order absorption processes. Depicted are regular (**A**) and semilogarithmic (**B**) plots of the percent remaining to be absorbed against time. Note the curvatures of the two processes on the two plots.

Extravascular Versus Intravenous Administration

Absorption delays and reduces the magnitude of **peak plasma concentration** compared with that seen after an equal intravenous bolus dose. These effects are portrayed for aspirin in Fig. 7-3.

The rise and fall of the drug concentration in plasma after extravascular administration are best understood by realizing that at any time,

$$\underset{\text{drug in body}}{\overset{\text{Rate of}}{\text{change of}}} = \underset{\text{absorption}}{\underset{\text{Rate of}}{k_a \cdot A_a}} - \underset{\text{elimination}}{\underset{\text{Rate of}}{k \cdot A}} \qquad \text{Eq. 7-3}$$

The scheme in Fig. 7-4, based on the reservoir model presented in Chapter 5 (Fig. 5-3) for disposition after a single intravenous bolus dose, illustrates the expectation. Drug enters the reservoir, not as a bolus (Chapter 5), but by a first-order process and is eliminated in the same manner as that following an intravenous dose.

Initially, with the entire dose at the absorption site (bucket) and none in the body (reservoir), rate of absorption is maximal and rate of elimination is zero. Thereafter,

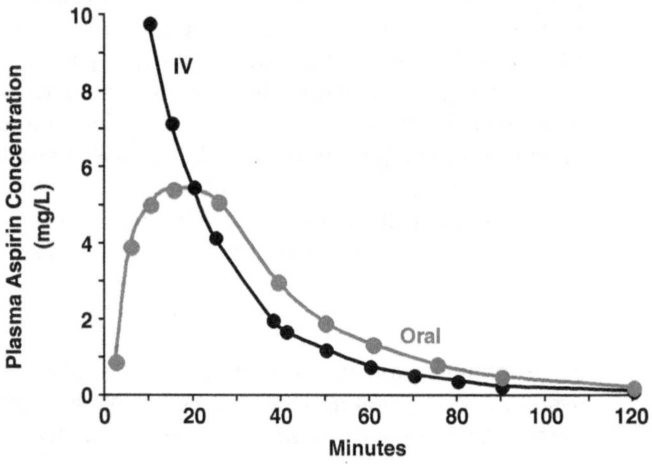

FIGURE 7-3 Aspirin (650 mg) was administered as an intravenous bolus (*black circle*) and as an oral solution (*colored circle*) on separate occasions to the same individual. Absorption causes a delay and a lowering of the peak concentration. (Modified from the data of Rowland M, Riegelman S, Harris PA, et al. Absorption kinetics of aspirin in man following oral administration of an aqueous solution. *J Pharm Sci* 1972;67:379–385. Adapted with permission of the copyright owner.)

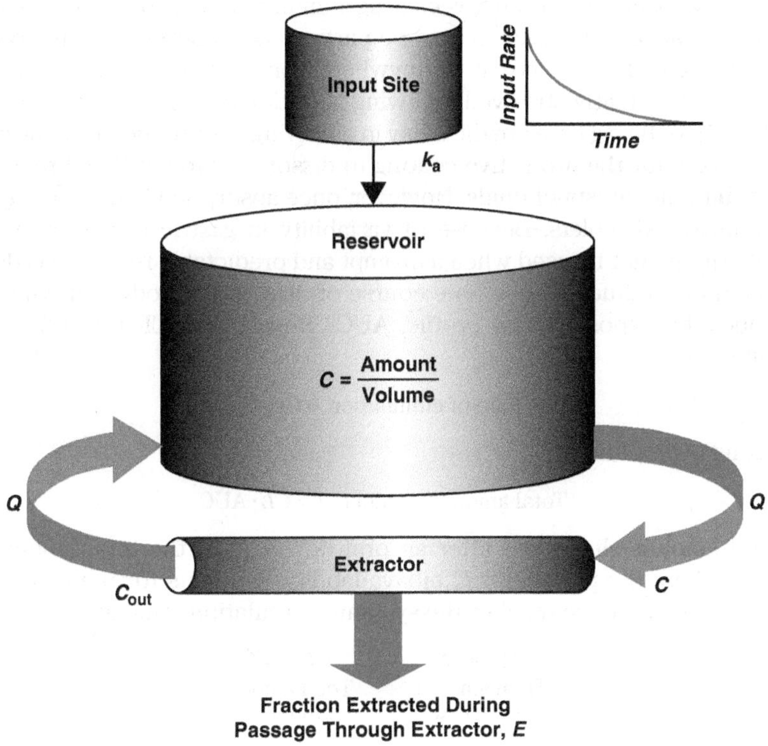

FIGURE 7-4 Scheme for the first-order systemic absorption and elimination of a drug after a single extravascular dose. The systemic absorption is simulated by the emptying of a water bucket (see Fig. 7-1). The rate constant for absorption k_a is the fractional rate of absorption, that is, the rate of absorption relative to the amount in the bucket. The elimination of the drug from the body (see Fig. 5-3) depends on the extent of its tissue distribution (volume of reservoir, V), and how well the drug is extracted from the fluid going to the eliminating organ (s) (as measured by clearance, CL). In this integrated model, the amount of water added to the reservoir from the bucket is negligible, as is the amount of drug in the extractor and in the fluid going to the extractor, relative to the amount in the reservoir.

as drug is absorbed, its rate of absorption decreases, whereas the concentration in the reservoir and, as a consequence, the rate of elimination ($CL \cdot C$) increases, making the difference between the two rates smaller with time. As long as the rate of absorption exceeds that of elimination, the concentration in the reservoir continues to rise. Eventually, a time, t_{max}, is reached when the rate of elimination matches the rate of absorption; the concentration is then at a maximum, C_{max}. Subsequently, the rate of elimination exceeds the rate of absorption and the concentration declines, as shown in Fig. 7-3 for the plasma concentration of aspirin after a single oral dose.

The peak plasma concentration is always lower following extravascular administration than the initial value following an equal intravenous bolus dose. In the former case, at the peak time, some drug remains at the absorption site and some has already been eliminated, whereas the entire dose is in the body immediately following a single intravenous bolus dose. Beyond the peak time, the plasma concentration is expected to exceed that following intravenous administration of the same dose, if the drug is fully bioavailable (completely absorbed). This occurs because of continuous absorption of drug. If bioavailability is low, the plasma concentration may remain below that after intravenous administration at all times. Frequently, the rising portion of the plasma concentration–time curve is called the **absorption phase,** and the declining portion, the **elimination phase.** As will subsequently be seen, while often true, this description may sometimes be misleading.

One may observe a delay between drug administration and the beginning of absorption. This is called a **lag time**; it may be particularly important when a rapid onset of effect is desired. The lag time can be anywhere from a few minutes to many hours. Long lag times are frequently observed following ingestion of enteric-coated tablets. Factors contributing to the lag time are the delay in emptying the product from the stomach and the time taken for the protective coating to dissolve or to swell and release the inner contents into the intestinal fluids. However, once absorption begins, it may be as rapid as with uncoated tablets. Because of variability in gastric emptying, enteric-coated products should not be used when a prompt and predictable response is desired.

Absorption influences the time course of drug in the body; but what of the total area under the exposure-time profile, AUC? Recall from Chapter 5 that the rate of elimination is:

$$\text{Rate of elimination} = CL \cdot C \qquad \text{Eq. 7-4}$$

Integrating over all time,

$$\text{Total amount eliminated} = CL \cdot \text{AUC} \qquad \text{Eq. 7-5}$$

The total amount eliminated after an oral dose equals the total amount absorbed, $F \cdot \text{Dose}$, where the parameter F, bioavailability, accounts for the fact that only this fraction of the oral dose reaches the systemic circulation. That is,

$$\underset{\substack{\text{Total amount}\\ \text{absorbed}}}{F \cdot \text{Dose}} = \underset{\substack{\text{Total amount}\\ \text{eliminated}}}{CL \cdot \text{AUC}} \qquad \text{Eq. 7-6}$$

Bioavailability

Systemic absorption is often incomplete when a drug is given extravascularly, for reasons to be discussed in the next chapter. Knowing the extent of absorption (bioavailability) helps to ensure that the correct dose is given extravascularly to achieve a therapeutic systemic exposure. Although dose is known and area can be determined following an extravascular dose, from Equation 7-6 it is apparent that clearance is needed to estimate bioavailability. Recall, from Chapter 5 (Equation 5-21), that to determine clearance, a drug must be given intravenously, as only then is the amount entering the systemic circulation known (the dose, $F = 1$). Therefore,

$$\text{Dose}_{iv} = CL \cdot \text{AUC}_{iv} \qquad \text{Eq. 7-7}$$

After an extravascular (ev) dose,

$$F_{ev} \cdot \text{Dose}_{ev} = CL \cdot \text{AUC}_{ev} \qquad \text{Eq. 7-8}$$

which, upon dividing Equation 7-8 by Equation 7-7 and knowing that clearance is unchanged, yields

$$F_{ev} = \left(\frac{\text{AUC}_{ev}}{\text{AUC}_{iv}}\right)\left(\frac{\text{Dose}_{iv}}{\text{Dose}_{ev}}\right) \qquad \text{Eq. 7-9}$$

For example, if the area ratio for the same dose administered orally and intravenously is 0.5, only 50% of the oral dose must have been absorbed systematically.

Relative Bioavailability

Relative bioavailability is determined when there are no intravenous data as part of the assessment, either because an IV dosage form is not available or, more commonly, because such data are not relevant to the assessment. The assessment involves comparing the fractions absorbed for different dosage forms (e.g., tablet vs. capsule), different routes of extravascular administration (e.g., oral vs. pulmonary), or different conditions (e.g., change in diet or coadministration with another drug).

Thus, taking the general case of two dosage forms:

Dosage Form A

$$\underset{\text{Total amount absorbed}}{F_A \cdot \text{Dose}_A} = \underset{\text{Total amount eliminated}}{CL \cdot \text{AUC}_A} \qquad \text{Eq. 7-10}$$

Dosage Form B

$$\underset{\text{Total amount absorbed}}{F_B \cdot \text{Dose}_B} = \underset{\text{Total amount eliminated}}{CL \cdot \text{AUC}_B} \qquad \text{Eq. 7-11}$$

So that,

$$\text{Relative bioavailability } (F_A/F_B) = \left(\frac{\text{AUC}_A}{\text{AUC}_B}\right) \cdot \left(\frac{\text{Dose}_B}{\text{Dose}_A}\right) \qquad \text{Eq. 7-12}$$

This relationship holds regardless of the extravascular route of administration, rate of absorption, or shape of the curve. Constancy of clearance is the only requirement.

CHANGES IN DOSE OR ABSORPTION KINETICS

The concentration–time profile following a change in dose or in the absorption characteristics of a dosage form can be anticipated.

Changing Dose

If all other factors remain constant, as anticipated intuitively, increasing the dose or the fraction of a dose absorbed produces a proportional increase in plasma concentration at all times. The value of t_{max} remains unchanged, but C_{max} and AUC increase proportionally with dose or fraction absorbed.

Changing Absorption Kinetics

Alterations in absorption kinetics, for example, by changing dosage form or giving the product with food, produce changes in the time profiles of the plasma concentration. This point is illustrated by the three situations depicted in the semilogarithmic plots of Fig. 7-5 (next page) involving only a change in the absorption half-life. All other factors (extent of absorption, clearance, and volume of distribution and hence elimination half-life) remain unchanged.

Disposition is Rate Limiting

In Case A of Fig. 7-5, the most common situation, absorption half-life is much shorter than elimination half-life. In this case, by the time the peak is reached, the majority of bioavailable drug has been absorbed and little of that has been eliminated. Thereafter, decline of the drug is determined primarily by the disposition of the drug, that is, disposition then becomes the rate-limiting step. The half-life estimated from the terminal decline is therefore that of elimination, not of absorption.

In Case B, absorption is a slower process (absorption half-life is longer) than in Case A, but still faster than the elimination process of the drug ($k_a > k$). The peak

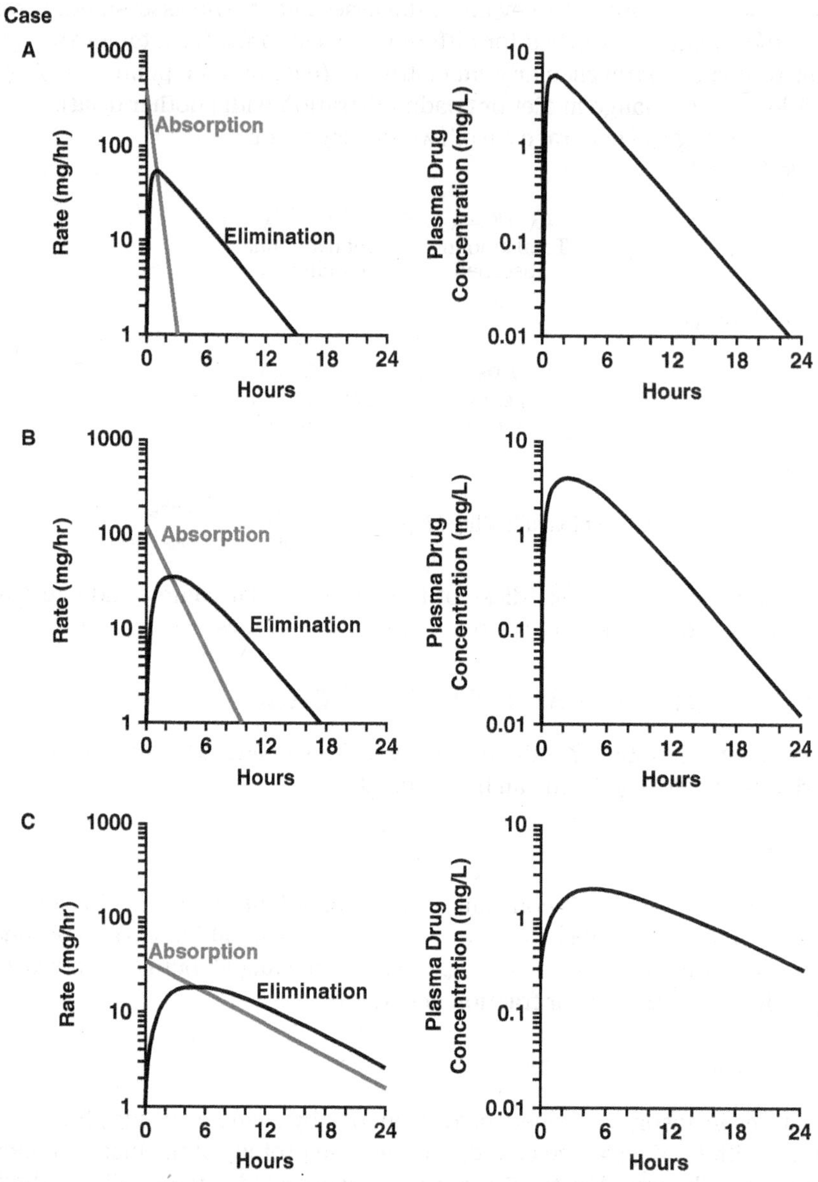

FIGURE 7-5 Rates of absorption and elimination with time (*graphs on left*) and corresponding plasma concentration–time profiles (*graphs on right*) following a single oral dose of drug under different input conditions. A slowing (from *top to bottom*) of drug absorption delays the attainment (t_{max}) and decreases the magnitude (C_{max}) of the peak plasma drug concentration. In Cases A and B (*top two sets of graphs*), the absorption process is faster than that of elimination, so disposition rate limits the decline of the concentration. In Case C (*bottom set of graphs*), absorption is so slow that it rate limits elimination so that the decline of drug in plasma now reflects absorption rather than elimination. Because there is always a net elimination of drug during the decline phase, the rate of elimination is slightly greater than the rate of absorption. In all three cases, bioavailability is 1.0 and clearance is unchanged. Consequently, the areas under the plasma concentration–time curves (corresponding linear plots of the top three graphs) are identical. The AUCs of the linear plots of the rate data are also equal because the integral of the rate of absorption, amount absorbed, equals the integral of the rate of elimination, amount eliminated.

occurs later (t_{max} increased) because it takes longer for the plasma concentration to reach the value at which rate of elimination ($CL \cdot C$) matches rate of absorption; the C_{max} is lower because less drug has been absorbed by that time. Even so, absorption is still essentially complete before the majority of absorbed drug has been eliminated. Consequently, disposition remains the rate-limiting step, and the terminal decline still reflects the elimination half-life.

Absorption Is Rate Limiting

Occasionally, absorption half-life is longer than elimination half-life, and Case C prevails (Fig. 7-5). The peak concentration occurs later yet and is lower than in the two previous cases, reflecting the slower absorption process. Again, during the rise to the peak, the rate of elimination increases and eventually, at the peak, equals the rate of absorption. However, in contrast to the previous situations, absorption is now so slow that considerable drug remains to be absorbed well beyond the peak time. Furthermore, at all times, most of the drug is either at the absorption site or has been eliminated; little of the dose is ever in the body. In fact, during the decline phase, drug is eliminated virtually as fast as it is absorbed. Absorption is now the rate-limiting or -controlling step ($k_a < k$). Under these circumstances, since the rate of elimination essentially matches the rate of absorption, the following approximation (≈) can be written:

$$\underset{\text{Rate of elimination}}{k \cdot A} \approx \underset{\text{Rate of absorption}}{k_a \cdot A_a} \qquad \text{Eq. 7-13}$$

That is,

$$\underset{\text{Amount in body}}{A} \approx \underset{\text{Amount remaining to be absorbed}}{\left(\frac{k_a}{k}\right) \cdot A_a} \qquad \text{Eq. 7-13}$$

Accordingly, the plasma concentration ($C = A/V$) during the decline phase is directly proportional to the amount remaining to be absorbed. For example, when the amount remaining to be absorbed falls by one-half, so does the plasma concentration. The time required for this to occur is the absorption half-life. That is, the half-life of decline of drug in the body now corresponds to the absorption half-life. **Flip-flop** is a common descriptor for this kinetic situation. An example of flip-flop kinetics is presented in Fig. 8-9 of the next chapter. When it occurs, the terms **absorption phase** and **elimination phase** for the regions where the plasma concentration–time curve rises and falls, respectively, are clearly misleading.

Distinguishing Between Absorption and Disposition Rate Limitations

Although disposition generally rate limits the decline of drug in the body, the preceding discussion suggests that caution should be exercised in interpreting the meaning of half-life determined from the decline phase following extravascular administration. Confusion is avoided if the drug is also given intravenously, although, as mentioned previously, this is not commonly done, especially if there is no clinical indication for this route of administration. Absorption and disposition rate limitations may still be distinguished by altering the absorption kinetics of the drug, and checking to see if the terminal half-life shortens (Fig. 7-5). This is most readily accomplished by giving the drug either in another dosage form such as a solution or by a different route. A longer half-life only indicates that absorption is the rate-limiting step for the decline by the new route or dosage form, but does not prove which is the rate-limiting step following administration of the original product.

ASSESSMENT OF PRODUCT PERFORMANCE

Formulation

Equality of drug content does not guarantee equality of response. The presence of different **excipients** (ingredients in addition to active drug) or different manufacturing processes may result in dosage forms containing the same amount of drug behaving differently in vivo. This is why testing for bioavailability of drug products is essential. Generally, the primary concern is with the extent of absorption. Variations in absorption rate with time may also be therapeutically important. **Biopharmaceutics** is a comprehensive term used to denote the study of pharmaceutical formulation variables on the performance of a drug product in vivo.

The major cause of differences in systemic absorption of a drug from various solid products is dissolution. There is, therefore, a strong need to control the content and purity of the numerous inactive ingredients used to stabilize the drug; to facilitate manufacture and maintain integrity of the dosage form during handling and storage; and to facilitate, or sometimes control, release of drug following administration of the dosage form. Intended or otherwise, each ingredient can influence the rate of dissolution of the drug, as can the manufacturing process. The result is a large potential for differences in absorption of drug among products. Indeed, a large variety of dosage forms of drugs are marketed in which release is intentionally delayed (lag in time when input starts) or extended (input over an extended time period). Such differences in release characteristics can be achieved without regard to the physicochemical properties of the drug. Key to the use of such products in vivo, however, is that the extent of absorption not be affected and that release rate limits systemic absorption. To maintain these properties for oral products, which move down the gastrointestinal tract with time, the permeability of the drug must be high in both the small and large intestines.

Assessment of absorption is useful not only to determine the effect of the formulation, but also to examine the effects of food, current drug administration, concurrent diseases of the alimentary canal, and other conditions that may alter systemic absorption. Many such assessments take the form of relative bioavailability. One unique kind of bioavailability assessment, which is widely used, is that of **bioequivalence** testing.

Bioequivalence Testing

The purpose of bioequivalence testing is to be able to predict the clinical (therapeutic) outcome of the use of a new product of a drug, when the clinical trials used for collecting efficacy and safety data were obtained with another product of the same drug. The basic idea is that if the products are pharmaceutically equivalent (they contain the same drug, at the same dose, and generally in the same dosage form, e.g., a tablet) and the pharmacokinetics, in terms of the exposure–time profile (which reflects rate and extent of absorption) are sufficiently similar, then the therapeutic outcome should be the same; that is, the products would show therapeutic equivalence. Another full clinical trial investigating efficacy and safety is thereby not necessary. In this sense, the bioequivalence trial serves as a surrogate for a full clinical trial. The major concern is prescribability, the expectation that pharmaceutically equivalent products will have the same therapeutic effect when therapy in a patient is started. Two products are considered to be bioequivalent if their concentration–time profiles are sufficiently similar so that they are unlikely to produce clinically relevant differences in either therapeutic or adverse effects. The common measures used to assess differences in exposure are AUC, C_{max}, and t_{max}.

In practice, C_{max} and t_{max} are estimated from the highest concentration measured and the time of its occurrence. As the plasma concentration–time curve is often flat near the peak, the value of C_{max} is generally reliable, but because of assay variability and infrequent blood sampling times, the value of t_{max} observed may not be a good representation of the actual time of its occurence. Furthermore, the accuracy of the t_{max} estimate is statistically limited by the discrete, and sometimes widely separated, sampling times. Emphasis in bioequivalence testing is therefore placed on AUC and C_{max}.

Bioequivalence testing arises in two basic situations. First, when a patent on an innovator's drug expires, other manufacturers may then wish to market a similar formulation of the drug. Formulations that are pharmaceutically equivalent and also bioequivalent to that of the innovator's product and bearing the generic name of the drug are called **generic products.** Second, bioequivalence testing is sometimes performed during the course of development of new drugs, for example, when a marketable tablet is developed but the original full clinical trial was conducted using another preparation, such as a capsule formulation. Capsules are used because it is relatively easy to adjust dose simply by filling the appropriate size capsule with different amounts of the granules or powder.

A typical bioequivalence trial is conducted with a crossover design (both treatments given to each subject on separate occasions and in random order). Usually about 24–36 healthy adult subjects are used and are often fasted to standardize conditions. The test and reference products are given in single doses. The AUC and C_{max} are examined statistically. If the 90% confidence interval for the ratio of the measures in the generic or new product (test product) to the innovator's product or product used in full clinical trials (reference product) is within the limits of 0.8 and 1.25 for both AUC and C_{max}, the test product is declared to be bioequivalent. The conclusion is not that their kinetics are the same, but simply that their kinetics are *sufficiently similar* to expect the same therapeutic outcome. The choice of the tolerance limits of 0.8 and 1.25 on either side of the reference is almost universal among national drug regulatory agencies, which evaluate such studies.

The statistical methods applied in bioequivalence testing are different from those applied in bioavailability assessment. In bioavailability studies, questions often asked are ones such as: "Is the oral bioavailability of Drug X in tablet Formulation 1 different from that in tablet Formulation 2?" "Is the peak exposure following an oral solution greater than that after a capsule dosage form?" "What is the oral bioavailability, and how confident are we in its estimate?" In bioequivalence testing, the question asked is: "Are the exposure measures (AUC and C_{max}) of the test product no less than 80% or no more than 125% of the reference product?" The question is not whether or not they are different, but whether or not they are sufficiently similar. The distinction between the two kinds of questions is emphasized in Fig. 7-6 (next page).

The terms bioequivalence and generic products tend to be restricted to products that contain conventional small molecular weight drugs. The situation is much more complex when considering protein drugs and other biologics (any medicinal product

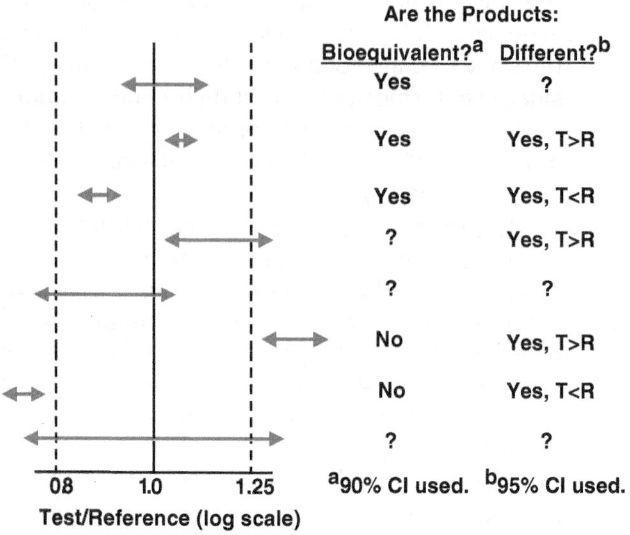

FIGURE 7-6 Declarations possible following the determination of confidence intervals (CI, *colored arrows*). In bioequivalence testing, the question is "Are the two products kinetically sufficiently similar to call them bioequivalent?" In bioavailability testing, the question is often "Do the products differ in their systemic delivery of the drug?" Note that the 90% CI is used in bioequivalence testing, whereas the 95% CI is typically used in difference testing. From a regulatory perspective, of the products tested only those that are bioequivalent to the innovator's product (reference) are permitted to be marketed and interchanged with it.

manufactured or extracted from biological sources, such as vaccines, blood products, and therapeutic serums). Some of these are produced by recombinant technology fermentation using microorganisms. Even though the product undergoes rigorous purification, there is always the possibility of some biological contamination, particular to the specific manufacturing process, which produces an adverse immunological response in some patients. Furthermore, subtle changes in the quaternary structure of the protein that can arise during fermentation and processing may affect its biological activity. For these and other reasons, in addition to undertaking a pharmacokinetic comparison, comparative assessment is also required of the pharmacodynamic, clinical, and safety profiles of protein or biologic drug products intended to be interchangeable. Test products that meet the regulatory requirements on all accounts are said to be **biosimilar**.

We now turn to the physiologic and physicochemical determinants of drug absorption after an extravascular dose, the topic of Chapter 8.

SUMMARY

- Systemic absorption after extravascular administration is often modeled as a first-order process.
- The plasma concentration–time profile after a single extravascular dose is characterized by a rise and a subsequent fall. The rise is a result of the rate of absorption being greater than the rate of elimination; the fall is the result of the converse.
- The peak concentration, and the time of its occurrence, is reached when the rate of elimination matches the rate of absorption.
- The bioavailability of a drug is determined from the areas under the curve after extravascular and intravascular administration, with correction for dose differences, if necessary.
- Bioequivalence testing is performed to determine whether the systemic exposure–time profiles following two different products of the same drug, dosage form, and dose are sufficiently similar to conclude that therapeutic equivalence is likely.
- For formulations of a protein drug intended to be biosimilar, equally prescribable as the marketed product, comparative assessment is required of the pharmacodynamic, clinical, and safety profiles in addition to pharmacokinetic comparison.

KEYTERM REVIEW

Absorption phase
Absorption rate constant
Absorption half-life
Absorption rate–limited elimination
Amount remaining to be absorbed
Area under the curve (AUC)
Bioavailability
Bioequivalence
Biopharmaceutics
Biosimilar
Delayed-release product
Disposition rate–limited elimination
Dosage forms
Drug product
Elimination phase
Excipients
Extravascular route
Extended-release product
First-order process
Flip-flop
Generic product
Immediate-release product
Lag time
Modified-release product
Peak plasma concentration
Rate-limiting step
Relative bioavailability
Systemic absorption
Time of peak plasma concentration
Zero order

KEY RELATIONSHIPS

$$\underset{\text{drug in body}}{\text{Rate of change of}} = \underset{\text{Rate of absorption}}{k_a \cdot A_a} - \underset{\text{Rate of elimination}}{k \cdot A}$$

$$\text{Rate of elimination} = CL \cdot C$$

$$F_{ev} = \left(\frac{AUC_{ev}}{AUC_{iv}}\right)\left(\frac{Dose_{iv}}{Dose_{ev}}\right)$$

$$\text{Relative bioavailability } (F_A / F_B) = \left(\frac{AUC_A}{AUC_B}\right) \cdot \left(\frac{Dose_B}{Dose_A}\right)$$

STUDY PROBLEMS

1. The effect of food and lying down on the bioavailability of an experimental antibiotic PJT483 was studied in 36 subjects using a three-way crossover design. Table 7-2 (next page) summarizes the results of the study. Which of the following statements is (are) consistent with the results of the study?
   I. Taking the drug while lying down decreased the extent of absorption of the drug.
   II. The speed of absorption was faster when the subjects were lying down than when they were upright.
   III. The high-fat breakfast caused the drug to be absorbed more rapidly and increased the amount systemically absorbed.
   A. I only
   B. II only
   C. III only
   D. I and II
   E. I and III
   F. II and III
   G. All
   H. None

TABLE 7-2 | Peak Concentration, AUC, and Peak Times After a 250-mg Oral Dose of PJT483 Under Various Conditions

Treatment (Drug Taken):	C_{max} (μg/L)[a]	AUC(0–24 hr) (μg-hr/L)[a]	t_{max} (hr)[a]
While fasting and upright	240 ± 65	2172 ± 514	0.82 ± 0.23
While fasting and lying down	142 ± 50[b]	1987 ± 763[c]	1.53 ± 0.40[b]
Just at the end of a high-fat breakfast	74 ± 33[b]	3214 ± 876[b]	2.67 ± 0.90[b]

[a]Values are expressed in mean ± standard deviation.
[b]Relative to fasting group, $P < 0.05$.
[c]Relative to fasting group, $P > 0.05$.

2. The 90% confidence intervals (CI) of three different products (Products A, B, and C) of a drug were compared with an innovator's product (Reference Product). The products were tested on separate occasions. The results of those studies, with respect to C_{max} only, were as follows:
   I. Product A versus Reference CI = 0.96–1.17
   II. Product B versus Reference CI = 0.78–1.15
   III. Product C versus Reference CI = 1.28–1.51

   Declaration of bioequivalence requires that both AUC and C_{max} measures be within the acceptable limits, 80–125% of the values of the reference product. For all three preparations, AUC was within those limits. Which *one, or more,* of the following conclusions is then valid?
   a. Products A and B both show bioequivalence.
   b. Product C is definitely not bioequivalent to the Reference Product.
   c. Product C is likely to be shown to be bioequivalent to the Reference Product if it is studied again in a new study with a much larger number of subjects.
   d. Product B is bioequivalent to the Reference Product.
   e. None of the three products can be declared to be bioequivalent to the Reference Product.
3. The absorption of a drug from an intramuscular site showed first-order kinetics and was fully bioavailable. The absorption rate constant after an injection into the deltoid muscle was 0.693/hr. Which *one, or more,* of the following statements is (are) correct?
   a. Ninety percent of the dose was systemically absorbed in 3.32 hours.
   b. The fraction of the dose remaining at the injection site at 2 hours was 0.125.
   c. The absorption half-life was 10 hours.
   d. Seventy-five percent of the dose was systemically absorbed at 3 hours.
   e. Had the drug been given as an intravenous bolus, 50% of the dose would have remained in the body at 1 hour.
4. First-order absorption is characterized by which of the following relationships?

   I. $-\frac{dA_a}{dT} = k \cdot A_a$

   II. $Aa = Aa(0) - k \cdot t$

   III. $-\frac{dA_a}{dT} = k$

   A. I only
   B. II only
   C. III only
   D. I and II
   E. I and III
   F. II and III
   G. All
   H. None

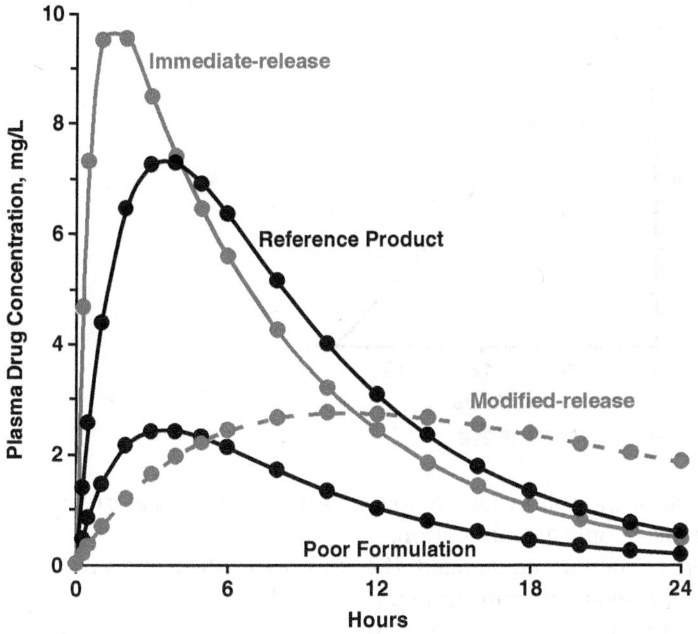

FIGURE 7-7

5. Fig. 7-7 is a composite of the observations for a drug that has been formulated in several different oral dosage forms: the original (Reference Product), an Immediate-release Product, a Modified-release Product, and what turned out to be a Poor Formulation (AUC reduced). Complete the table below by inserting the appropriate word (*increase, decrease, not changed*) describing the change observed in each of the absorption parameters, k_a and F, relative to that of the Reference Product. Qualify any answer for which you feel it appropriate.

Formulation	k_a	F
Immediate-release		
Modified-release		
Poor Formulation		

6. The concentration–time profile following a single 25-mg oral dose of a drug is shown in Fig. 7-8 (next page). Draw on the semilogarithmic plot the expected concentration–time profiles (rough approximations) when:
   a. The extent of absorption (bioavailability) is halved, but there is no change in clearance or in absorption kinetics, that is, k_a is constant.
   b. The absorption process is slowed (k_a becomes 10 times smaller than before and is now 2 times smaller than k), but the extent of absorption (F) is the same and the disposition kinetics (CL,V) is unchanged. This situation might occur when the dosage form is changed, such as from a rapid-release to a slow-release product. Modified-release dosage forms of theophylline and many other drugs are examples.

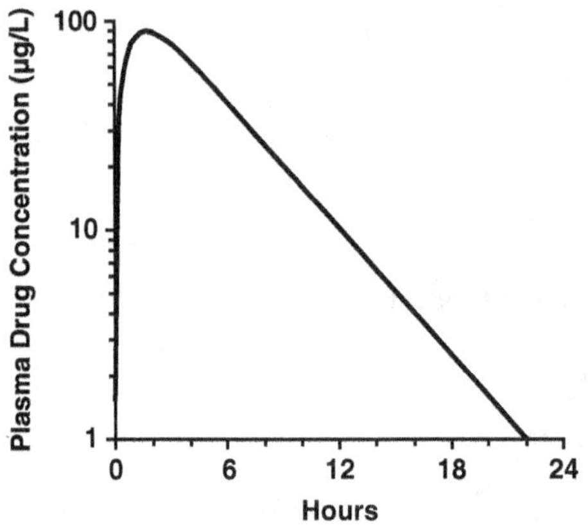

FIGURE 7-8

7. Briefly determine which of the following statements are correct or incorrect. For those that are ambiguous, supply a qualification.
   a. All other parameters remaining unchanged, the slower the absorption process, the higher is the peak plasma concentration after a single oral dose.
   b. For a given drug and subject, AUC is proportional to the amount of drug absorbed systemically.
   c. The absorption rate constant (k_a) is smaller than the elimination rate constant (k). Therefore, the terminal decline of the plasma concentration versus time curve reflects absorption, not elimination.
   d. After a single oral dose, an increase in the extent of absorption leads to a shortening of the peak time.
   e. Zero-order absorption is characterized by a constant rate of drug input until no more drug remains to be absorbed.
8. The pharmacokinetics of sumatriptan, a serotonin receptor agonist used in treating migraine headaches, has been compared following subcutaneous, oral, rectal, and intranasal administration. Table 7-3 lists key observations following these four routes of administration.
   a. Calculate the relative bioavailability of sumatriptan following the oral tablet, rectal suppository, and nasal spray (relative to that following subcutaneous administration).

TABLE 7-3 | Total Systemic Exposure (AUC), Peak Exposure (C_{max}), Time of Peak Exposure (t_{max}), and Terminal Half-life of Sumatriptan Following Administration by the Subcutaneous, Oral, Rectal, and Intranasal Routes

	Subcutaneous	Oral	Rectal	Intranasal
Dose administered (mg)	6	25	25	20
AUC (µg-hr/L)	90.3	52.2	71.6	47.8
C_{max} (µg/L)	69.5	16.5	22.9	12.9
t_{max} (hr)	0.17	1.5	1.0	1.5
Terminal $t_{1/2}$ (hr)	1.9	1.7	1.8	1.8

Adapted from Duquesnoy C, Mamet JP, Sumner D, et al. Comparative clinical pharmacokinetics of single doses of sumatriptan following subcutaneous, oral, rectal, and intranasal administration. *Eur J Pharm Sci* 1998;6:99–104.

b. Complete the table below by comparing the maximum plasma concentrations (C_{max}) and the ratios of the maximum concentration to the area under the curve (C_{max}/AUC) observed following an equivalent 25-mg dose of drug by the four routes of administration.

Observation	Subcutaneous Solution	Oral Tablet	Rectal Suppository	Nasal Spray
C_{max} (μg/L)[a]				
C_{max}/AUC (hr^{-1})[b]				

[a]Per 25 mg of sumatriptan.
[b]C_{max}/AUC has also been used as a measure of the kinetics of drug input when comparing across formulations and routes of administration for the same drug.

c. How would you explain the much higher values of C_{max} and C_{max}/AUC following the subcutaneous route without a change in half-life?

9. Channer and Roberts (1985) studied the effect of delayed esophageal transit on the absorption of acetaminophen. Each of 20 patients awaiting cardiac catheterization swallowed a single tablet containing acetaminophen (500-mg) together with barium sulfate, a radio-opaque compound. The first 11 subjects swallowed the tablet while lying down; in 10 of these subjects, transit of the tablet was delayed, as visualized by fluoroscopy. In the other 9 subjects who swallowed the tablet while standing, it entered the stomach immediately. In both groups, the tablet was taken with a sufficient volume of water to ease swallowing. Table 7-4 lists the average plasma

TABLE 7-4 | Mean Acetaminophen Concentrations in Subjects Standing and Lying Down after a Single 500-mg Oral Dose

	Mean Plasma Acetaminophen Concentration (mg/L)	
Time (min)	**Subjects Standing**	**Subjects Lying Down**
0	0	0
10	2.1	0.1
20	5.6	0.3
30	5.8	1.1
40	6.3	1.9
50	4.1	2.8
60	3.5	3.2
90	2.8	3.9
120	2.2	3.1
150	1.7	2.9
180	1.4	2.0
210	1.5	1.7
240	0.75	1.0
360		0.7

Abstracted from Channer, KS, Roberts CJC. Effect of delayed esophageal transit on acetaminophen absorption. *Clin Pharmacol Ther* 1985;37:72–76. The AUC values (to time infinity) for the subjects who were standing and lying down were 697 mg-min/L and 773 mg-min/L, respectively.

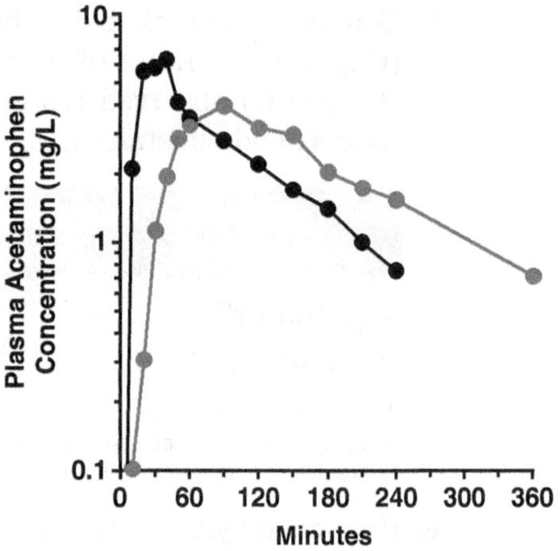

FIGURE 7-9 Mean acetaminophen concentration in subjects standing (black) and lying down (color) after a single 500-mg orql dose. (Data abstracted from Channer, K.S. and Roberts, C.J.C. Effect of delayed esophageal transit on acetaminophen absorption. *Clin Pharmacol Ther* 1985;37:72–76.)

acetaminophen data obtained over 6 hours after swallowing the tablet. Fig. 7-9 is the corresponding semilogarithmic display of the data in Table 7-4.

a. What effect does delayed esophageal transit have on the speed and extent of absorption of acetaminophen?

b. What process, absorption or disposition, rate limits the decline in plasma drug concentration?

c. Acetaminophen is used for the relief of pain. Do the findings of this study affect the recommendation for the use of this drug?

CHAPTER 8

Physiologic and Physicochemical Determinants of Drug Absorption

OBJECTIVES

The reader will be able to:

- Describe the sequence of events and processes involved in systemically absorbing a drug after extravascular administration generally and specifically after oral administration.
- List five factors influencing dissolution rate of a drug.
- Distinguish between dissolution-rate and permeability-rate limitations in systemic absorption after oral administration.
- State the mean transit times of materials in the fasted stomach, small intestine, and large intestine.
- State the role of gastric emptying and intestinal transit in the systemic absorption of a drug given orally with particular reference to the physicochemical properties of the drug and its dosage form.
- Discuss how food can influence the rate and extent of systemic absorption of a drug given orally.
- Anticipate for which compounds intestinal permeability is likely to be the reason for incomplete oral bioavailability for a drug absorbed by passive diffusion.
- List possible competing reactions responsible for low oral bioavailability of drugs, together with one example of each possibility.
- State why protein drugs must generally be given parenterally.
- State why the systemic absorption of antibody drugs often continues for days, sometimes even weeks, when they are administered in solution by the intramuscular or subcutaneous routes.

Before a drug can pass through the membranes dividing the absorption site from the blood at any site of extravascular administration, it must be in solution. Yet most drugs are administered as solid preparations, such as tablets and capsules. However, before addressing the issues involving drug release from a solid dosage form, let us consider the physiologic and physicochemical events that result in systemic absorption after administration of a drug in solution. We begin with oral administration.

ABSORPTION FROM SOLUTION

Systemic absorption is favored after oral administration because the body acts as a sink, producing a concentration difference between the diffusible unbound concentrations at the absorption site and in systemic blood. The concentration gradient across the absorptive membranes is maintained by distribution of absorbed drug to tissues and by its elimination. Physiologic and physicochemical factors that determine movement of drug through membranes in general were presented in Chapter 4. Included among them were the molecular size and physicochemical properties of the drug, the nature of the membrane involved, perfusion, pH, and the presence of transporters. These factors and others are now considered with respect to drug passage through gastrointestinal membranes. In this context, gastrointestinal absorption is the term that is subsequently used for this process.

Gastrointestinal Absorption

The first potential site for absorption of orally administered drugs is the stomach. In accordance with the prediction of the pH partition hypothesis, weak acids are absorbed more rapidly from the stomach at pH 1.0 than at pH 8.0, and the converse holds for weak bases. Absorption of acids, however, is much faster from the less acidic small intestine (pH 6.6–7.5) than from the stomach. These apparently conflicting observations can be reconciled. Surface area, permeability, and, when perfusion rate-limits absorption, blood flow are important determinants of the rapidity of absorption. The intestine, especially the small intestine, is favored on all accounts. The total absorptive area of the small intestine, produced largely by microvilli, has been calculated to be about 200 m^2, and an estimated 1 L of blood passes through the intestinal capillaries each minute. The corresponding estimates for the stomach are only 1 m^2 and 150 mL/min. The permeability of the intestinal membranes to drugs is also greater than that of the stomach. These increases in surface area, permeability, and blood flow more than compensate for the decreased fraction of un-ionized acid in the intestine. Indeed, the absorption of all compounds—acids, bases, and neutral compounds—is faster from the small intestine than from the stomach. Because absorption is greater in the small intestine, systemic absorption is no faster than the rate of gastric emptying which is often the controlling step in the speed of drug absorption even when given orally in solution. In the following discussion, the examples chosen are either drugs administered as solutions or where there is reason to expect, based on solubility considerations for example, that the drug dissolves within the time it spends within the stomach, usually about 30 minutes or less prior to entering the intestine. This is especially the case when an oral dosage form is taken on an empty stomach with a glass of water.

Gastric Emptying

Food, especially fat, slows gastric emptying, which is one reason why drugs are frequently recommended to be taken on an empty stomach when a rapid onset of action is desired. Drugs that influence gastric emptying also affect the speed of absorption of other drugs, as shown in Fig. 8-1 for acetaminophen, a common analgesic/antipyretic, when remifentanil, a potent ultra–short-acting opioid, is concurrently administered by intravenous infusion. The observed slowing of systemic absorption of acetaminophen is a result of slowed gastric emptying by remifentanil, and is common to all opioids, which contributes to the constipation seen with this class of drugs. The figure also

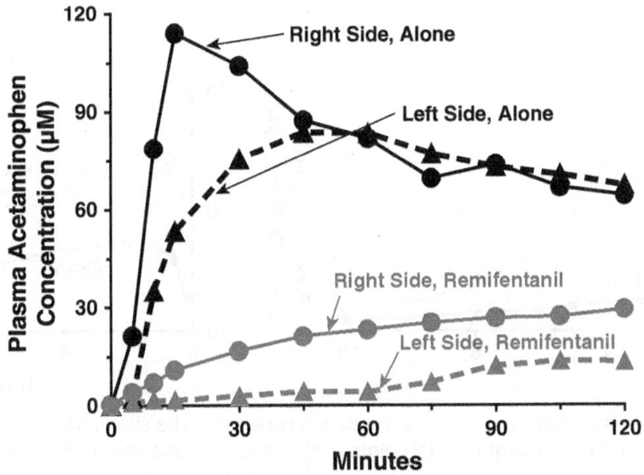

FIGURE 8-1 Gastric emptying can rate-limit systemic drug absorption. Remifentanil, an ultra-short-acting opioid narcotic analgesic, has a major effect on gastric emptying as observed by the mean systemic exposure-time profiles of acetaminophen after its oral administration (1.5 g dissolved in 200 mL of water) to 10 healthy volunteers in the presence and absence of the narcotic. The drug was given alone (*black lines*) and 10 minutes after the start of a constant-rate intravenous infusion of remifentanil of 0.2 μg/kg/min (*colored lines*). Posture was also shown to influence gastric emptying as observed when acetaminophen was taken while the subjects were lying on their left side with the head lower than the feet by 20° (*dotted lines*) than when the subjects were on their right side with the head higher than the feet by 20° (*solid lines*). (Data from Walldén J, Thorn S-E, Wattwil M. The delay of gastric emptying induced by remifentanil is not influenced by posture. *Anesth Analg* 2004;99:429–434.)

suggests that gastric emptying is faster when lying on the right than on the left side, but the differences were not statistically significant. Although at first glance it would appear that the extent of absorption (area under the curve) is affected by remifentanil or the position of the body, one cannot be certain because of the limited time over which blood samples were taken in the study. The total area under the curve, not provided, is needed. Clearly, it is unlikely that a patient would get a rapid onset of response to a drug when gastric emptying is so slowed. However, for this analgesic, the slowing of gastric emptying is immaterial as the anesthetic effect of remifentanil predominates. In general, the stomach may be viewed as a repository organ from which pulses of drug are ejected by peristalsis onto the absorption sites in the small intestine, and slowing the process delays the onset of drug response.

Intestinal Absorption and Permeability

Throughout its length, the intestine varies in its multifaceted properties and luminal composition. The intestine may be broadly divided into the small and large intestines separated by the ileocecal valve. Surface area per unit length decreases from the duodenum to the rectum. Electrical resistance, a measure of the degree of tightness of the junctions between the epithelial cells, is much higher in the colon than in the small intestine. Proteolytic and metabolic enzymes, as well as active and facilitated transport systems are distributed variably along the intestine, often restricted to specific regions. The colon abounds with anaerobic microbiota. The mean pH, 6.6, in the proximal small intestine rises to 7.5 in the terminal ileum, and then falls sharply to 6.4 at the start of the cecum before finally rising again to 7.0 in the descending colon.

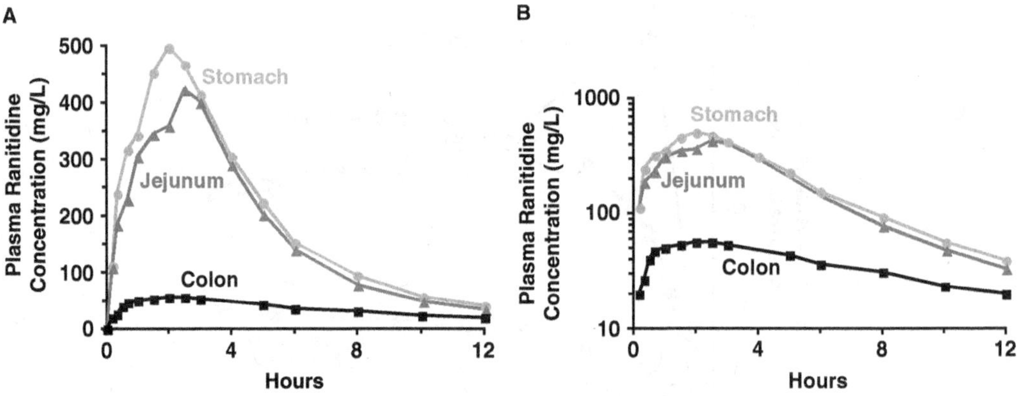

FIGURE 8-2 The gastrointestinal absorption of ranitidine varies with the site of its administration. The variation is shown in linear (**A**) and semilogarithmic (**B**) plots of the mean plasma concentration–time profiles of ranitidine observed after placing an aqueous solution (6 mL) containing 150 mg of ranitidine hydrochloride into the stomach (*faint colored line with circles*), jejunum (*colored line and triangles*), and colon (*black line with squares*) of eight volunteers via a nasoenteric tube. The much less extensive absorption of this small (MW = 313 g/mol) polar molecule from the colon is consistent with the idea that the permeability–surface area (*P·SA*) product of this drug is much lower in the colon than in the small intestine. Notice that absorption of ranitidine effectively ceases (in terminal decline phase) by 3 hours when placed in the stomach or jejunum, even though the drug is incompletely bioavailable (*F* = 0.6; data not shown). This suggests that the small intestine is the major site of absorption when ranitidine is taken orally. Also, notice in B that the terminal half-life of the decline in the plasma concentration is longer when the drug is administered into the colon, because absorption there is rate-limiting (see Chapter 7, p. 129). (Adapted from Williams MF, Dukes GE, Heizer W, et al. Influence of gastrointestinal site of drug delivery on the absorption characteristics of ranitidine. *Pharm Res* 1992;9:1190–1194.)

The permeability–surface area product (*P*·SA, see Chapter 4) tends to decrease progressively from duodenum to colon. This applies to all drug molecules traversing the intestine epithelium by non–carrier-mediated processes, whether via the transcellular (through cell) or paracellular (around cells) routes, when drug solutions are placed in different parts of the intestine, as illustrated in Fig. 8-2 for ranitidine. The extent of this drug's absorption is dramatically decreased when it is administered into the colon, as reflected by the reduced AUC (Fig. 8-2A). Its absorption kinetics is also affected as reflected by an increased terminal half-life (Fig. 8-2B), indicating that its absorption has now become rate-limiting.

How much of this decrease in absorption is due to a decrease in permeability, and how much is due to a decrease in surface area between small and large intestine are not known for certain. For permeable drugs, absorption is rapid and probably complete within the small intestine. Even if some drug were to enter the large intestine, the permeability there would still be sufficiently high to ensure that all that entered would be absorbed. For these drugs, although absorption across the intestinal epithelia may be perfusion rate–limited, as mentioned above, the overall rate-limiting step in systemic absorption from solution is likely to be gastric emptying.

As discussed in Chapter 4, molecular size is a particularly important determinant of permeability. Small polar substances, such as the antiviral acyclovir (250 g/mol), the H_2-antagonist cimetidine (252 g/mol), and atenolol (266 g/mol), primarily move paracellularly across the epithelium, although there is evidence of some involvement of transporters. Permeability, in general, and paracellular permeability, in particular, appear to drop off sharply with molecular weights above 350 g/mol, a value at which compounds appear to approach the molecular dimensions of the tight junctions between intestinal cells.

In general, drugs that are not reliably active systemically when given orally because of their poor absorption must be given parenterally. This is not so much because of their low oral bioavailability, but because of their excessively variable oral absorption, both among patients and, from time to time, within the same patient, and sometimes because there is a need for very large doses to adequately achieve a therapeutic systemic exposure. But there are exceptions, such as the bisphosphonates, for example, alendronate, ibandronate, and zoledronic acid. These stable drugs, used to increase bone mineral density and reduce the frequency of factures in the elderly, are given orally in spite of their very low bioavailabilities (about 0.5%–0.7%). They are relatively safe and so can be administered in high enough doses that the small fraction that is absorbed is sufficient to achieve therapeutic benefit. Despite its low oral bioavailability, pyridostigmine is also given orally to treat myasthenia gravis. Although oral administration is ruled out for many antimicrobial agents, such as the aminoglycosides, because of poor and variable intestinal permeability, they do have utility in treating some infections and diseases of the alimentary canal itself. The use of vancomycin in treating pseudomembranous colitis is an example.

An additional determinant of permeability, and hence absorption is the presence of transporters, particularly those on the apical side of the epithelial cells, that is, facing the intestinal lumen. Uptake transporters, such as PEPT1 and OATP3, facilitate the absorption of amoxicillin, L-dopa, and the antiepileptic/analgesic gabapentin, all of which would otherwise be poorly absorbed. Indeed, as discussed in Chapter 4, it is because the inherent passive permeability of such molecules is low that transporters exert an influence. In contrast, systemic absorption of some drugs is reduced by the presence of efflux transporters, for example, P-glycoprotein. Drug examples include: fexofenadine, an antihistamine; paclitaxel, an anticancer drug; and saquinavir, an antiretroviral agent. Low apparent permeability results, not so much from inability to cross the apical intestinal membranes, but from the action of this efflux transporter.

Concurrent administration of inhibitors of a transport system (e.g., erythromycin, an antibiotic; itraconazole, an antifungal agent; quinidine, used in atrial fibrillation; and ritonavir, a protease inhibitor) can increase the oral absorption of these transported substrates, while coadministration of inducers of this efflux transporter (e.g., rifampin, an antitubercular drug, and St. John's Wort, alleged to be useful for treatment of depression and other mental disorders) have the opposite effect. This is clearly illustrated by the effect of rifampin on digoxin pharmacokinetics (Fig. 8-3 on next page). Digoxin, a large (781 g/mol) molecule containing three sugar groups, is absorbed and predominantly renally eliminated unchanged; bioavailability is usually quite high (about 60–70%), and most absorption appears to occur within the first 4 hours after administration, in keeping with limited absorption beyond the small intestine. Rifampin pretreatment has no material effect on the disposition kinetics of digoxin but, rather, reduces its oral bioavailability (based on decreased total AUC). A slowing in the speed of its absorption is also clearly indicated by the decrease in C_{max} and the increase in t_{max}. The mechanism is an increase in the intestinal expression of P-glycoprotein, for which digoxin is a substrate. The absorption of digoxin is permeability rate–limited. Therefore, a decrease in its effective permeability owing to increased P-glycoprotein efflux decreases both the speed and the extent of its absorption.

An additional consideration is that distribution of transporters along the gastrointestinal tract varies. Certainly, this is true for P-glycoprotein, with activity increasing down the intestinal tract, being highest in the large intestine. This higher activity may, in part, explain why such drugs as ranitidine have such a significantly lower permeability in the colon than in the small intestine (Fig. 8-2).

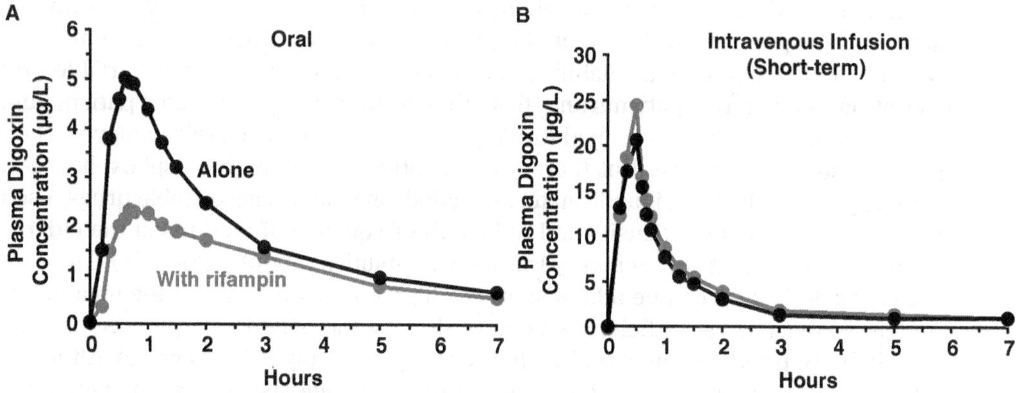

FIGURE 8-3 Rifampin pretreatment reduces the absorption of digoxin. Shown are plots of mean plasma digoxin concentration–time profiles after oral **(A)** and intravenous **(B)** administration (as a 30-minute infusion) of 1-mg digoxin alone (*black circles*) and after 10 days' of rifampin pretreatment (600 mg daily, *colored circles*) to seven healthy adults. A clear depression in the oral absorption of digoxin is inferred by the lower concentrations after oral but not intravenous administration after rifampin pretreatment. This was corroborated by a 30% decrease in total AUC (0–144 hours) (from 54.8 to 38.2 µg-hr/L), corresponding to a fall from 63% to 38% in oral bioavailability. (Redrawn from Greiner B, Eichelbaum M, Fritz P, et al. The role of intestinal P-glycoprotein in the interaction of digoxin and rifampin. *J Clin Invest* 1999;104:147–153.)

Insufficient Time for Absorption

Absorption of drug following oral administration is often reduced because of the limited time within the alimentary canal, and specifically at the sites where absorption is favored by its physicochemical properties or by the presence of transporters. The time for transiting the areas where absorption occurs is a major limitation. The transit time for the small intestine is about 3–4 hours, while that of the large intestine is from 10 to 36 hours or occasionally longer. Drugs with poor permeability characteristics show low oral bioavailability for this reason. If they remained longer at the absorption sites, permeability would be much less of an issue. Recall that, when ranitidine is given orally, only 60%, on average, of a dose is absorbed, and virtually all within the first 3–4 hours after administration when it is in the small intestine. The relationship between fraction absorbed intestinally and the jejunal (the segment between duodenum and ileum) permeability of many drugs is shown in Fig. 8-4. Clearly, low-permeability drugs (examples in Table 8-1) are likely to be

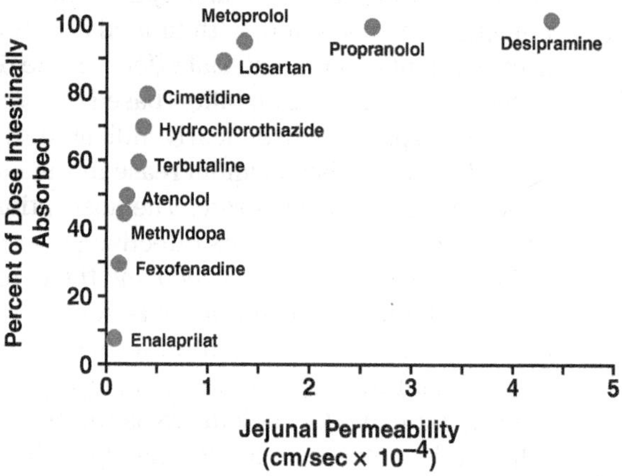

FIGURE 8-4 The fraction of a dose absorbed intestinally after oral administration correlates with human jejunal permeability. Drugs with permeabilities less than 1.0 cm/sec × 10^{-4} are likely to be incompletely absorbed. The lower the permeability below this value, the greater is the likelihood of incomplete absorption. (Adapted from Petri N, Lennernäs H. In vivo permeability studies in the gastrointestinal tract. In: van der Waterbeemd H, Lennernäs H, Artusson P, eds. *Drug Bioavailability, Estimation of Solubility, Permeability, Absorption and Bioavailability.* Berlin, Germany: Wiley-VCH, 2003:345–386.)

TABLE 8-1 | Examples of Drugs Showing Low Oral Bioavailability Due to Low Intestinal Permeability

Alendronate	Gentamicin
Amikacin	Ibandronate
Carbenicillin	Neomycin
Cefamandole	Pyridostigmine
Ceftazodime	Streptomycin
Flumazenil	Vancomycin

All of the drugs listed are antimicrobial agents, except the following: alendronate and ibandronate, agents used to treat and prevent osteoporosis; flumazenil, an agent used to reverse the sedative effects of benzodiazepines; and pyridostigmine, an agent used to treat myasthenia gravis and poisoning by certain nerve gases.

poorly absorbed. Unless degraded in the alimentary canal, the balance of an oral dose of such drugs is recovered unchanged in feces, as is the case for ranitidine. Needless to say, such drugs are generally poor candidates for oral extended-release dosage forms, given that much of the release from such products is within the large intestine (see below for further discussion).

The lack of absorption because of the limited time within the gastrointestinal tract applies to drugs at the other extreme of the permeability scale as well, but for another reason. A drug that is highly permeable but with very low water solubility may also be poorly absorbed because the concentration of released drug is limited by its aqueous solubility, resulting in little drug being available for absorption within the contact time available. Griseofulvin, an antifungal agent, is an example. Formulation is key to increasing its systemic absorption after oral administration by increasing its dissolution.

Causes of Changes in Oral Bioavailability

The oral bioavailability (F) of drugs is commonly less than one, even when administered in solution. There are many reasons for the reduced systemic absorption, in addition to low intestinal permeability. Recall from Chapter 2 that a drug must pass sequentially from the gastrointestinal lumen, through the gut wall, and through the liver, before entering the general circulation (Fig. 8-5 on next page). This sequence is an anatomic requirement because blood perfusing virtually all gastrointestinal tissues drains into the liver via the hepatic portal vein. Drug may also be lost by decomposition in the lumen; the fraction entering the intestinal tissues, F_F, is then the fraction neither lost in the feces nor decomposed in the lumen. Of this permeating drug, only a fraction, F_G, may escape destruction within the intestinal tissues, thereby reducing the fraction of dose reaching the portal vein further to $F_F \cdot F_G$. If drug is also eliminated in the liver, then only a fraction, F_H, of that reaching it escapes extraction there. Accordingly, the measured overall oral systemic bioavailability, F, is given by

$$F = F_F \cdot F_G \cdot F_H \quad \text{Eq. 8-1}$$

For example, if 50% of the drug is lost at each step, the oral bioavailability of the drug, measured systematically, would be 0.5 × 0.5 × 0.5 = 0.125, or 12.5%. Note that the drug can be rendered totally unavailable systemically at any one of these steps.

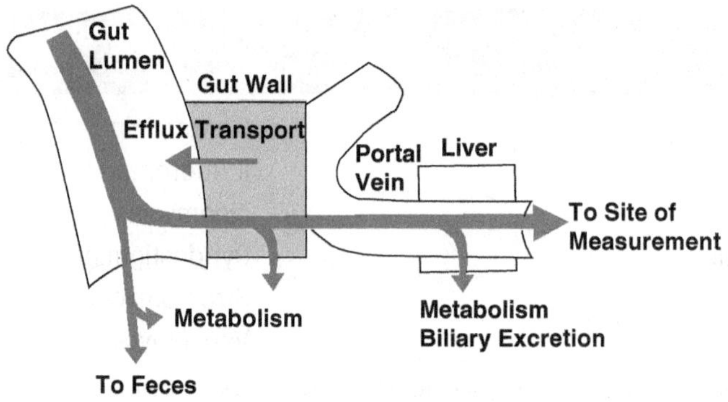

FIGURE 8-5 A drug, given as a solid or a solution, encounters several barriers and sites of loss in its sequential movement (*colored arrows*) from the gastrointestinal tract to the systemic circulation. Dissolution, a prerequisite to movement across the gut wall, is the first step. Incomplete dissolution, slow penetration of the gastrointestinal membranes, decomposition in the gut lumen, and efflux transporters in the gut wall are some causes of poor bioavailability. Removal of drug as it first passes through the gut wall and the liver further reduces the systemic bioavailability , so that the overall oral bioavailability becomes $F = F_F \cdot F_G \cdot F_H$.

First-Pass Loss

As briefly considered in Chapter 2, metabolism during passage across the intestinal wall and through the liver reduces the amount reaching the general circulation following oral administration; the first-pass effect. A few examples to illustrate this first-pass loss follow.

The gut contains many of the enzymes found in the liver, in particular CYP3A4 and several of the glycosyltransferases (1A8 and 1A10). Table 8-2 lists drugs of moderate to low oral bioavailability due primarily to first-pass metabolic loss. All of these drugs are metabolized predominantly by CYP3A4. Despite this commonality, notice that for some, such as tacrolimus and buspirone, there is a substantial gut wall loss, while for others, such as triazolam and nifedipine, it is modest. The differences among them are

TABLE 8-2 | Availabilities of Various Substrates of CYP3A4 Across the Gut Wall and the Liver

CYP3A4 Substrate	F^a	$F_F{}^b$	F_G	F_H
Tacrolimus	0.14	1	0.14	0.96
Buspirone	–	–	0.21	0.24
Atorvastatin	0.14	1	0.24	0.58
Cyclosporine	0.22–0.36	0.86	0.33–0.48	0.75–0.88
Felodipine	0.14	1	0.45	0.34
Midazolam	0.25–0.41	1	0.40–0.79	0.49–0.74
Triazolam	0.55	0.85	0.75	0.75
Nifedipine	0.41	1	0.78	0.53
Quinidine	0.78	0.95	0.90	0.86
Alprazolam	0.84	0.92	0.94	0.97

[a] $F = F_F \cdot F_G \cdot F_H$.
[b] $F_F = 1$ for those drugs for which no other data are available.
Abstracted from Galetin A, Hinton LK, Burt H, et al. Maximum inhibition of intestinal first-pass metabolism as a pragmatic indicator of intestinal contribution to the drug-drug interaction of CYP3A4 cleared drugs. *Curr Drug Metab* 2007;8:685–693.

probably due to a combination of intestinal permeability, intrinsic intestinal metabolic activity, and for some, intestinal transporters, discussed below. Notice also that there is relatively little correlation between F_G and F_H. Thus, for nifedipine $F_G > F_H$, for tacrolimus $F_H > F_G$, while for midazolam F_G and F_H contribute almost equally to the low oral bioavailability.

Another example of a drug showing first-pass loss is orlistat (Xenical). Still another is aspirin. Apart from both having a first-pass loss, one in the gastrointestinal wall (orlistat) and the other primarily in the liver (aspirin), orlistat and aspirin have little in common. They have different chemical structures and possess different pharmacologic activities. Aspirin (MW = 190 g/mol) is a simple acetyl ester of salicylic acid, whereas orlistat is a larger (MW = 496 g/mol) more complex molecule. Aspirin is an anti-inflammatory agent through its active metabolite, salicylic acid, while orlistat acts locally as a lipase inhibitor within the gastrointestinal tract to slow fat absorption and help control obesity. The almost complete first-pass metabolism of the small fraction of orlistat that permeates the intestine has, therefore, little impact on its efficacy.

When metabolites formed during the first pass through the intestinal wall and the liver are inactive or less potent than the parent drug, the oral dose may need to be larger than the equivalent intravenous or intramuscular dose if the same therapeutic effect is to be achieved. Any drug with a high hepatic extraction ratio (see examples listed in Table 6-5) has a low and often highly variable oral bioavailability. Being physiologically determined, no amount of pharmaceutical manipulation can improve on this value for an oral dosage formulation. Sometimes, the problem is so severe that either the drug must be given parenterally, or it must be discarded in favor of another drug candidate. Flumazenil, a benzodiazepine receptor antagonist, and naloxone, an opioid antagonist, are examples. These drugs are so highly extracted by the liver that they must be given parenterally to be effective.

This feature of naloxone has been advantageously used in therapy. A combination product of naloxone, a potent narcotic analgesic antagonist, and pentazocine, a potent narcotic agonist with abuse potential, is effective as an analgesic when administered orally because naloxone, but not pentazocine, is very extensively metabolized during the first pass through the liver. However, when the product is administered parenterally, a common procedure of addicts, the mixture is inactive because of the antagonistic effect of naloxone. The advantage of the combination in the oral product is to prevent its intravenous injection by drug abusers.

Competing Gastrointestinal Reactions

Any reaction (examples listed in Table 8-3 on next page) that competes with gastric or intestinal absorption reduces the oral bioavailability of a drug. They can be either enzymatic or nonenzymatic in nature. Acid hydrolysis in the stomach is a common nonenzymatic one. Enzymatic reactions include those caused by digestive enzymes, metabolic enzymes within the gastrointestinal epithelium, and enzymes in the microbiota, residing predominately in the large bowel. Complexation reactions with other drugs also occur; the result may be low drug bioavailability. For example, coadministration of activated charcoal or cholestyramine reduces the absorption of a number of drugs, including: leflunomide, an agent used to treat rheumatoid arthritis; cephalexin, an antibiotic; and piroxicam, an analgesic agent. When both an adsorbent and an adsorbable drug are concurrently used, their administration must be appropriately timed to avoid their concurrent presence in any region of the gastrointestinal tract. Otherwise, the bioavailability of the drug may be greatly reduced.

TABLE 8-3 | Representative Reactions Within the Gastrointestinal Tract that Compete With Drug Absorption From Solution

Reaction	Drug	Comment
Adsorption	Sumatriptan	Adsorption to charcoal; adsorbed material is not absorbed.
Conjugation		
Sulfoconjugation	Ethinyl estradiol	Concurrent administration of inhibitors of sulfoconjugation (e.g., ascorbic acid and acetaminophen) increase bioavailability of this drug.
Glucuronidation	Morphine	Two glucuronides are formed. The 6-glucuronide has analgesic activity; the 3-glucuronide is inactive.
Decarboxylation	Levodopa	*Loss of activity:* Given with a peripheral L-dopa decarboxylase inhibitor to reduce gastrointestinal metabolism.
Efflux transport	Fexofenadine	Efflux transporters, such as P-glycoprotein, reduce absorption of this drug.
Hydrolysis		
Acid	Penicillin G	*Loss of activity:* Product is inactive.
	Erythromycin	*Loss of activity:* Product is inactive.
	Digoxin	Products (digitoxides) have variable activity.
Enzymatic	Aspirin	Salicylic acid, an active anti-inflammatory compound is formed.
	Pivampicillin	*Active ampicillin formed:* Pivampicillin (ester) is inactive.
	Insulin	*Loss of activity:* Product is inactive.
Oxidation	Cyclosporine	*Loss of activity:* Products are less active or inactive.
Reduction (microbiota)	Olsalazine	Intended for local (colon) anti-inflammatory action; parent drug not systemically absorbed, but is reduced to two molecules of the active metabolite, 5-aminosalicylic acid.

The complexities that occur in vivo make quantitative prediction of the contribution of a competing reaction to decreased bioavailability difficult. Sometimes, the problem of incomplete absorption can be circumvented by physically protecting the drug from destruction in the stomach or by synthesizing a more stable derivative, which is converted to the active molecule within the gastrointestinal tract or within the body. Similarly, to enhance absorption, more permeable derivatives are made, which are rapidly converted to the active molecule, often during passage through the intestinal wall. For example, absorption of the polar antibiotic ampicillin is incomplete. The systemic delivery of this acidic drug is improved substantially by administering it as a more lipophilic and permeable inactive ester prodrug, pivampicillin, which is quickly hydrolyzed within the gut wall to ampicillin, which is then absorbed systemically. Another example is that of valganciclovir, an antiviral agent. The hydrolysis of this compound by esterases within the gut wall and liver is so rapid that only ganciclovir is detected in the systemic circulation. Valganciclovir is therefore, by design, a prodrug as well.

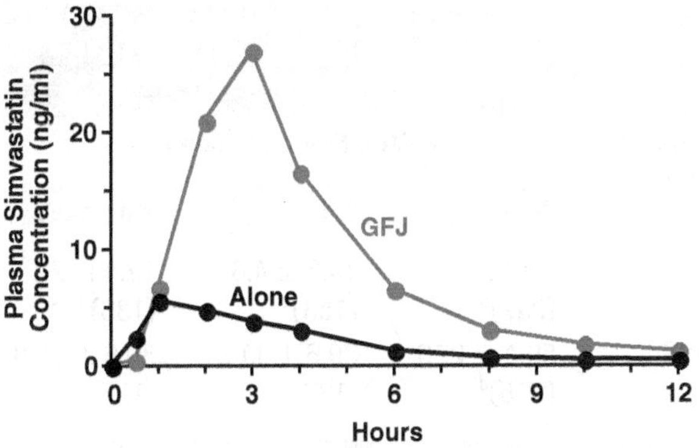

FIGURE 8-6 The mean plasma simvastatin concentration with time after administration of a single 40-mg dose of simvastatin with 200 mL of either water (*black circles*) or grapefruit juice (GFJ, *colored circles*) daily for 3 days. Note the large (3.6-fold) increase in AUC when grapefruit juice is concurrently given. (Figure adapted from Fig. 1 in Lilja JJ, Neuvonen M, Neuvonen PJ. Effects of regular consumption of grapefruit juice on the pharmacokinetics of simvastatin. *Br J Clin Pharmacol* 2004;58:56–60.)

For drugs that undergo extensive first-pass metabolism in the gut wall and the liver, there is often a very large effect of induction or inhibition on their bioavailability. The sequential loss in these organs may partially explain the large effect. For example, consider a drug for which the extraction ratios in the gut wall and liver were both 0.7 and that an inducer is given that increases these values to 0.9. The bioavailability would then be decreased from 0.09 (0.3×0.3) to 0.01 (0.1×0.1), a nine-fold reduction. The reduction would only be three-fold if the metabolism occurred only in the liver.

The concurrent administration of grapefruit juice and simvastatin is an example of a food–drug interaction due to reduced first-pass metabolism (Fig. 8-6). The oral bioavailability of simvastatin is normally about 5%, but when one glass of grapefruit juice is taken once daily for 3 days and concurrently with 40 mg of simvastatin on day 3, its systemic exposure (as reflected by AUC) is increased 3.6-fold. This effect is caused by the presence, within grapefruit juice, of inhibitors of the drug's metabolism, primarily within the gut wall. Hence, such inhibition is expected to have greater impact on the oral bioavailability of those drugs mentioned above, such as tacrolimus, for which most of the first-pass metabolic loss occurs in the gut wall, than others, such as nifedipine, for which the liver is the primary cause of loss.

The degree of inhibition of simvastatin first-pass intestinal metabolism is a function of how much, as well as when, grapefruit juice is ingested, as illustrated by the data shown in Table 8-4 (next page), when "high-dose" grapefruit juice (200 mL of double strength) is given three times a day for 3 days. The falloff in the inhibition of the metabolism after discontinuing grapefruit juice is examined by waiting 1, 3, and 7 days before giving the drug. Notice that the "high-dose" grapefruit ingestion increases the exposure of simvastatin 13.5-fold (compared with 3.6-fold when only one standard glass of grapefruit juice is given daily, Fig. 8-6). Also note that 24 hours after stopping grapefruit juice intake, the increase in AUC is only about 10% of that observed when currently administered, and that the AUC has essentially only returned to the control value 1 week later. The therapeutic impact of this interaction is tempered by the fact that several metabolites of simvastatin are also active such that the increase in exposure systemically and within the liver, the site of action, to all active species is less than that observed for simvastatin itself.

Another example is budesonide, a synthetic corticosteroid used in treating Crohn's disease of the ileum and ascending colon. The drug is given in a modified-release dosage form, which releases drug in the region of the alimentary canal where the disease is common. Drug easily permeates the intestinal wall, but, owing to extensive

TABLE 8-4 | Mean (± SD) Peak Concentrations (C_{max}) and Total Area Under the Curve (AUC) After a Single 40-mg Dose of Simvastatin With and Without Grapefruit Juice (GFJ)

Measure	Control (Water Only)	Administration Concurrent of GFJ	Time After Discontinuing GFJ		
			24 hr	3 d	7 d
C_{max} (ng/mL)	9.3 ± 4.5 (100)[a]	112 ± 44.8 (1200)[a]	22.0 ± 9.7 (237)[a]	14.2 ± 4.6 (153)[a]	12.4 ± 7.2 (133)[a]
AUC (ng-hr/mL)	28.9 ± 14.5 (100)[a]	390 ± 126 (1350)[a]	59.4 ± 27.6 (206)[a]	39.6 ± 11.9 (137)[a]	30.6 ± 15.8 (106)[a]

The drug was administered with 200 mL water alone (part 1 of study) or following administration of double-strength grapefruit juice (GFJ) 3 × daily at 7:00 AM, noon, and 8:00 PM for 3 days and at 0.5 and 1.5 hours after simvastatin intake (part 2 of study). In part 3, subjects received the GFJ as above, but the dose of simvastatin was withheld for 24 hours, 3 days, or 7 days after discontinuing GFJ.
[a]Percent of the control value.

CYP3A4-catalyzed first-pass metabolism in gut wall and liver, systemic availability is low, thereby reducing the adverse systemic effects of the corticosteroid. Coadministration of drugs that inhibit CYP3A4, however, reduces the first-pass loss and increases systemic exposure and therefore adverse events. Coadministration of ketoconazole, a potent inhibitor of CYP3A4 at conventional doses, for example, has been reported to increase by eight-fold the AUC of budesonide.

Some drugs are substrates for both luminal efflux transporters and metabolic enzymes, within the intestinal cells, as shown schematically in Fig. 8-7. Together, they reduce the oral bioavailability to a greater extent than if only one of the two processes was involved. Drug examples that appear to include this coupling effect are: HIV-1 protease inhibitors, indinavir, nelfinavir, saquinavir, and ritonavir; the chemotherapeutic agent, paclitaxel; the cholesterol lowering drug, simvastatin; and the immunosuppressive agent, cyclosporine. The extent to which inhibitors of the enzyme activity and/or the transport system increase systemic availability depends on the contributions of metabolism and transport to first-pass intestinal loss.

Saturable First-Pass Metabolism

When absorption is rapid and the dose is relatively large, some extensively metabolized drugs show a disproportional increase in C_{max} and AUC on increasing the oral dose,

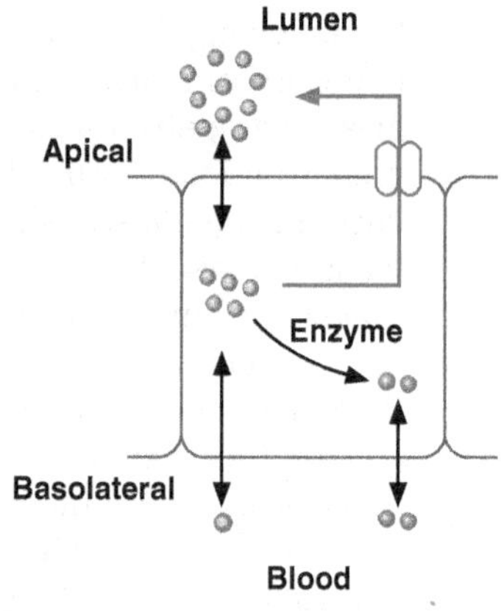

FIGURE 8-7 For some drugs, systemic absorption after oral administration depends on both enzymatic metabolism and efflux transporters (*depicted in color*) in the intestinal epithelium. The presence of efflux transporters on the apical side in concert with the intracellular metabolism may diminish the movement of drug from the intestinal lumen to mesenteric blood. Inhibition of either the metabolic activity or the efflux transport leads to an increase in the net movement of unchanged drug into the systemic circulation. In the figure, drug appears as black molecules and metabolite as colored ones.

TABLE 8-5 | Examples of Drugs Showing Saturable First-Pass Metabolism in the Gut Wall, Liver, or both After Oral Administration of Therapeutic Doses

Drug	Indication	Drug	Indication
Alprenolol	Hypertension, angina, and cardiac arrhythmia	Niacin	Hyperlipidemia
Atorvastatin	Hyperlipidemia	Nicardipine	Hypertension
Darifenacin	Overactive bladder	Omeprazole	Duodenal ulcers
5-Fluorouracil	Certain cancers	Propafenone	Atrial fibrillation
Fluvastatin	Hyperlipidemia	Propranolol	Hypertension
Hydralazine	Hypertension	Rivastigmine	Alzheimer's Disease
Isosorbide dinitrate	Angina	Verapamil	Angina and cardiac arrhythmias

examples of which are listed in Table 8-5. These are drugs that have a low bioavailability at low doses, because of extensive first-pass metabolic loss (high extraction ratio) either in the gut wall or in the liver, or both. At higher doses, metabolism approaches saturation. Evidence supporting this conclusion is that in many cases, no change in the elimination half-life is observed. This behavior can be understood by realizing that, given the small volume of intestinal fluid, the concentration of drug entering the gut wall and entering the liver via the portal vein can be much higher than that of the systemically circulating drug, owing to a combination of hepatic extraction and subsequent dilution of absorbed drug by its distribution to the tissues of the body. So once absorption is complete, the plasma concentrations entering the gut wall and the liver are too low to cause saturation of the metabolic enzymes, especially in the terminal phase of decline where the half-life is measured. When saturable first-pass metabolism occurs, product formulation can have an impact on the bioavailability of orally administered drugs. Generally, the slower the release, as in modified-release products, the lower is the expected bioavailability of the drug.

Absorption From Intramuscular and Subcutaneous Sites

Small Molecular Weight Drugs

In contrast to the gastrointestinal tract, absorption of most drugs in solution from muscle and subcutaneous tissue is perfusion rate–limited. For example, consider the data in Table 8-6 (next page) for the local anesthetic lidocaine. Shown are the peak plasma concentrations observed when the same dose of lidocaine is administered parenterally at different sites of the body. Recall from Fig. 7-5, for a given dose, when C_{max} is higher, drug absorption is faster. Large differences in speed of absorption are clearly evident, the speed increasing from subcutaneous tissue to intercostal muscle (between the ribs), in line with an increasing tissue perfusion rate.

The dependence of rapidity of absorption on local blood flow is taken advantage of when lidocaine is used as a local anesthetic for local surgical procedures. The addition of epinephrine, a vasoconstrictive agent, reduces the blood flow and, as a consequence, reduces bleeding and prolongs the local anesthetic effect.

In some conditions, such as hemorrhagic shock, perfusion of skeletal muscle tissue is drastically reduced, in this case because of extensive blood loss. It is then

TABLE 8-6 | Influence of Site of Injection on the Peak Venous Lidocaine Concentration Following Injection of a 100-mg Dose

Injection Site	Peak Plasma Lidocaine Concentration (mg/L)	Perfusion Rate
Intercostal	1.46	↑
Paracervical	1.20	
Caudal	1.18	
Lumbar epidural	0.97	
Brachial plexus	0.53	
Subarachnoid	0.44	
Subcutaneous	0.35	

Taken from Covino BG. Pharmacokinetics of local anaesthetic drug. In: Prys-Roberts C, Hug CC, eds. *Pharmacokinetics of Anaesthesia.* Oxford, UK: Blackwell Scientific Publications, 1984:270–292.

inappropriate to give drugs requiring a rapid onset of action by the intramuscular as well as subcutaneous routes—the intravenous route is then used. Reduced tissue perfusion in this condition becomes a major disadvantage to pharmacotherapy.

This dependence of absorption on perfusion may be explained by the nature of the barrier (capillary membrane) between the site of injection (interstitial fluid) and blood. This membrane, a much more loosely knit structure than the epithelial lining of the gastrointestinal tract (see Chapter 4), offers little impedance to the movement of drugs from the intestinal lumen to blood, even for polar ionized drugs. For example, gentamicin, a relatively large (MW = 1486 g/mol), water-soluble, ionized, polar base, is poorly absorbed when given orally because it has great difficulty penetrating the gastrointestinal mucosa. It also does not pass the blood–brain barrier, nor is it reabsorbed in the renal tubule. However, it is rapidly and completely absorbed systemically from an intramuscular site. This low impedance by the capillary membrane in muscle and subcutaneous tissue applies to all small drugs, independent of charge or degree of ionization.

Macromolecules and Lymphatic Transport

In contrast to small molecules, size, polarity, and charge are important for administration of proteins and large polypeptide drugs; their transport across many membranes is hindered. Furthermore, because of their polarity and decomposition by proteolytic enzymes in the gastrointestinal tract, their oral absorption is often low and erratic. Most of the information on these kinds of drugs has been obtained following nonvascular parenteral administration. For the subcutaneous and intramuscular routes, drug reaches the systemic circulation by two parallel mechanisms: diffusion through the interstitial fluids into blood capillaries and convective flow of the interstitial fluids into and through lymphatic channels. Molecular size is of primary importance for passage across the capillary membranes. Polypeptides of less than approximately 10,000 g/mol, such as insulin (6000 g/mol), primarily reach the systemic circulation by this pathway. Polypeptides of greater than about 20,000 g/mol are less able to traverse the capillary membranes; by default, they primarily reach the blood via the lymphatic system. Some drug, of course, is still moving across the capillary membrane, just at a slower rate. A diagrammatic representation of the lymphatic system is shown in Fig. 8-8.

Lymph flow is very slow (movement of interstitial fluid into lymphatic vessels is 500 times, and return of lymph to blood is 5000 times, slower than blood flow) and causes absorption from nonvascular parenteral sites to continue for many hours, as

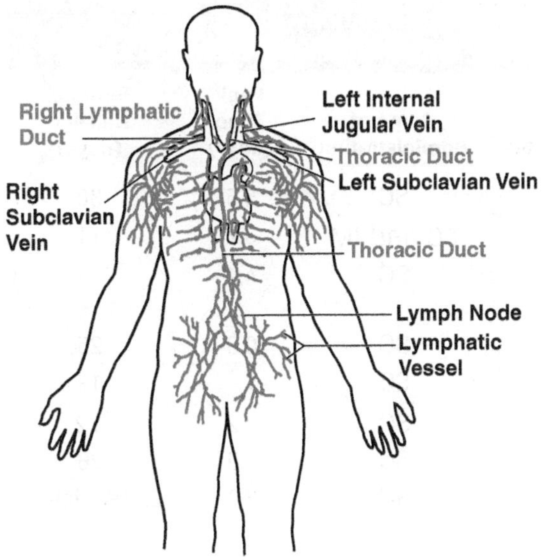

FIGURE 8-8 A sketch of the lymphatic system. Note that drug in the interstitial fluids of subcutaneous or muscular tissue, placed there by injection, moves through the lymphatic vessels and one or several lymph nodes before reaching the systemic circulation. Lymph returns drug to the bloodstream from a portion of the right side of the body via the right lymphatic duct and from the tissues of the rest of the body via the thoracic duct. These ducts empty into the right and left subclavian veins, respectively.

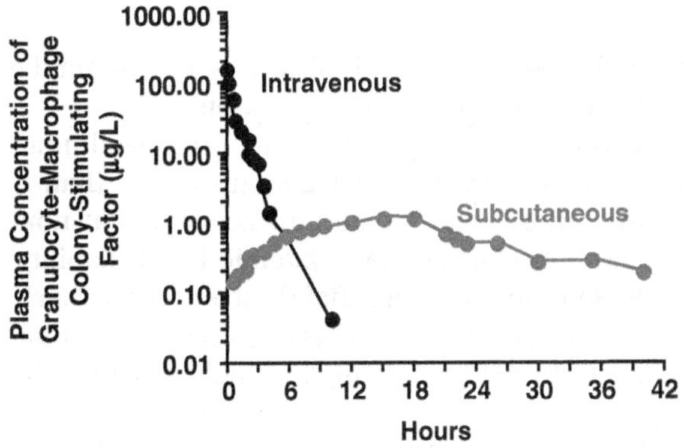

FIGURE 8-9 Plasma concentrations of glycosylated recombinant human granulocyte-macrophage colony-stimulating factor following intravenous (*black circle*) and subcutaneous (*colored circle*) bolus injections of 8 µg/kg on separate occasions. (Adapted from Hovgaard D, Mortensen BT, Schifter S, et al. Clinical pharmacokinetic studies of a human haemopoietic growth factor, GM-CSF. *Eur J Clin Invest* 1992;22:45–49.)

shown in Fig. 8-9 for filgrastim. Filgrastim (Neupogen) is a glycosylated recombinant human granulocyte-macrophage colony-stimulating factor (MW = 15,000–34,000 g/mol) used to decrease the incidence of infection, as manifested by febrile neutropenia in patients with nonmyeloid malignancies receiving myelosuppressive anticancer drugs. This drug has a half-life of 68 minutes after intravenous administration of a single dose, but after subcutaneous administration, the plasma concentration is prolonged for at least 42 hours, with a rate of decline indicating continuing input even at this time. Elimination of this protein drug after subcutaneous administration is clearly rate-limited by its systemic absorption.

Many new therapeutic agents are monoclonal antibodies (MW = 150,000 g/mol). These are predominantly absorbed lymphatically following subcutaneous or intramuscular administration, and much more slowly (as indicated by t_{max} values on the order of days, Table 8-7, next page) than small proteins and polypeptides, showing that the speed of absorption through the lymphatics is related in an inverse fashion to molecular size. Nonetheless, at therapeutic doses, many monoclonal antibodies have

TABLE 8-7 | Bioavailability of Selected Monoclonal Antibody Drugs After Subcutaneous and Intramuscular Administration of a Single Dose[a]

Antibody	Molecular Weight (kg/mol)	Bioavailability	Route of Administration	Peak Time (days)	Terminal Half-life (days)
Adalimumab	148	0.64	SC	5.5	30
Alefacept	91	0.80	SC and IM	3.2[b]	11
Certolizumab pegol	91	0.79	SC	4.7	14
Denosumab	147	0.62	SC	10.0	25
Efalizumab	150	0.50	SC	–	17
Etanercept	150	0.67	SC	2.2	4.2
Omalizumab	149	0.62	SC	7.5	26
Palivizumab	148	–	SC	2.0	20 (Pediatric)

The IM and SC curves were virtually superimposed.
[a]From *Physician's Desk Reference(PDR)*, 62nd edition. Montvale, NJ: Medical Economics Co., 2008.
[b]From Sweetser MT, Woodworth J, Swan S, et al. Results of a randomized open-label crossover study of the bioequivalence of subcutaneous and intramuscular administration of alefacept. *Dermatol Online J* 2006;3:12(3):1.

disposition half-lives on the order of weeks, so despite their slow absorption, unlike that seen with filgrastim, absorption still does not rate-limit elimination.

Nonvascular parenteral routes offer the advantage of providing prolonged input for short half-life proteins. This may allow for less frequent administration than is required by the intravenous route. However, one must take into account that nonvascular parenteral administration often results in reduced systemic bioavailability. Proteolytic enzymes are known to be present, in the interstitial fluid and particularly in lymph nodes, through which the protein drugs must pass. This is in contrast to small molecular weight drugs, which are almost always completely available systemically when given by these routes.

The speed of absorption, after both intramuscular and subcutaneous administration and for both small molecules and macromolecules, has been shown to be highly dependent on the site of injection, local temperature, and rubbing at the injection site, which increases movement of drug into both the vasculature and the lymphatic system.

For all routes of administration, consideration should be given to both the particular properties of the site of administration and the drug itself. For example, when given rectally, a drug may not be retained long enough for absorption to be complete. Nonetheless, the factors influencing absorption from this less conventional site are in common with those generally influencing absorption from oral, intramuscular, and subcutaneous sites.

ABSORPTION FROM SOLID DOSAGE FORMS

When a drug is taken orally in a solid dosage form, such as a tablet or a capsule, a number of processes must occur before it can be systemically available. The dosage form must disintegrate and deaggregate, and the drug must dissolve to be absorbed, as shown in Fig. 8-10. Dissolution is a key factor, but not the only one. Table 8-8 summarizes factors that determine the release of a drug from a solid dosage form, and the rate and extent

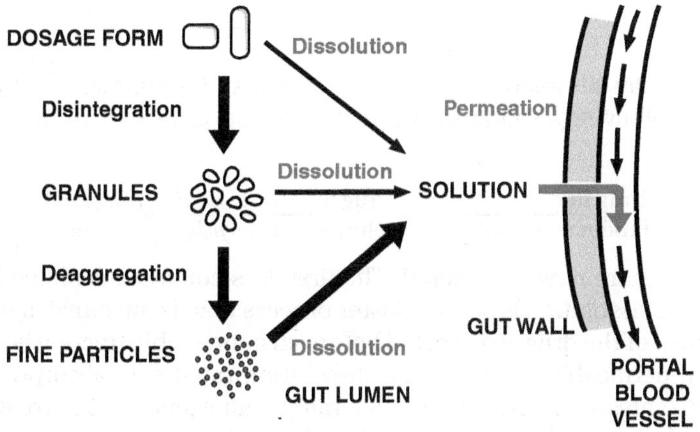

FIGURE 8-10 After oral administration of a typical immediate-release solid dosage form, tablet or capsule, the product undergoes disintegration to granules. These granules further deaggregate to fine particles. Dissolution of drug occurs at all stages, but usually that from fine particles predominates (see *thickness of arrows*). The drug, now in solution, permeates the membranes of the gastrointestinal tract (*colored arrow*) to reach the mesenteric blood vessels that carry the drug via the portal vein and liver to the systemic circulation.

TABLE 8-8 | Factors Determining the Release and Absorption Kinetics of a Drug Following Oral Administration of a Solid Dosage Form

Release Characteristics of Dosage Form
Disintegration/deaggregation
Dissolution of drug from granules (also dependent on inactive ingredients [excipients] and formulation variables)
Physicochemical Properties of Drug
Ionization (acid/base)
Partition coefficient (n-octanol/water)
Solubility in water
Physiology of Gastrointestinal Tract
Colonic retention
Gastric emptying
Intestinal motility
Perfusion of the gastrointestinal tract
Permeability of gut wall
Gastrointestinal Tract Abnormalities and Diseases
Crohn's disease
Gastric resection (e.g., in obesity)
Diarrhea

of systemic absorption after an oral dose. The factors are classified into four groups, namely, release characteristics of the dosage form, physicochemical properties of drug, physiology of the gastrointestinal tract, and presence of gastrointestinal tract abnormalities and diseases.

Dissolution

The reason why dissolution is so important may be appreciated by realizing that absorption following a solid requires drug dissolution, as only drug in solution can be absorbed.

$$\text{Drug in Product} \xrightarrow[\textit{Dissolution}]{} \text{Drug in solution} \xrightarrow[\textit{Absorption}]{\textit{Intestinal}} \text{Absorbed drug} \qquad \textbf{Eq. 8-2}$$

Two situations are now considered. The first, less common, depicted in Fig. 8-11A, is one in which dissolution is a much faster process than is intestinal absorption. Consequently, most of the drug is dissolved before an appreciable fraction is absorbed. Here, commonly, permeability rather than dissolution rate-limits absorption. An example is the gastrointestinal absorption of sucralfate, an agent used in treating gastric and intestinal ulcers, when given as a tablet. This polar drug dissolves rapidly from the tablet, but has difficulty penetrating the gastrointestinal epithelium. Hence, little drug is absorbed. The systemic input is **rate-limited by intestinal absorption** due to poor permeability. Within limits, differences in rates of dissolution of sucralfate from different tablet formations have relatively little or no effect on the speed of systemic absorption of this drug.

In the second, and more common, situation shown in Fig. 8-11B, dissolution proceeds relatively slowly, and any dissolved drug readily traverses the gastrointestinal epithelium. Systemic absorption cannot proceed any faster, however, than the rate at which the drug dissolves. That is, absorption is **dissolution rate–limited.** In this

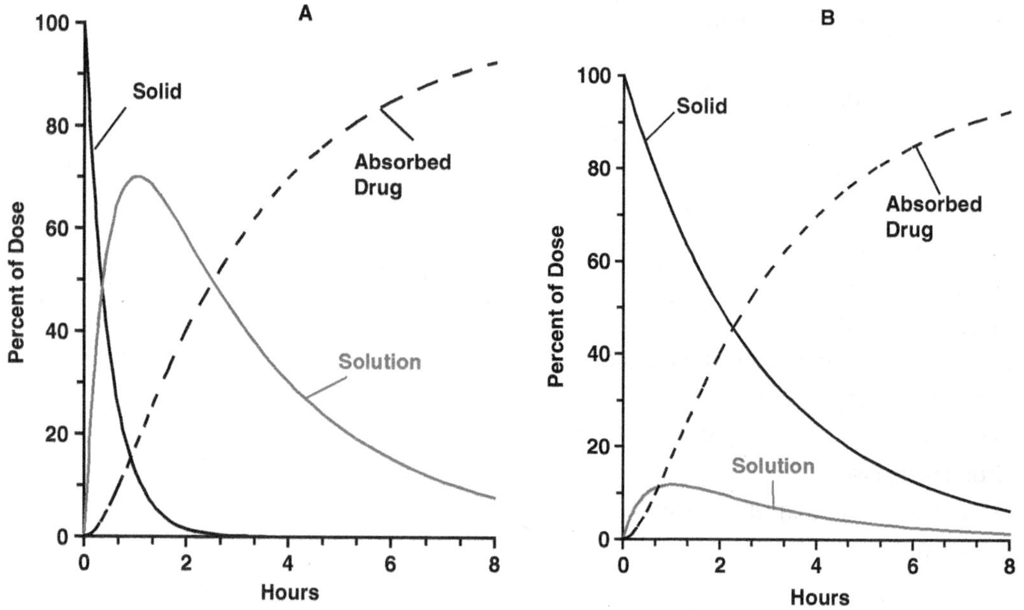

FIGURE 8-11 When absorption is permeability rate-limited **(A)**, most of the drug has dissolved (*colored line*) in the gastrointestinal tract before an appreciable fraction has been absorbed after a single oral dose. In contrast, when dissolution rate-limits absorption **(B)**, very little drug is in solution (*colored line*) at the absorption site at any time; drug is absorbed almost as soon as it dissolves. Notice that, except during the early stages of absorption, the majority of drug yet to be absorbed is always found just before the rate-limiting step: in solution in Case A and as solid in Case B.

case, changes in dissolution profoundly affect the rate, and sometimes the extent, of drug absorption. Evidence supporting dissolution rate–limited absorption comes from the noticeably slower systemic absorption of most drugs from solid dosage forms than from a simple aqueous solution after oral administration. It also comes from modified-release dosage forms in which release, and therefore dissolution, is intentionally prolonged.

Gastric Emptying and Intestinal Transit

Before discussing the role of gastric emptying on absorption of drugs given as solids, consider the information provided in Fig. 8-12. Shown are the mean transit times in the stomach and small intestine of small nondisintegrating pellets (diameters between 0.3 and 1.8 mm) and of large, single nondisintegrating units (either capsules, 25 mm by 9 mm; or tablets, 8–12 mm in diameter).

During fasting, gastric emptying of both small and large solids is seen, on average, to be rapid, with a mean time of around 1 hour, although somewhat longer than the 30 minutes typical of a solution. In this state, the stomach displays a complex temporal pattern of motor activity with alternating periods of quiescence and moderate contraction of varying frequency, the "housekeeping wave," which moves material into the small intestine. The exact ejection time of a solid particle therefore depends on its

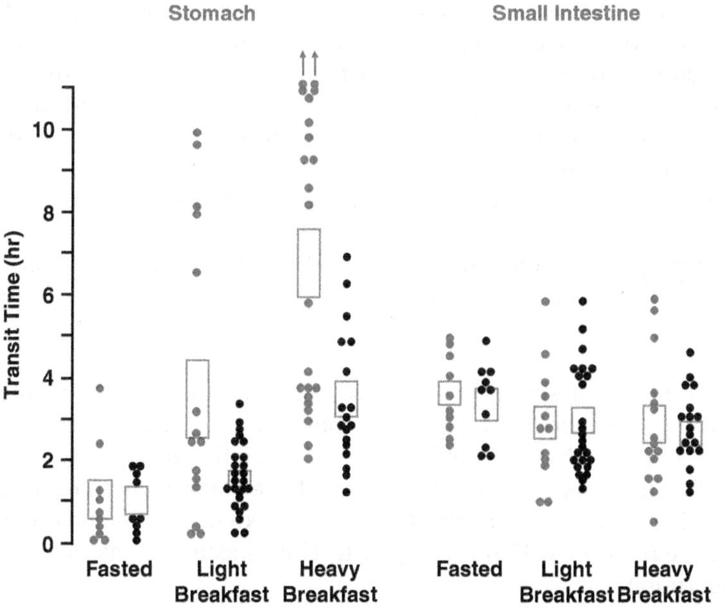

FIGURE 8-12 Food, particularly a heavy meal, increases the gastric transit time of small pellets (*black circles*) and, even more markedly, of large single pellets (*colored circles*). In contrast, neither food nor the physical size of the solid affects the small intestine transit time. The data (*individual points, black* or *colored circles,* and the range encompassing the mean ± one SE, indicated by the *rectangles*) were obtained in healthy young adults using drug-free nondisintegrating materials. The points with an arrow indicate the solid was still in the stomach at the time of the last observation, 16 hours. The pellets were labeled with a γ-emitting isotope and monitored externally by gamma scintigraphy. (Adapted from Davis SS, Hardy JG, Fara J. Transit of pharmaceutical dosage forms through the small intestine. *Gut* 1986;27:886–892.)

size, when it is ingested during the motor activity cycle, and where it is located within the stomach. The likelihood of ejection is greatest when the solid particle is in close proximity to the pyloric sphincter when the housekeeping wave occurs. Thus, even for small solid particles and fasting conditions, gastric emptying can vary from minutes to several hours.

The situation is very different after eating. As shown in Fig. 8-12, when taken on a fed stomach, the gastric transit time of solids is increased. This increase is greater after a heavy meal than after a light one and is much greater for a large single unit than for small pellets. For example, the mean gastric transit time among subjects for large single-unit systems is now almost 7 hours, with some pellets still in the stomach in some subjects 11 hours after ingestion. These observations are explained by the sieving action of a fed stomach. Solids with diameters greater than 7–10 mm pass into the small intestine more slowly and less predictably than those of smaller diameter. Some individuals consistently show prolonged gastric emptying of large pellets in the fed state, whereas for others, it is much less apparent. These differences have largely been ascribed to interindividual differences in the size of the pyloric sphincter. This retention of large pellets is generally consistent with the physiologic role of the stomach, that is, to retain larger food particles until they are reduced in size to facilitate further digestion. With conventional tablets, rapid disintegration, and deaggregation into fine particles achieves the same objective. As long as the stomach remains in a fed state, the conditions above prevail. For those persons who eat three hearty meals a day with several snacks in between, gastric emptying of large pellets may be slowed most of the waking hours of the day.

In contrast to events in the stomach, the transit time of solids within the small intestine varies little among subjects, appears to be independent of either the size of a solid or the presence of food in the stomach, and is remarkably short, an average of approximately 3 hours (Fig. 8-12), a time similar to that found for the transit of liquids. Both solids and liquids appear to move down the small intestine as a plug with relatively little mixing. As the mouth-to-anus transit time is typically 1–3 days, these data on gastric and small intestinal transit times indicate that, for the majority of this time, unabsorbed materials are in either the large bowel or the rectum. Given the physiologic information above, we can now understand the possible role of gastric emptying and intestinal transit on the absorption of drugs administered in solid dosage forms. Consider the following situations.

Rapid Dissolution in Stomach

This is the common situation seen with many permeable and soluble drugs, such as ibuprofen and acetaminophen, in conventional immediate-release tablets and capsules. Drug dissolves so rapidly in the stomach that most of it is in solution before much of the drug has entered the intestine. Here, gastric emptying clearly influences the rate of drug absorption, but only to the extent that liquids and deaggregated particles are retained within the stomach. Thus, hastening gastric emptying quickens drug absorption.

Rapid Dissolution in Intestine

Sometimes, drug does not materially dissolve within the stomach, whereas in the intestine it rapidly both dissolves and moves across the intestinal wall. Gastric emptying then also affects the speed of drug absorption. An enteric-coated product is an extreme example of this situation. Proton pump inhibitors, such as omeprazole, lansoprazole, and pantoprazole, and didanosine, an antiviral agent, are examples of drugs that are rapidly hydrolyzed to inactive products in the acidic environment of the stomach. Aspirin, sulfasalazine, used to treat ulcerative colitis, and bisacodyl, a laxative, are gastric irritants. A solution to both types of problems has been to enterically coat these drug products with a material resistant to acid but not to the intestinal fluids. When an enteric-coated product such as a large single tablet is tested, the time for it to pass from the stomach into the intestine varies unpredictably from 20 minutes to several hours when taken on an empty stomach, and up to 12 hours or even more when taken on a fed stomach (see Fig. 8-12). Accordingly, such enteric-coated products cannot be used when rapid and reliable absorption is required. A product composed of enteric-coated small granules is an improvement because the delivery of the granules to the intestine is expected to be more reliable, being less dependent on a single event, a "housekeeping wave," and on food intake.

Poor Dissolution

Some drugs, such as the oral antifungal broad-spectrum anthelmintic, albendazole, are sparingly soluble or almost insoluble in both gastric and intestinal fluids. When these drugs are administered as a solid, there may already be insufficient time for complete dissolution and absorption. With a fixed short time within the small intestine, slow release from the stomach increases the time for drug to dissolve there before entering the intestine, thereby favoring increased bioavailability. As mentioned, food—fat in particular—delays gastric emptying. This delay may be one of the explanations for the observed five-fold increase in the plasma concentration of albendazole sulfoxide, its primary metabolite, when parent drug is taken with a fatty meal. Subsequently, intestinal fluid and contents move from the small into the large intestine, and water is reabsorbed. The resulting compaction of the solid contents may severely limit further dissolution and hence absorption of such drugs.

Absorption From Other Sites

Drugs may be administered at virtually any site on or within the body. Inhalation is exploited as a means of local delivery of drugs for the treatment of pulmonary diseases. To minimize systemic exposure, and side effects, many drugs administered by this route have a high systemic metabolic clearance, which not only ensures rapid clearance of any pulmonary absorbed drug but also low bioavailability of any swallowed drug, due to high first-pass hepatic loss. An example in this class is the steroid beclomethasone, with a very high clearance (150 L/hr), short half-life (30 minutes), and very low oral bioavailability (1%–2%). There is also considerable interest in exploiting some of the less conventional sites, such as nasal and buccal cavities, as a means of delivering drugs systemically. Polypeptide and protein drugs have received particular attention, as shown in Table 8-9 (next page). Transdermal application has become popular for systemic delivery of small, generally lipophilic, potent molecules that require low input rates to achieve effective therapy. Examples of transdermal and other transmembrane delivery systems are listed in Table 8-10 (next page).

We have now covered the critical determinants of the pharmacokinetics of drugs after a single dose administered intravenously and extravascularly. Such information now needs to be placed within the context of the responses produced following administration by these routes, the content of the next chapter, *Response Following a Single Dose.*

TABLE 8-9 | Examples of Unconventional Sites and Methods of Administration of Polypeptide and Protein Drugs

Polypeptide/Protein	Therapeutic Use[a]	Site and Method of Administration
Bacitracin zinc and polymyxin B sulfate (anti-infective agent)	Superficial ocular infections (local effect)	Eye: Application of ointment.
Calcitonin-salmon (thyroid hormone that acts primarily on bone)	Postmenopausal osteoporosis (systemic effect)	Nasal spray: The relative bioavailability (compared with IM dose) is 3%.
Desmopressin (synthetic form of antidiuretic hormone)	Primary nocturnal enuresis and diabetes insipidus (systemic effect)	Intranasal: Administered through a soft, flexible, plastic rhinal tube; also nasal spray.
Dornase alfa (recombinant human deoxyribonuclease)	Cystic fibrosis (local effect)	Oral: Also, inhalation using nebulizer.
Gladase (papain, a proteolytic enzyme, plus urea)	Removal of necrotic tissue (local effect)	Topical: Ointment applied directly to wound.
Leuprolide acetate (naturally occurring gonadotropin-releasing hormone)	Advanced prostatic cancer (systemic effect)	Implant: Inserted subcutaneously on inner side of upper arm. Product constantly releases 120 μg/day and is replaced once yearly.
Pancrelipase powder (lipase, protease, and amylase–digestive enzymes)	Cystic fibrosis (local intestinal effect)	Taken orally with meals.

[a]Therapeutic use and note on whether the effect is obtained locally or systemically.

TABLE 8-10 | Examples of Transdermal Delivery Systems

Drug	Use	Delivery
Clonidine	Treatment of hypertension	Delivery of 0.1, 0.2, or 0.3 mg clonidine per day for 1 week.
Estradiol	Estrogen replacement, menopause	Constant rate of delivery applied twice weekly to once weekly with 14–16 days off, depending on indication.
Fentanyl	Continuous pain relief	Applied every 3 days.
Nicotine	To help cessation of smoking	Various dose strengths designed to be applied daily for 2–8 weeks
Norelgestromin/ethinyl estradiol	Prevention of pregnancy	Weekly change of patch for 3 weeks. One week no patch.
Oxybutynin	Treatment of overactive bladder	Applied every 3–4 days.
Progesterone	Progesterone supplementation, secondary amenorrhea	Vaginally, twice daily for progesterone supplement, every other day for treating amenorrhea.
Scopolamine	Motion sickness	Effect lasts for 3 days (1.0 mg delivered).
Testosterone	Testosterone replacement therapy, male hypogonadism	Once daily application.
Patch	–	–
Gel	–	–
Buccal system	–	–

SUMMARY

- Systemic absorption after oral administration requires that drug dissolves in the gastric and luminal fluids and traverses across gastrointestinal membranes.
- Gastric emptying plays a major role in determining the rate and extent of systemic absorption after oral administration. Dissolution, surface area, membrane permeability, and intestinal blood flow are additional primary determinants of systemic absorption.
- Low oral bioavailability can result from limited transit time in the gastrointestinal tract. This result applies to both highly polar (permeability rate–limited) and nonpolar (dissolution rate–limited) drugs. Decomposition due to low gastric pH, digestive enzymes, or enzymes of the colonic microbiota also reduce systemic absorption. Metabolism within the gut wall and liver during the first-pass through these organs further reduces oral bioavailability.
- Systemic absorption from intramuscular and subcutaneous sites of administration is rapid for small molecules (<10,000 g/mol), whether polar or not, whereas macromolecules (>20,000 g/mol) primarily reach the systemic circulation via the lymphatics. This occurs, by default, because movement across blood capillary membranes becomes slower than movement through the lymphatics.
- Absorption via the lymphatics can be very slow with systemic absorption half-lives for monoclonal antibodies in the order of days.
- Bioavailability is usually 100% following subcutaneous and intramuscular administration for small molecules, but can be greatly reduced for protein drugs because of proteolytic activity at the absorption site and within the lymphatic system.

KEY TERM REVIEW

Area under the curve (AUC)
Bioavailability
Dissolution
Extravascular route
Gastric emptying
Hepatic extraction
Intramuscular injection
Lymphatic system
Macromolecules
Paracellular transport
Permeability
Permeability rate–limited absorption
Permeability–surface area product
pH
Prodrugs
Rate-limiting step
Solubility
Subcutaneous absorption
Systemic absorption
Time of peak plasma concentration
Transcellular transport
Transit time

KEY RELATIONSHIPS

$$F = F_F \cdot F_G \cdot F_H$$

$$\begin{matrix}\text{Drug in} \\ \text{Product}\end{matrix} \xrightarrow[\textit{Dissolution}]{} \begin{matrix}\text{Drug in} \\ \text{solution}\end{matrix} \xrightarrow[\textit{Absorption}]{\textit{Intestinal}} \begin{matrix}\text{Absorbed} \\ \text{drug}\end{matrix}$$

STUDY PROBLEMS

1. The systemic absorption of drug following the administration of an immediate-release tablet dosage form is influenced by many factors. Which *one* of the following factors is most closely associated with the absorption kinetics of a drug taken in tablet form during fasting conditions?
   a. Disintegration of the tablet
   b. Time of day the tablet is taken
   c. Elimination half-life of the drug
   d. Dissolution of the drug
   e. pH of the colonic lumen
2. Studies with nondisintegrating pellets have shown that gastric emptying is slowed by eating a meal, especially a fatty one. Which *one* of the following statements is the most accurate reflection of the results of those studies?
   a. Large pellets tend to be retained for a shorter time in the stomach than small ones after a meal.
   b. The transit time of large pellets in the small intestine tends to be longer than that for small pellets when they are taken with a fatty meal.
   c. Small pellets tend to be held in the stomach longer than large ones under fasting conditions.
   d. Both large and small pellets are typically retained in the alimentary tract for 24–72 hours.
   e. The typical transit time in the small intestine for small pellets after a heavy breakfast is 6 hours.
3. Which of the following statements about systemic absorption of drugs from intramuscular and subcutaneous sites is (are) correct?
   I. The systemic absorption of small molecules injected intramuscularly in solution is perfusion rate–limited—the more rapid the perfusion rate of the site of injection, the quicker is the absorption process.
   II. For polypeptides greater than 20,000 g/mol in size, systemic absorption primarily occurs via the lymphatics after both intramuscular and subcutaneous administrations.
   III. The site of an injection, the temperature of the skin, and rubbing at the injection site can all influence the speed at which a drug is systemically absorbed following a subcutaneous injection.

   A. I only　　**E.** I and III
   B. II only　　**F.** II and III
   C. III only　　**G.** All
   D. I and II　　**H.** None
4. The release of a drug from a tablet formulation can greatly influence its rate and extent of systemic absorption and its duration in the body after oral administration. Consider the following sequence of steps to address this question: dissolution, intestinal absorption, elimination from the body. Which of the following statements is (are) correct?
   I. When dissolution rate-limits absorption, at all times there is very little drug in solution within the gastrointestinal tract compared with that yet to be dissolved.
   II. When intestinal permeation rate-limits absorption, the amount in solution in the gastrointestinal tract quickly becomes greater than that still undissolved, and remains so thereafter.

III. When release from the dosage form rate-limits the overall process, the terminal decline of the plasma drug concentration with time reflects the speed of the dissolution step.

A. I only	**E.** I and III
B. II only	**F.** II and III
C. III only	**G.** All
D. I and II	**H.** None

5. List at least five reasons why oral bioavailability of drugs is often less than 100%.
6. Comment on the likely influence of a heavy fat meal, relative to the fasting state, on the speed and extent of oral absorption of a drug (i.e., AUC, C_{max}, t_{max}) in each of the following cases. All of the drugs, except the one in Part C, are chemically stable in the gastrointestinal tract.
   a. A water-soluble highly permeable drug is administered in an immediate-release tablet.
   b. A sparingly soluble lipophilic drug is administered as an intended immediate-release capsule dosage form. Oral bioavailability is typically only 26% due to low aqueous solubility.
   c. An acid-labile drug is taken as a single enterically coated (resistant to acidic gastric pH) 0.8-g tablet.
7. Dexmedetomidine, a relatively selective α_2-adrenergic agonist for sedation of initially intubated and mechanically ventilated patients during treatment in an intensive care setting, was studied in 12 healthy male subjects. Fig. 8-13 shows the concentration–time profiles after intravenous injection (over 5 minutes) and oral administration (drug solution ingested with 150 mL of water). The doses were the same, namely, 2 μg/kg. The AUC was 4.44 μg-hr/L and 0.566 μg-hr/L after IV and oral administration, respectively. The drug is extensively metabolized.
   a. Is the decline of dexmedetomidine after its oral administration rate-limited by its absorption or elimination? Briefly describe how you come to your conclusion.
   b. Calculate the oral bioavailability and clearance of dexmedetomidine in the group studied, mean weight 70 kg.
   c. Knowing that the plasma-to-blood concentration ratio of this drug is 0.8 and that $fe \leq 0.01$, calculate the expected oral bioavailability, assuming that metabolism

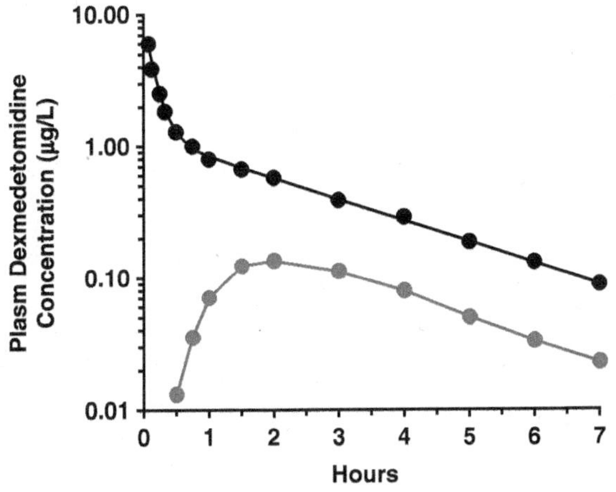

FIGURE 8-13 Mean curves of dexmedetomidine concentrations in plasma with time after intravenous (IV) (*black circle*) and oral administration (*colored circle*) of a single 2.0 μg/kg dose. (Data taken from Anttila M, Penttila J, Helminen A, et al. Bioavailability of dexmedetomidine after extravascular doses in healthy subjects. *Br J Clin Pharmacol* 2003;56:691–693.)

occurs only in the liver and all orally administered drug reaches the liver intact ($F_F = F_G = 1.0$). Mean hepatic blood flow in a 70-kg adult is 1.35 L/min.

d. Does the observed value for oral bioavailability correspond to that calculated in B? If not, how might you explain the difference, and should alternative routes of administration be considered?

8. Discuss the primary factors determining the speed and extent of systemic absorption of protein drugs following their subcutaneous and intramuscular administration.

9. Kampf et al. studied the pharmacokinetics of recombinant human erythropoietin, a glycosylated protein (MW = 34,000 g/mol) used to increase red blood cell formation in patients with end-stage renal disease, after single IV and SC injections of 40 units/kg on separate occasions. Table 8-11 lists the salient findings of these studies. The mean weight of the patients was 60 kg.

TABLE 8-11 | Mean AUC, Maximum Plasma Concentration, and Terminal Half-life of Erythropoietin in End-Stage Renal Disease Patients Following Intravenous and Subcutaneous Administration

Injection	AUC (unit-hr/L)	Maximum Concentration (Units/L)	Time of Maximum Concentration	Terminal Half-life (hr)
Intravenous	3010	417	5 min[a]	6.7
Subcutaneous	1372	40.5	12 hr	16.1

[a]Time of first sample.
Abstracted from Kampf D, Echardt KU, Fischer HC, et al. Pharmacokinetics of recombinant human erythropoietin in dialysis patients after single and multiple subcutaneous administration. *Nephron* 1992;61:393–398.

a. Determine the clearance and volume of distribution of this drug.

b. Calculate the bioavailability of erythropoietin after subcutaneous administration in these patients. How might you explain your answer?

c. The maximum concentration observed was much lower, and the terminal decline phase much slower, after the subcutaneous, than the intravenous, dose. How do you explain these observations?

CHAPTER 9

Response Following a Single Dose

OBJECTIVES

The reader will be able to:

- Define the following terms: effect compartment, effective half-life, hysteresis, pharmacokinetic–pharmacodynamic modeling, time delay.
- Show graphically how one can readily detect when response lags behind the plasma drug concentration after a single extravascular dose, and give at least two explanations for the delay.
- Give two examples each of situations in which measured response is rate-limited by pharmacokinetics and pharmacodynamics.
- Explain why a graded response tends to decline linearly with time after a single dose when response lies between 80% and 20% of its maximum.
- Give two approaches taken to reveal the direct concentration–response relationship from response–time data following a single dose of drug.
- Explain why duration of response is often proportional to the logarithm of dose, and when it is, be able to calculate both the apparent minimum effective dose and effective half-life.

In Chapter 3, we considered the relationship between systemic exposure and response, that is, the pharmacodynamics of a drug, without much consideration of time. In practice, time always needs to be considered. In this chapter, we integrate pharmacokinetics with response over time following a single dose of drug. Given the many complexities determining the temporal pattern of response, concepts that have universal application do not exist. The subsequent discussion is generally restricted to drugs that act reversibly and directly at the site of action to produce a response. Furthermore, in this chapter metabolites are considered to be inactive or, at the least, not to reach a sufficiently high concentration to contribute to response.

It is important to realize that the amount of drug involved in producing a response at the site of action is usually only a minute fraction of the total amount in the body. Consequently, drug so involved generally has little to no effect on its own pharmacokinetics. Recall, from Chapter 6, exceptions are drugs, particularly monoclonal antibodies, that exhibit target-mediated disposition.

TIME DELAYS BETWEEN CONCENTRATION AND RESPONSE

Drug response often lags behind its plasma concentration. Let us examine how such delays are detected and how they come about.

Detecting Time Delays

A striking example of a delay in effect is seen after an intravenous bolus dose of digoxin (Fig. 9-1). The left ventricular ejection time index, an electrocardiographic measure of effect on the heart, rises while its plasma concentration falls during the first 4 hours. Certainly, these data do not mean that less drug is needed to produce a greater response. Rather, distribution of digoxin into cardiac tissue with subsequent binding to the target receptor is slow. Therefore, to use plasma concentration as a guide to drug effect, one should wait until distribution equilibrium of drug between plasma and cardiac tissue is reached, which is about 6 hours after a dose of digoxin. On relating response to concentration before 6 hours, an absurd relationship is observed. The response is lowest when the concentration is highest, and the converse is true. We would be foolish to conclude that what is needed for a substantial effect is a low concentration or no drug at all.

In contrast to an intravenous bolus dose, plasma drug concentration first rises and then falls after a single oral dose. This may lead to **hysteresis** in the concentration–response relationship, a useful diagnostic of the temporal features of drug response. Hysteresis refers to the response taking a path, relative to the concentration, that is different when the concentration rises from that when it falls. An example of such a curve is shown in Fig. 9-2 after the oral administration of naproxen, an analgesic, antipyretic, and anti-inflammatory agent. Shown in Fig. 9-2A are the plasma concentration and the mean pain relief in a dental pain model with time after a single 500-mg dose of naproxen. Although a time lag between plasma concentration and response is suggested from this graph, a delay is much more apparent when response is plotted directly against the corresponding plasma concentration (Fig. 9-2B), yielding a characteristic hysteresis loop. Initially, during the absorption phase, response lags behind the rise of naproxen in plasma. Subsequently, while the plasma concentration starts to fall, response continues to rise. Only after 5 hours does response follow the fall in plasma concentration. Notice that the chronologic sequence of the paired concentration–response observations moves in a counterclockwise direction.

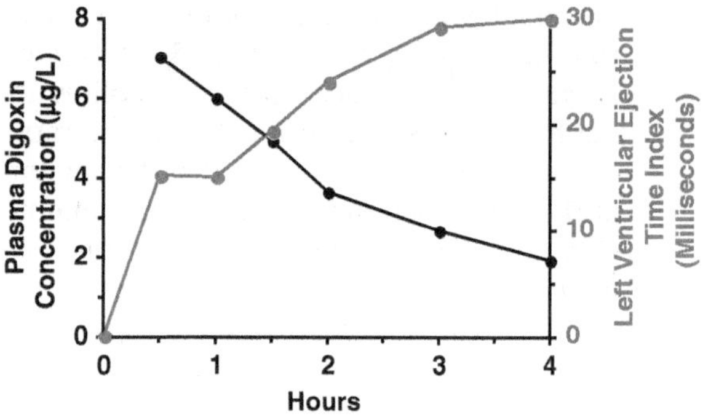

FIGURE 9-1 The prolongation in the left ventricular ejection time index (*colored line*), a measure of cardiac effect, increases as the plasma digoxin concentration (*black line*) declines for 4 hours after IV administration of a 1-mg dose of digoxin. Average data from six normal subjects. (Redrawn from data of Shapiro W, Narahara K, Taubert K. Relationship of plasma digitoxin and digoxin to cardiac response following intravenous digitalization in man. *Circulation* 1970;42:1065–1072. Reproduced by permission of the American Heart Association, Inc.)

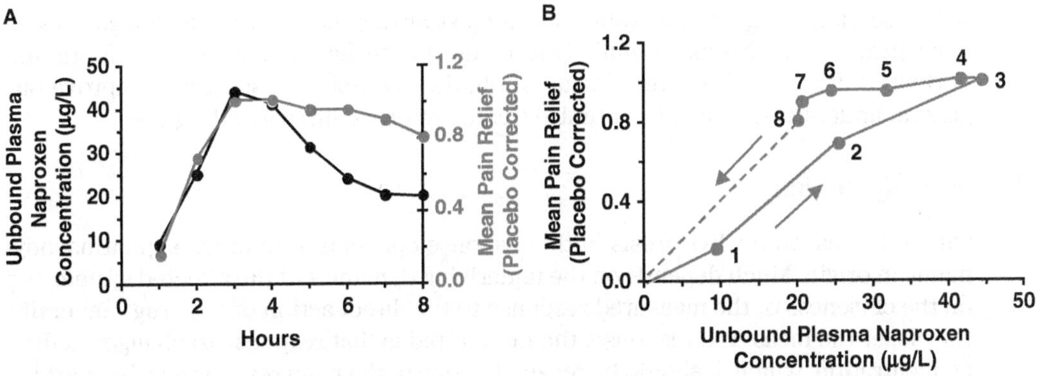

FIGURE 9-2 **A.** Plot of unbound plasma naproxen concentration (*black line*) and of associated mean pain relief (corrected for placebo response, *colored line*) in a dental pain model with time after an oral 500-mg dose of naproxen. **B.** Pain relief clearly shows a hysteresis when plotted directly against the unbound plasma concentration of naproxen, in that different responses are apparent at the same unbound plasma concentration on the rising and declining parts of the plasma concentration–time profile. The time of sampling from 1 to 8 hours is noted next to each point. Notice that the hysteresis is counterclockwise. The extrapolation beyond 8 hours indicates that eventually no benefit is achieved as the plasma naproxen concentration falls toward zero. (Drawn from data kindly provided by Syntex, USA Inc., 1994.)

CAUSES OF TIME DELAY

There are many reasons, both kinetic and dynamic, for a counterclockwise hysteresis. One reason is that, although plasma concentration of the drug is monitored, response may be primarily due to an active metabolite, which takes time to reach its peak concentration. Obviously, in this case, the wrong compound is being monitored. Other reasons include time for distribution to the target site, the occurrence of several events or reactions between the initial interaction with the target and the measured response, and when the drug affects either the production or removal of the target itself or the species being monitored.

Tissue Distribution

With naproxen, as with many drugs, this counterclockwise hysteresis is caused by delayed distribution to the site of action. The therapeutic consequence of such delays depends on the clinical setting. Recall that distribution kinetics depends on tissue perfusion, membrane permeability, and tissue affinity for drug. Many drugs are small lipophilic molecules that equilibrate rapidly across well-perfused tissues, such as the heart and brain, which are often target organs, that is, organs containing the site of action. Under these circumstances, because the period of observation in clinical practice is often hours, if not days, a delay in effect is likely to be minimal and drug in plasma can be correlated directly with effect. This was the case in the study from which the propranolol data in Chapter 3 (Fig. 3-6) were obtained. Propranolol was given orally, and measurements were made over several hours, particularly after the peak plasma concentration had been reached. The previous statements apply even if distribution throughout the body has not been achieved; all that is required is that distribution equilibrium of drug between plasma and target organ be reached.

Emergency admissions and surgical procedures are special settings during which responses are frequently measured in minutes rather than hours. Here, delays in response after drug administration are almost always noticed. Even though plasma concentration monitoring is unlikely to be used in these circumstances, it is still important to delineate the determinants of the time course of response to improve our general understanding and to optimize treatment procedures and drug use.

Pharmacodynamics

Often, the reason for hysteresis in the response-concentration curve is pharmacodynamic in origin. Much depends on the underlying dynamics of the affected system and on the closeness of the measured response to the direct action of the drug. Generally, the closer the measured response, the more rapid is that response to changes in drug concentration, which, it should be recalled, is one of the main reasons why biomarkers are used as early signals of therapeutic outcome. The only drug-specific characteristic is its interaction with the receptor. All steps subsequent to occupation are a property of the affected system within the body and are the same for all drugs acting on this receptor by the same mechanism. The kinetics of this cascade of events varies greatly. Sometimes, relative to the kinetics of the drug, response is virtually instantaneous. In such cases, we have a **pharmacokinetic rate–limited response**, and hysteresis may not be seen except, perhaps, at the very earliest moments after drug administration. An example, previously considered, is the β-blockade produced by propranolol in which response rises and falls in time with plasma concentration. This is essentially the case also with the benzodiazepines, producing central nervous effects, such as sedation, by interacting with its receptor. Their time courses of response, which differ markedly, are determined primarily by their pharmacokinetics, varying from the ultra-short-acting hypnotic midazolam with a half-life of 3 hours to the long-acting hypnotic diazepam, with a half-life in the order of 2 days.

At other times, the kinetics of the cascade of pharmacodynamic events is relatively slow. This is the case with corticosteroids such as prednisolone and methylprednisolone. These drugs interact with a cytosolic receptor within the cell; the complex then migrates to the nucleus and triggers a complex series of events, which ultimately leads to a decrease in synthesis of endogenous cortisol, subsequently expressed as a decrease in the plasma concentration of this steroid hormone. When the pharmacodynamics of the system is slower than the pharmacokinetics of the drug, we then have a **pharmacodynamic rate–limited response.** Then, changes in the pharmacokinetics of the drug will have only a modest or minimal effect on the kinetics of response, unless the pharmacokinetics of the drug for some reason becomes very much slower (as might occur if its elimination is drastically reduced owing to coadministration of a strong inhibitor of its elimination). Some examples and additional reasons for the delay in measured response follow.

As our first example, consider the antipyretic effect on administering ibuprofen to 36 febrile children. The mean fall in rectal temperature is noted in Fig. 9-3A relative to the concentration of drug. The relationship implies that the drug has little effect at early times when the concentration is high and maximal effect when the concentration has dropped to 15 mg/L.

Actually, ibuprofen acts directly in the brain to affect the heat control mechanism, thereby causing decreased heat production. With rapid entry into the brain, the effect of ibuprofen is greatest at early times and has partially worn off by the time the temperature is minimal, reflecting maximal measured response to the drug (Fig. 9-3B). Temperature is an integrated response that measures the cumulative effect of the drug. The rate of change in body heat, reflected by temperature, is then

$$\text{Rate of change in body heat} = \text{Rate of heat production} - \text{Rate of heat loss} \quad \textbf{Eq. 9-1}$$

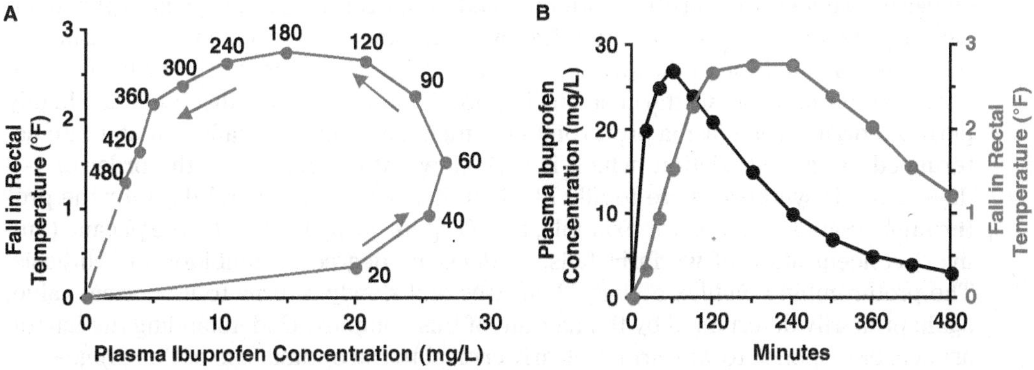

FIGURE 9-3 The fall in rectal temperature (observation minus baseline in degrees Fahrenheit, 1.8°F = 1.0°C) in 36 febrile children from 6 months through 11 years of age after a 6-mg/kg oral dose of ibuprofen. **A.** Relationship between the fall in temperature and plasma ibuprofen concentration. Note the large degree of hysteresis present. The time of sampling (minutes) is indicated next to each point. **B.** Plasma ibuprofen concentration (*black line*) and fall in temperature (*colored line*) as a function of time after dosing. (Redrawn from Kelley MT, Walson PD, Edge JH, et al. Pharmacokinetics and pharmacodynamics of ibuprofen isomers and acetaminophen in febrile children. *Clin Pharmacol Ther* 1992;52:181–189.)

Even if heat production were instantly reduced, time is required for body heat to dissipate and body temperature to fully reflect the reduction. Note that as the concentration of ibuprofen falls, so does its effect, and gradually, the body temperature returns, in this example, toward the preexisting value.

The second example is that of the oral anticoagulant warfarin, used in the treatment of deep vein thrombosis. The response to warfarin is monitored clinically by prolongation in the clotting time of blood, a function of the prothrombin complex activity in plasma. This complex is continuously being formed and degraded. Fig. 9-4 shows a

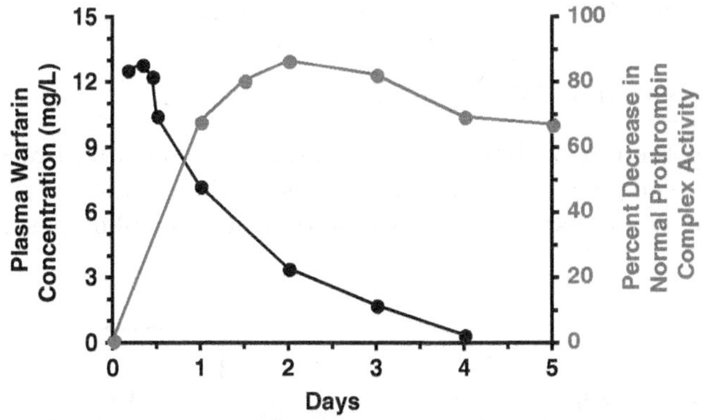

FIGURE 9-4 The sluggish response in the plasma prothrombin complex activity (*colored line*) to inhibition of its synthesis in the liver by warfarin reflects the indirect nature of the measurement and the slow elimination of this complex. For the first 2 days after giving a single oral 1.5-mg/kg dose of sodium warfarin, response (defined as the percent decrease in the normal complex activity) steadily decreases. During the first day, at this dose, the concentration of warfarin is sufficient to almost completely block complex synthesis. As warfarin concentration (*black line*) falls, the synthesis rate of the complex increases, and by 48 hours equals the rate of degradation of the complex; the measured response is then at a maximum. Thereafter, as the plasma concentration falls further, with the synthesis rate exceeding the rate of degradation, the response falls. Eventually, when all the warfarin has been eliminated, the plasma prothrombin complex activity concentration returns—sluggishly—to the normal baseline value. The data points are the averages of 5 male volunteers. (From Nagashima R, O'Reilly RA, Levy G. Kinetics of pharmacologic effects in man: the anticoagulant action of warfarin. *Clin Pharmacol Ther* 1969;10:22–35.)

sluggish response–time profile, with the maximum occurring 1–2 days after the much earlier peak warfarin concentration following an oral dose of warfarin. Warfarin's direct effect is inhibition of the synthesis of the prothrombin complex in the liver, which occurs very rapidly as warfarin, a small lipophilic molecule, readily enters this highly perfused organ. The plasma prothrombin complex activity then falls, but at a rate determined by its degradation, which is very slow with a half-life on the order of 1–3 days. Even if synthesis were totally blocked, it would take several days for the prothrombin complex to fall, for example, to 25% of its normal value. As the plasma (and liver) concentration of warfarin falls, so does the degree of inhibition of synthesis. The prothrombin complex activity then rises and slowly returns to its normal value, again primarily determined by the half-life of this complex. Understanding the kinetic aspects of response to warfarin is clearly critical to the optimal use of this drug.

Generalizing, the level of many substances or measured quantities in the body depends on the difference between rates of input and loss, or formation and elimination, as depicted in Fig. 9-5 and expressed in Equation 9-2.

$$\text{Rate of change in body} = \text{Rate of input} - \text{Rate of loss} \qquad \text{Eq. 9-2}$$

Normally, input and loss are balanced so that the level of the substance or measured quantity remains relatively stable with time, thereby ensuring an internal homeostasis. In addition to body heat, and prothrombin complex, other examples are body water content, white and red cell counts, and the concentrations of many proteins, such as albumin, and other endogenous compounds, including hormones, enzymes, and serum electrolytes. Drugs act directly by either increasing or decreasing the rates of input or output, thereby changing the level of the quantity being measured. Normally, the effect is a graded response, which can be adequately characterized by Equation 3-2, Chapter 3.

The delay between attainment of a peak plasma drug concentration and maximal measured response varies widely. Full response in blood pressure to a change in peripheral resistance or in cardiac output occurs within minutes, whereas the maximal response of the prothrombin complex activity to warfarin, as shown in Fig. 9-4, is not seen for 1–2 days after a single oral dose of this anticoagulant.

DECLINE OF RESPONSE WITH TIME

After peaking, the response to a drug declines with time after oral administration of a single dose. The most common reason is the decline in the exposure to the drug at the target site. When response is rate-limited by pharmacokinetics, response declines

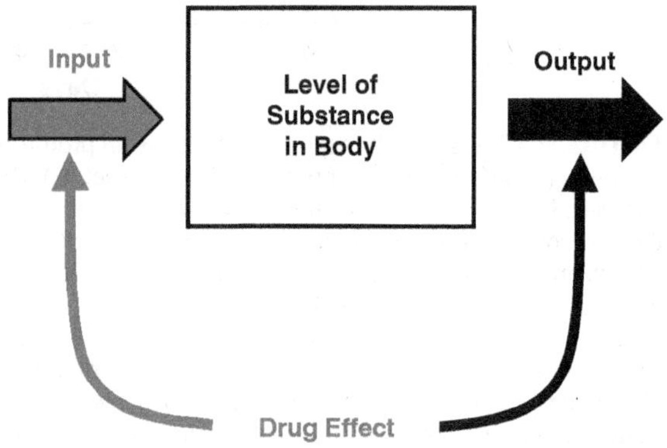

FIGURE 9-5 The level of many systems and endogenous compounds in the body is normally relatively constant, reflecting the balance between the rates of input and output. A drug may act directly to increase or decrease either input or output, thereby perturbing the level. Measurement of the level of the substance in plasma reflects the state of that system at any point in time. The time scale of response can vary from minutes to months; it is often determined by the output rate constant of the monitored system or endogenous compound.

with plasma drug concentration. Sometimes, however, the response falls more slowly than the plasma drug concentration, a pharmacodynamic rate limitation. Each of these situations is now considered.

When Response Changes in Line With Plasma Concentration: A Pharmacokinetic Rate Limitation

How the intensity of response varies with time depends, as does the duration of effect, on dose and on rate of drug removal from the site of action. It also depends on the region of the concentration–response curve covered during the decline. Here, discussion is limited to the situation in which the concentration–response relationship is maintained at all times and drug distributes rapidly to and from the site of action.

To appreciate the relationships among dose, intensity of response, and time, consider the events depicted in Fig. 9-6A, which follow the intravenous administration of a 10-mg bolus dose of a drug with a half-life of 1 hour. A plot of intensity of response against logarithm of the plasma concentration is shown in Fig. 9-6B.

For didactic purposes, the plot is divided into three regions. In **Region 1,** up to 20% maximal response, intensity of response is directly proportional to the plasma concentration; in **Region 2,** covering 20%–80% of maximal response, intensity is proportional to the logarithm of concentration; and in **Region 3,** response gradually approaches the maximal value despite large changes in concentration. Because the initial concentration lies in Region 3, and despite a rapid fall in concentration in the first hour, intensity of response remains almost constant and maximal. Only after 3 hours, when concentration falls below 2 mg/L and response falls below 80% of the maximal value, does response begin to decline more rapidly. Then, for the next 5 hours, on passing through Region 2, *response declines almost linearly with time.* Beyond 8 hours, when the concentration falls below 0.1 mg/L and enters Region 1, the fall in response parallels that of drug.

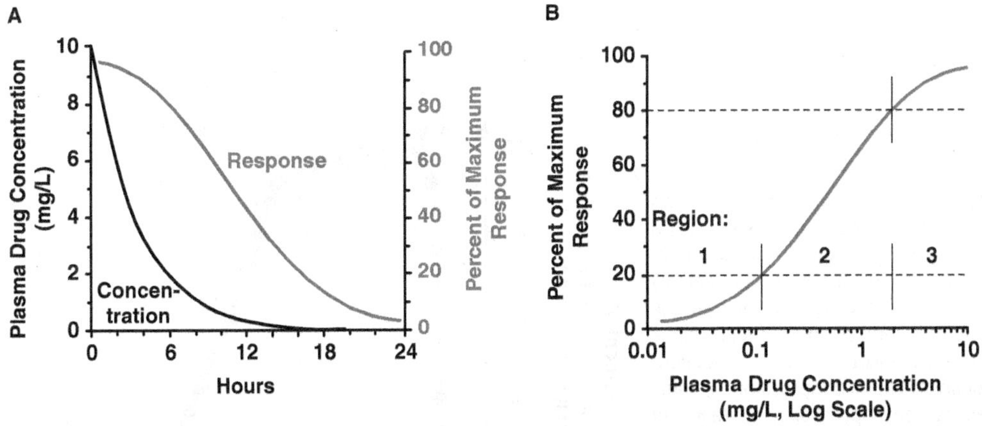

FIGURE 9-6 The decline in the intensity of pharmacologic effect with time (*colored line,* **A**) after a single large intravenous bolus dose of a drug displaying monoexponential decline (*black line,* graph **A**) depends on the region of the concentration–response curve (**B**). Initially, in Region 3, the response remains almost maximal despite a 75% fall in concentration. Thereafter, as long as the concentration is within Region 2, intensity of response declines approximately linearly with time. Only when concentration falls into Region 1 does decline in response parallel that of drug in plasma. The concentration–response relationship is defined by: $E = E_{max} \cdot C^{\gamma}/(C_{50}^{\gamma} + C^{\gamma})$ with $E_{max} = 100\%$, $C_{50} = 0.5$ μg/L, and $\gamma = 1$.

The reason for the essentially constant rate of decline in response in Region 2 (Fig. 9-6A, between 80% and 20% of maximum response), while the plasma concentration declines exponentially, is apparent in Fig. 9-6B. In this region.

$$\text{Response} = m \cdot \ln C + b \qquad \text{Eq. 9-3}$$

where m and b are the slope and intercept of the relationship. Substituting $\ln C(80\%) - k \cdot t$ for $\ln C$ in Eq. 9-3, where $C(80\%)$ is the concentration upon entering Region 2 from Region 3, t is the time since entering the region, and k is the elimination rate constant of the drug. Collecting terms therefore yields:

$$\text{Response} = (m \cdot \ln C(80\%) + b) - m \cdot k \cdot t \qquad \text{Eq. 9-4}$$

Letting $E(80\%)$ be the intensity of response $(m \cdot \ln C(80\%) + b)$ when the concentration is $C(80\%)$, gives

$$\text{Response} = E(80\%) - m \cdot k \cdot t \qquad \text{Eq. 9-5}$$

Note, in this simple scheme, that the rate of decline, $m \cdot k$, depends on both slope of the intensity versus ln concentration relationship and the half-life of the drug.

These concepts are now illustrated with degree of muscle paralysis produced by the neuromuscular blocking agent succinylcholine. Changes in degree of muscle paralysis with time, following a 0.5-mg/kg bolus dose of succinylcholine to a patient, are shown in Fig. 9-7. The 1-minute delay before onset of effect is probably accounted for by the time required for blood to circulate from injection site to muscle and, in part, by the time for succinylcholine to diffuse into the neuromuscular junction. Once at the site, however, full response ensues promptly. Total paralysis is then maintained for a full 2 minutes despite the continual rapid inactivation, by hydrolysis, of this agent (elimination half-life = 3.5 minutes). Subsequently, the effect subsides. As predicted, between 80% and 20% of maximal response, the effect declines at a constant rate—in this instance, 22% per minute. The reason for this very rapid decline in response is a combination of its short half-life of elimination and a steep concentration–response curve. Changes in muscle paralysis can therefore be produced within a few minutes

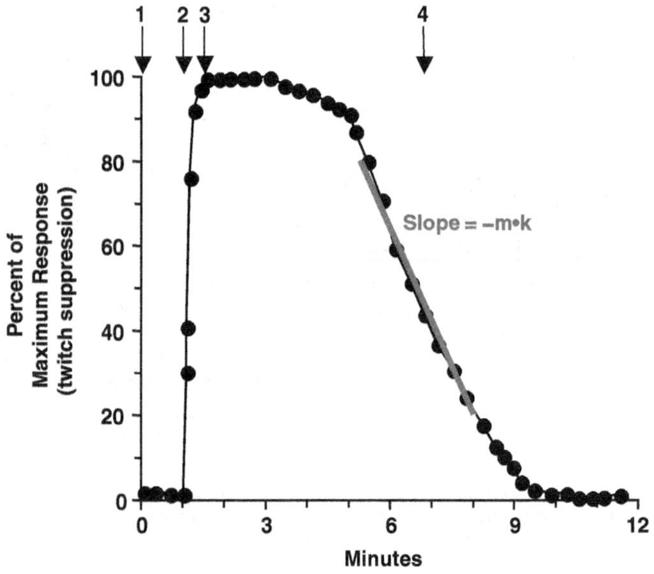

FIGURE 9-7 Changes in the degree of muscle paralysis (assessed as the suppression of a twitch produced in response to ulnar nerve stimulation) with time following an intravenous bolus dose of 0.5 mg/kg succinylcholine to a subject. *1,* Time of injection; *2,* onset of twitch suppression; *3,* complete twitch suppression; *4,* recovery of twitch to 50% (T_{50}) of the maximum twitch height. Note that response declines essentially linearly with time between 20% and 80% of maximum effect (*declining colored line*). (Modified from Walts LF, Dillon JB. Clinical studies on succinylcholine chloride. *Anesthesiology* 1967;28:372–376.)

of changing administration, and once administration is stopped, the patient promptly recovers, both desirable characteristics.

When Response Changes More Slowly Than Plasma Concentration: A Pharmacodynamic Rate Limitation

We have seen that response does not track plasma concentration and stays essentially constant and maximal so long as the concentration remains in Region 3 of the concentration–response curve. However, there are other situations in which response declines more slowly than plasma concentration for pharmacodynamic reasons. One such situation arises when a drug consumes the target receptor or enzyme, which then has to be resynthesized, thus taking time. This explains one action of aspirin. In addition to its long use as an analgesic and anti-inflammatory agent, in more recent years, it has gained widespread use as a prophylactic to reduce the chances of the occurrence of thromboembolic complications, such as recurring myocardial infarction, by inhibiting platelet aggregation. Recall from Chapter 5 that, with a half-life of only 15 minutes, almost the entire ingested dose of aspirin (acetylsalicylic acid) has been eliminated within 2 hours of ingestion (see Fig. 9-8A). Elimination of this ester occurs almost entirely by hydrolysis to form salicylic acid. This metabolite is devoid of antiplatelet activity, yet antiplatelet activity remains for many days. Aspirin affects platelet aggregation by rapidly and irreversibly inhibiting, by acetylation, prostaglandin cyclo-oxygenase. This effect lasts for the lifetime of the platelet and prevents the formation of thromboxane B_2, which, when platelet cells are fractured, promotes platelet adhesion and subsequent clot formation. Thromboxane B_2, and hence platelet adhesion activity, returns to normal only with the production of new platelets, a very slow process with activity not fully restored for at least a week after a single 650-mg dose of aspirin (Fig. 9-8B).

A similar situation is seen with omeprazole, but the explanation is somewhat more complicated. Omeprazole, an inhibitor of the proton pump within the acid-secreting parietal cells of the stomach, is used in the treatment of heartburn and gastric

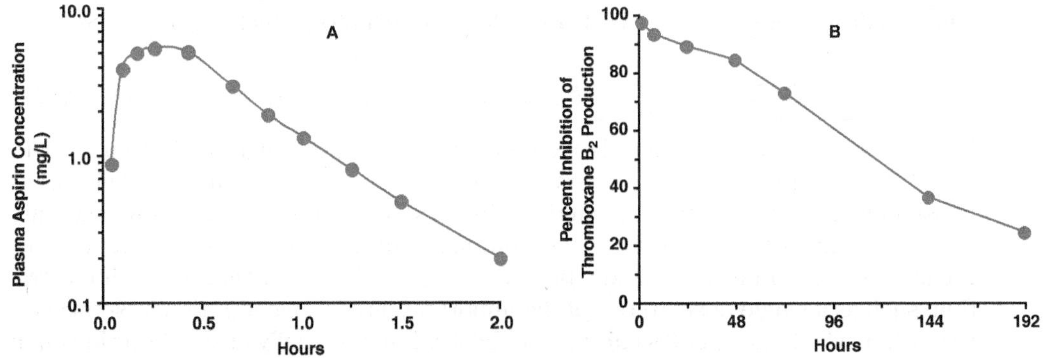

FIGURE 9-8 A. Upon oral administration of 650 mg, aspirin is both rapidly absorbed and eliminated from the body owing to rapid hydrolysis, such that little remains after 2 hours. **B.** Despite this, its effect as an inhibitor of platelet thromboxane B_2 persists for many days, owing to aspirin covalently binding and inactivating cyclooxygenase, which prevents the formation of thromboxane B_2, which then has to be resynthesized, a slow process. Note the almost 100-fold difference in the time scales. (Adapted from Ali M, MacDonald JW, Thiessen JJ, et al. Plasma acetylsalicylate and salicylate and platelet cyclooxygenase activity following plain and enteric coated aspirin. *Stroke* 1980;11:9–13).

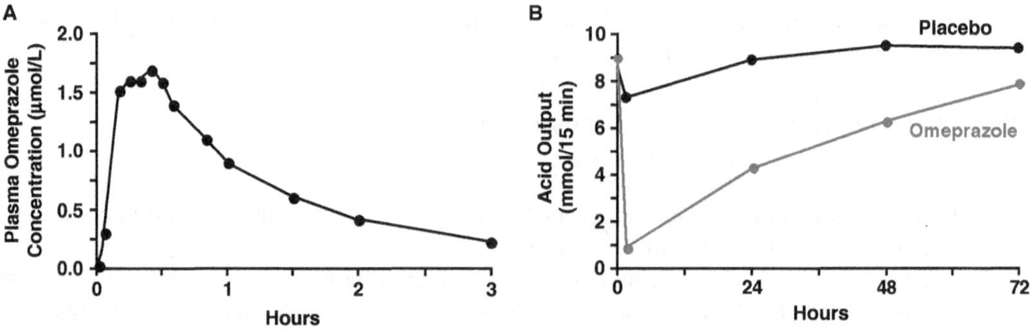

FIGURE 9-9 Despite being very rapidly metabolized within the body, such that little remains in plasma after 3 hours following a 40-mg oral dose of omeprazole (**A**), the inhibition of gastric acid secretion (*colored line*) continues for several days (**B**). Also shown is the response after a placebo dose (*black line*). The response (expressed as a decrease in acid output over 15 minutes following a 1-hour infusion of intravenous pentagastrin, which maximally induces gastric acid secretion) was assessed before administration of drug or placebo at 2 hours postadministration, and again at 1, 2, and 3 days. This slow restoration of gastric acid secretion after omeprazole administration is due to a combination of very slow dissociation of tightly bound omeprazole-derived compounds to the proton pump receptor within the parietal cells of the stomach, together with the covalent binding and inactivating by omeprazole of this receptor, requiring synthesis of new receptor, which takes time. (A composite figure taken from data provided in Lind T, Cederberg C, Ekenved G, et al. Effect of omeprazole-a gastric proton pump inhibitor on the pentagastrin simulated secretion in man. *Gut* 1983;24:270–276.)

and duodenal ulcers. This widely prescribed drug is rapidly absorbed, reaching a peak plasma concentration within 1 hour of oral dosing, and rapidly eliminated, largely by conversion to inactive metabolites, with a half-life of just under 1 hour. Gastric acid production promptly falls, but the return to baseline is very slow, over days (Fig. 9-9). Like aspirin, omeprazole covalently binds and inactivates its receptor—in this case the proton pump—which takes time to be resynthesized. However, this fails to explain completely the observed temporal pattern of gastric acid secretion. It appears that part of the explanation lies in the extremely tight affinity of locally formed omeprazole-derived compounds for the proton pump, with a very slow dissociation of the formed drug–receptor complex. In this situation, the plasma concentration rapidly falls below the limit of measurement, giving the impression that response persists when no drug is present in the body including the receptor, which is not the case.

REVEALING THE DIRECT CONCENTRATION–RESPONSE RELATIONSHIP

Single-dose administration is relatively uncommon in drug therapy. In Chapters 11 and 12, we discuss the more common situation of chronic therapy, achieved via either constant-rate administration or multiple dosing. Often, the objective is to maintain response by maintaining plasma concentrations relatively constant. In such situations, it can be useful to unravel the kinetics of response following acute drug administration, such as a single dose, to reveal the important direct concentration–response relationship, which then guides chronic administration, especially in situations in which the relationship does not vary on chronic drug administration. The approach taken depends on the reason for the delay in response with time after giving drug. Two common situations are considered.

When a delay in achieving a response is due to slow distribution to the active site, a pharmacodynamic model with an **effect compartment** linked to the plasma concentration has been used, as depicted in Fig. 9-10, to reveal the direct

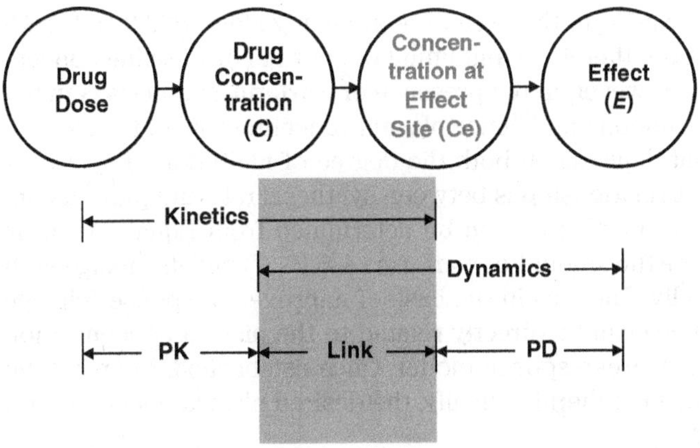

FIGURE 9-10 The concept of an effect compartment linking plasma concentration (PK) with response (PD) helps to accommodate the frequently observed delay in time between plasma concentration and response. The delay is due to the time needed to distribute into the site of action. By accommodating for and thus effectively removing this delay, it is possible to reveal the underlying direct relation between effect site concentration (Ce) and response.

concentration–response relationship. The time course of the delay can vary from minutes to hours. This procedure has been applied to naproxen, which was previously shown to exhibit hysteresis (Fig. 9-2). This hysteresis disappears when an effect compartment is added, exposing the direct relationship between response and concentration in the effect compartment (Fig. 9-11), which can be adequately summarized by the exposure–response model of Equation 3-2.

In situations in which the drug affects either the production or loss of a body constituent, the approach taken is different. To illustrate the approach, consider the case of warfarin, which, as mentioned, lowers the concentration of the prothrombin complex by inhibiting its synthesis. In common with other endogenous substances, the amount of each clotting factor in the complex, A, is a result of a difference between its rates of synthesis, R_{syn}, and degradation. Often, as in this case, degradation is a first-order process, with the rate of degradation given by $k_t \cdot A$, where k_t is the degradation-rate constant of the clotting factor. Thus, at any moment,

$$\underset{\text{Rate of change of clotting factor}}{\frac{dA}{dt}} = \underset{\text{Rate of synthesis}}{R_{syn}} - \underset{\text{Rate of degradation}}{k_t \cdot A} \qquad \text{Eq. 9-6}$$

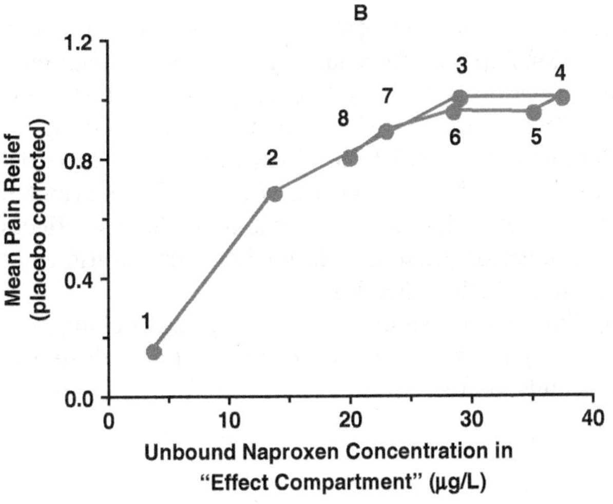

FIGURE 9-11 Mean pain relief (corrected for placebo response) in a dental pain model plotted as a function of the unbound plasma concentration of naproxen within the effect compartment following an oral 500-mg dose. Notice that when an effect compartment is used, the counterclockwise hysteresis, seen when pain relief is plotted against unbound plasma concentration of naproxen (Fig. 9-2B), disappears. The response can now be related to the effect site concentration at all times. The time of sampling from 1 to 8 hours is noted next to each point. (Drawn from data kindly provided by Syntex, USA Inc., 1994.)

Normally, in the absence of warfarin, the system is at steady state, $dA/dt = 0$, with synthesis matching degradation, thereby maintaining the normal or baseline concentration of the clotting factor. However, in the presence of warfarin, synthesis is inhibited without affecting k_t. The amount, and hence plasma concentration, of the clotting factor then falls at a rate that depends on both the degree of inhibition of synthesis by warfarin and k_t. The direct relationship is between synthesis rate and plasma concentration of warfarin. The synthesis rate can be determined from Equation 9-6 by knowing or estimating k_t, since the amount of warfarin ($A = V \cdot C$) and its change with time are known experimentally. Then, as in the case of naproxen, response (change in synthesis rate from baseline) can be directly related to the plasma concentration of warfarin by a suitable exposure–response model. Once established, knowing the reduction in synthesis rate needed therapeutically, the desired plasma concentration of warfarin can be predicted.

The response by patients to a drug may change when, for example, other drugs are coadministered. Then it is helpful to know whether this is caused solely by a change in its pharmacokinetics, pharmacodynamics, or both. Analyzing data along the lines discussed above to provide the direct concentration–response relationship helps to clarify the situation.

ONSET AND DURATION OF RESPONSE

Onset of Effect

After a single dose, an effect can be said to begin when the concentration at the site of action reaches a critical value. The time of onset of effect is governed by many factors including route of administration, absorption, distribution to target site, and other time delays of pharmacodynamic origin, as discussed previously in this chapter and elsewhere in the book. Additional factors affecting time of onset are dose and the exposure–response relationship, that is, whether response is pharmacokinetically or pharmacodynamically rate limited.

Increasing the dose usually shortens the time of onset of effect by shortening the time required to achieve the critical concentration at the site of action.

Duration of Effect

For a drug with no delays in response, relative to drug at the site of action, and showing a fixed exposure–response relationship, an effect lasts as long as the minimum effective concentration at the site of action is exceeded. After an intravenous bolus dose, the duration of effect is therefore a function of both dose and rate of drug removal from the site of action. Removal can result from either elimination or redistribution from the site to more slowly equilibrating tissues. When a drug distributes rapidly to all tissues, including the site of action, and response immediately reflects the concentration of drug at the site of action, then the relation between duration and kinetics is readily conceived following a single bolus dose.

Consider, for example, a drug that distributes into a volume V, and is eliminated by first-order kinetics, characterized by the rate constant k. After a bolus dose, the plasma concentration falls exponentially, that is,

$$C = \frac{\text{Dose}}{V} e^{-k \cdot t} \qquad \text{Eq. 9-7}$$

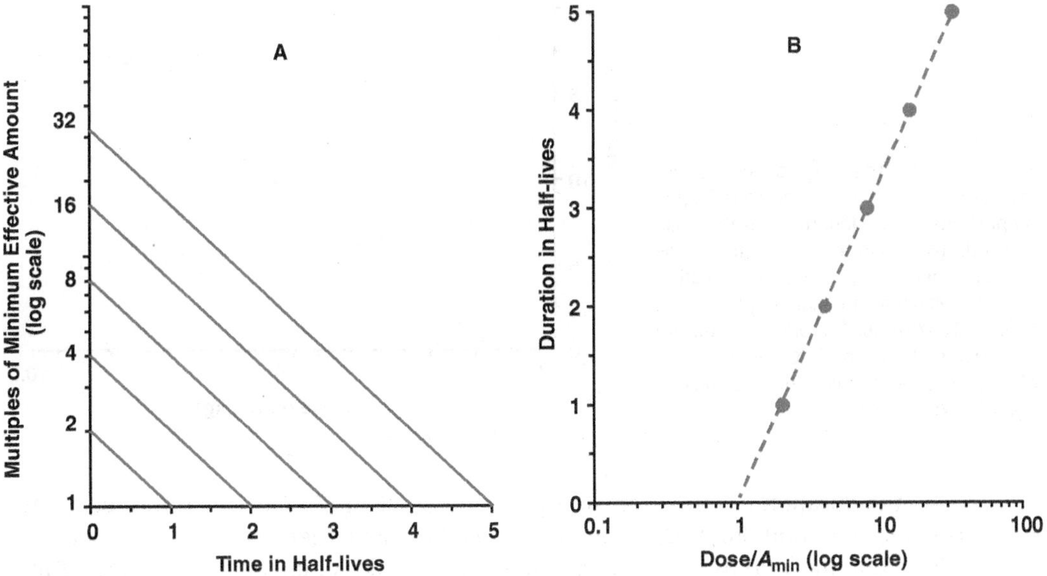

FIGURE 9-12 **A.** The duration of effect increases by one half-life with each doubling of the dose. **B.** Duration is also proportional to the logarithm of the dose. Note in these figures that time is expressed in multiples of half-life, and dose is expressed in multiples of the minimum amount of drug needed to produce the desired effect, A_{min}.

Eventually, a time is reached, the duration of effect (t_D), when the plasma concentration falls to a value (C_{min}) below which the response is less than that minimally desired (Fig. 9-12). The relationship between C_{min} and t_D is given by appropriately substituting into the preceding equation; thus:

$$C_{min} = \frac{\text{Dose}}{V} e^{-k \cdot t_D} \quad \text{Eq. 9-8}$$

Upon rearrangement and taking logarithms, an expression for t_D is obtained,

$$t_D = \frac{1}{k} \ln\left(\frac{\text{Dose}}{C_{min} \cdot V}\right) \quad \text{Eq. 9-9}$$

where $C_{min} \cdot V$ is the minimum amount needed in the body, A_{min}. According to Equation 9-9, a plot of duration of effect against the logarithm of dose should yield a straight line with a slope of $1/k$ and an intercept, at zero duration of effect, of $\ln A_{min}$ (Fig. 9-12B). For example, the duration of effect of many local anesthetics is proportional to the logarithm of the injected dose. The muscle relaxant effect of succinylcholine also conforms to this last equation. Fig. 9-13 shows the times to 50% (T_{50}) recovery of muscle twitch (a measure of neuromuscular block after stimulation of a nerve) following intravenous injections of 0.5-, 1-, 2-, and 4-mg/kg bolus doses of succinylcholine. The value of k, estimated from the slope, is 0.2 /min; the half-life is about 4 minutes, as mentioned previously.

To further appreciate the last equation, consider the following statement: "Duration of effect increases by one half-life with each doubling of dose." This must be true. To prove that it is, let a given dose D_O produce a duration of effect, t_D. When twice the dose ($2 \cdot D_O$) is given, the amount in the body falls by one-half in one half-life, that is,

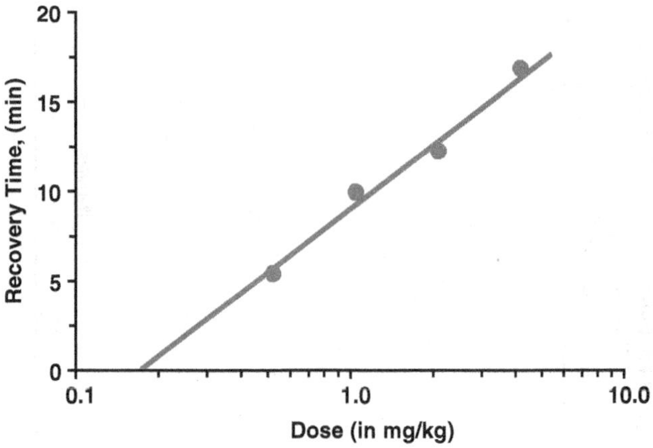

FIGURE 9-13 The time to 50% recovery from succinylcholine paralysis (T_{50}) is proportional to the logarithm of the dose injected. (Redrawn from the figure by Levy G. Kinetics of pharmacologic action of succinylcholine in man. *J Pharm Sci* 1967;56:1687–1688. The original data are from Walts LF, Dillon JB. Clinical studies of succinylcholine chloride. *Anesthesiology* 1967;28:372–376.)

to D_O; the duration of effect remaining beyond one half-life must therefore be t_D. Accordingly, the total duration of effect produced by the larger dose is $t_{1/2} + t_D$. Hence, it follows that the increase in the duration of effect on doubling the dose is one half-life. For example, as 0.5 mg/kg of succinylcholine results in a T_{50} of approximately 6 minutes, the duration of effect following 1 mg/kg is 10 minutes (Fig. 9-13). The increase in the time to recover, 4 minutes, is the half-life of succinylcholine at the site of action. By inspecting the T_{50} curve in Fig. 9-13, it is apparent that the increase in duration (Δt_D) is the same with each further doubling of the dose.

In the case of succinylcholine, the half-life estimated from the dose–duration of action relationship is the elimination half-life of the drug. For some other drugs such as omeprazole, it is the loss of drug from the site of action. To cover these and other situations, the half-life so estimated from pharmacologic data is sometimes referred to as the **effective half-life** of the drug.

Raising dose to extend duration of effect is not without risks, however, especially for a drug with a short half-life and a narrow window of therapeutic concentrations. For example, to extend the duration of effect by two half-lives, the quadrupled dose required may produce too great an initial response or may substantially increase the chance of toxicity. An alternative and safer approach may well be to slow the input of drug, creating a flatter exposure–time profile. The plasma concentration then remains above the C_{min} for an extended time, and the peak concentration is reduced (see Fig. 7-5), both aims of some modified release dosage forms (see Chapter 12). Extending the duration of effect is also, and mainly, achieved by chronically inputting drug into the body by means of constant-rate release systems or multiple dosing, topics of much of the next section: Therapeutic Regimens.

SUMMARY

- Time delays between plasma concentration and response are evident when hysteresis is seen on plotting response directly against plasma concentration after extravascular administration.
- Time delays in the response vs. plasma concentration relationship may be due to slow distribution of drug to the site of action, a pharmacokinetic consideration, or to sluggishness of the response following direct action of drug at the target site, a pharmacodynamic consideration.

- A pharmacodynamic rate limitation in response arises when the dynamics of response is slower than the pharmacokinetics of the drug.
- A common situation in which pharmacodynamics rate-limits the change in measured response is one in which drug acts directly on either input or output of an endogenous system that turns over slowly and the measured response reflects the state of that system at any point in time.
- Often the intensity of a graded response declines linearly with time between 80% and 20% of the maximum response.
- Sometimes, response declines more slowly than plasma concentration owing to drug remaining in Region 3 of the concentration–response relationship, to slow dissociation of drug from its receptor, or to irreversible interaction with its receptor, which then has to be resynthesized.
- The underlying direct relationship between response and drug concentration can be revealed, given response with time observations after a single dose of drug, when the reason for time delay in response is known.
- The duration of response increases by one terminal half-life for each doubling of a dose of a drug. This is true whether a bolus iv dose or a dose of a modified release dosage form (when terminal decline is governed by half-life of drug release) is administered.
- The duration of a graded response is often proportional to the logarithm of the dose. Duration may be extended for a given dose by prolonging the input of drug into the body.

KEY TERM REVIEW

Decline of response with time
Direct response
Duration of response
Effect compartment
Effective half-life
Hysteresis
Intensity of response
Onset of effect
Pharmacodynamic rate–limited response
Pharmacokinetic rate–limited response
Pharmacokinetic–pharmacodynamic modeling
Target organ
Time delay

KEY RELATIONSHIPS

$$\text{Rate of change in body} = \text{Rate of input} - \text{Rate of loss}$$

$$t_D = \frac{1}{k}\ln\left(\frac{\text{Dose}}{C_{min} \cdot V}\right)$$

STUDY PROBLEMS

1. Which of the following statements is (are) correct?
   I. After the concentration reaches a peak, the response to a drug declines with time after administration of a single extravascular dose. The most common reason for the decline is a decrease in exposure to the drug at the target site.
   II. When response changes in line with plasma concentration in the terminal phase, pharmacokinetics is the rate-limiting step. Although the actual rate of

decline in the response depends on where the concentrations are with respect to C_{50}, it is particularly slow when the peak concentration greatly exceeds C_{50}.

III. If the plasma concentration of a drug after an intravenous bolus declines by a first-order process with a half-life of 2 hours, yet the measured response has decreased by only 50% 7 days later, the decline of the response must be pharmacokinetically rate-limited.

A. I only **E.** I and III
B. II only **F.** II and III
C. III only **G.** All
D. I and II **H.** None

2. Which *one* of the following statements is the *most* accurate?
   a. When the response to a drug is delayed with respect to its systemic exposure, a plot of the response as a function of the plasma concentration after an oral dose produces a clockwise hysteresis loop.
   b. The response to a drug is positively and directly proportional to the concentration of a key body constituent. The response to the drug should therefore increase with either an increase in the production rate or a hastening of the loss of the key body constituent.
   c. When a delay in achieving a response is due to slow distribution to the active site, a pharmacodynamic model with an effect compartment linked to the plasma concentration can be useful.
   d. For a drug that shows first-order kinetics and for which its response is predicted at all times by its systemic exposure, the duration of its response above some minimum value is expected to increase by 50% for every doubling of an intravenous dose.
3. Which of the following statements is (are) correct?

I. Hysteresis in a response-versus-plasma concentration curve cannot be observed after intravenous bolus administration of the drug.

II. Between 80% and 20% of maximum effect, a graded response is expected to decline exponentially with time after intravenous administration of a single bolus dose.

III. For a drug showing first-order disposition kinetics and producing a graded response, the duration of its response increases linearly with dose.

A. I only **E.** I and III
B. II only **F.** II and III
C. III only **G.** All
D. I and II **H.** None

4. Fig. 9-14 shows the degree of lowering of the mean arterial pressure (MAP) produced by minoxidil in a hypertensive patient with a baseline MAP of 157 mm Hg.

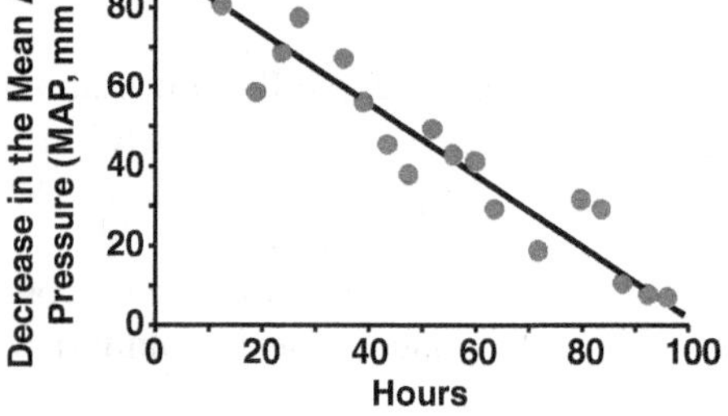

FIGURE 9-14 The degree of lowering of the mean arterial blood pressure (MAP), in a patient with a baseline MAP of 157 mm Hg, falls at a constant rate following a single oral 25-mg dose of minoxidil. (From Shen, D, O'Malley, K, Gibaldi, M, McNay, JL. Pharmacodynamics of minoxidil as a guide to individualizing dosage regimens in hypertension. *Clin Pharmacol Ther* 1975;17:593–598.)

The effect appears to decline linearly with time after a single 25-mg dose of the drug. The plasma minoxidil concentration following this dose peaked at 1 hour and then declined with a half-life of 4.2 hours, so that almost no drug remained at 20 hours. Using the line as the response-time function, which of the following statements is (are) consistent with, and would explain, these observations?

I. A metabolite with a longer half-life is responsible for the hypotensive action of the drug.
II. The response to the drug is pharmacodynamically rate-limited.
III. Administration of the drug once daily should be adequate to maintain its hypotensive action.

A. I only
B. II only
C. III only
D. I and II
E. I and III
F. II and III
G. All
H. None

5. Fig. 9-15 shows the relationship between reduction in systolic blood pressure and plasma drug concentration for a drug under steady-state conditions. The line shown is the best fit of the parameters of the graded response model below to the data in an individual subject.

$$\text{Reduction in systolic blood Pressure, mm Hg} = \frac{E_{max} \cdot C^{\gamma}}{C_{50}^{\gamma} + C^{\gamma}}$$

a. Estimate the values for E_{max}, C_{50}, and γ.
b. Given that the half-life of the drug (which exhibits one-compartment characteristics) is 6 hours, estimate the time after a single dose for the response (reduction in blood pressure) to drop from the initial value of 25 mm of Hg to a value of 5 mm of Hg.
c. Would you expect the response (reduction in blood pressure) to decline exponentially or linearly during the time frame given in Part B? Show how you come to your conclusion.

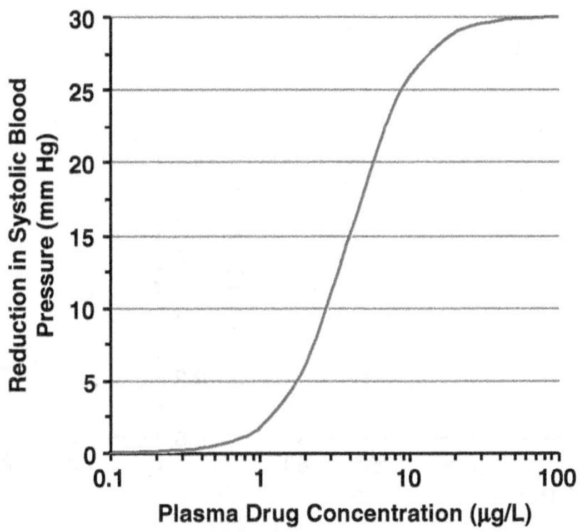

FIGURE 9-15

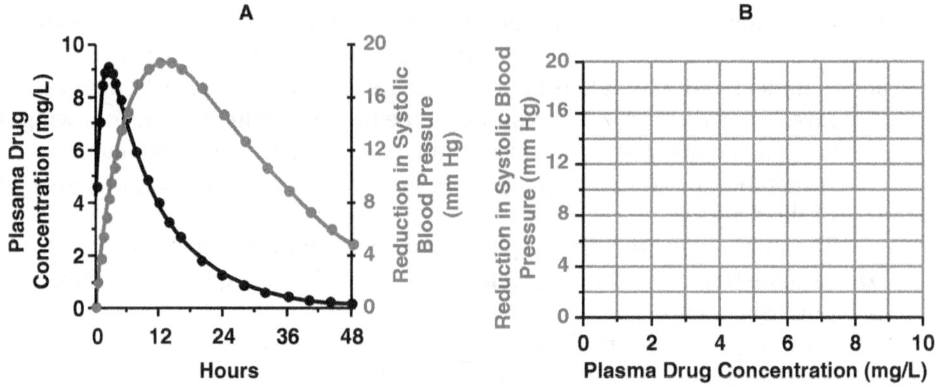

FIGURE 9-16 **A.** Plasma drug concentration (*black*) and reduction in systolic blood pressure (*color*) with time after a single oral dose. **B.** Reduction in systolic blood pressure as a function of the plasma drug concentration.

6. The following observations displayed in Fig. 9-16A were made for a drug. Clearly, the blood pressure–lowering effect (color) and the plasma concentration–time profile (black) do not match.
   a. Draw on Fig. 9-16B the relationship you anticipate between effect and the plasma concentration. Be sure to identify whether the hysteresis is clockwise or counterclockwise.
   b. Give two possible explanations (mechanisms) for the observations in Fig. 9-16.
7. a. Give two examples of a situation in which changes in response with time are rate-limited by the kinetics of a drug, and two examples that are rate-limited by the dynamics of an affected system.
   b. A common and clinically significant toxicity of many anticancer drugs is leukopenia, an abnormal fall in the number of leukocytes in blood. Leukocytes are important in the immunologic defense of the body. Most focus clinically is on the lowest leukocyte count after chemotherapy treatment, but the time course of the fall in count is also important. Shown in Fig. 9-17 are the plasma

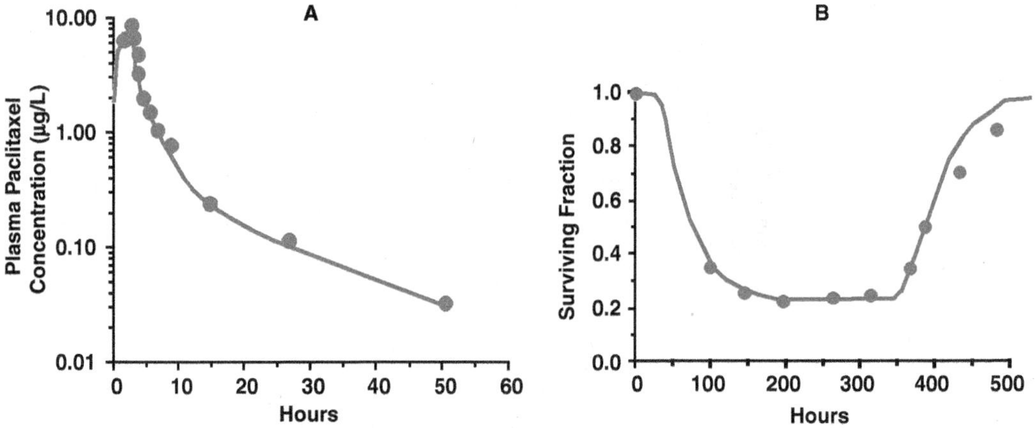

FIGURE 9-17 Plasma paclitaxel concentration-time profile **(A)** and the fraction of leukocytes in blood (relative to baseline) with time **(B)** in a patient receiving an intravenous dose of paclitaxel. The continuous lines are the best line fits of respective models to the data. (From Minami H, Sasaki Y, Saijo N et al. Indirect-response model for the time course of leukopenia with anticancer drugs. *Clin Pharmacol Ther* 1998;64:511–521.)

concentration–time course of one anticancer compound, paclitaxel (A), and the corresponding time profile of leukocyte count (B) in a patient after a single administration of the drug.

Knowing that paclitaxel inhibits the production of leukocytes, discuss the disparity between the relatively rapid elimination of the drug and the sluggish changes in the percentage of leukocytes surviving in blood in the patient, only returning to the baseline value 3 weeks after drug administration.

8. Propranolol, a β-adrenergic blocking agent, is used in the treatment of hypertension and angina. One rapid test of its activity is its ability to decrease the heart rate for a given workload, that is, reduce exercise tachycardia. DG McDevitt and DG Shand (*Clin Pharmacol Ther* 1975;18:708–715) observed a linear relationship between percent reduction in exercise tachycardia and the logarithm of plasma concentration of propranolol. The slope of the line is +11.5%. The table below lists the effect with time after intravenous bolus administration of 20-mg propranolol. These data are also plotted in Fig. 9-18.

Time (hr)	0.25	1	2	4	6
Reduction in exercise tachycardia (%)	28	25.5	22	15	8

a. Why does the response decline linearly with time? Furthermore, satisfy yourself that the slope of the relationship is $-m \cdot k$, where k is the elimination rate constant of the drug. HINT: What are the expected relationships between plasma concentration and time, and between response and plasma concentration?

b. From the plot of the data in Fig. 9-18, estimate the slope of the response with time and hence the apparent half-life of propranolol in plasma.

c. Calculate the minimum amount of propranolol needed in the body to achieve a 15% reduction in exercise tachycardia.

d. Calculate how long the reduction in exercise tachycardia is expected to remain above 15% after:

(1) A 40-mg IV bolus dose

(2) A 70-mg IV bolus dose

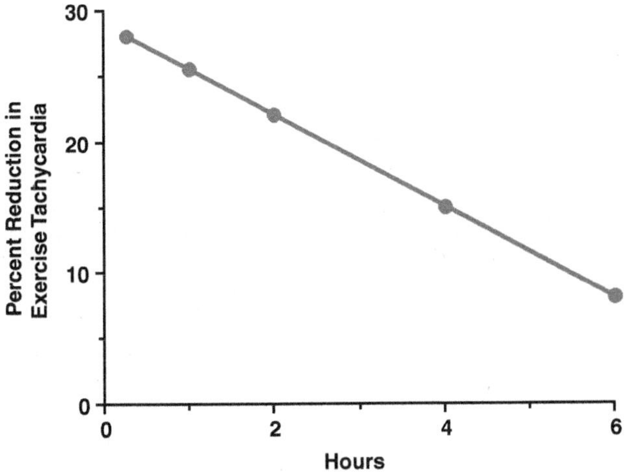

FIGURE 9-18 Percent reduction in exercise tachycardia with time following a 20-mg intravenous dose of propranolol. (Data from McDevitt DG and Shand DG. Plasma concentration and the time-course of beta-blockade due to propranolol. *Clin Pharmacol Ther* 1975;18:708–715.)

9. A compound is given as an IV bolus to a patient requiring a minimum plasma concentration of 4 mg/L for a therapeutic effect. Given that Dose = 100 mg; $k = 0.10$/h; $V = 8$ L, and assuming a one-compartment model,
   a. Calculate how long the clinical effect is expected to last with this dose.
   b. Calculate how long the clinical effect lasts following a 200-mg dose.
   c. Determine the duration of effect following a 100-mg dose, if $k = 0.05$/hr and the change in k is a result of
      (1) A twofold decrease in clearance; and
      (2) A doubling of the volume of distribution by increased nonspecific tissue binding.
   d. Does doubling the dose of a drug under the initial conditions ($k = 0.10$/hr; $V = 8$ L) yield the same change in duration of clinical effect as doubling the half-life?

SECTION III

Therapeutic Regimens

CHAPTER 10

Therapeutic Window

OBJECTIVES

The reader will be able to:

- List the factors that determine a therapeutic dosage regimen of a drug.
- Define the terms: dosage regimen, therapeutic index, therapeutic utility, therapeutic utility curve, therapeutic window.
- Explain the strategy behind the establishment of a therapeutic window.
- List the range of plasma concentrations associated with therapy within the patient population for common indications of five of the drugs listed in Table 10-1.
- Discuss briefly three circumstances in which response to a drug may not correlate well with its systemic exposure.

DOSAGE REGIMENS

Treatment of patients with various diseases or conditions with a drug often requires the maintenance of an appropriate systemic exposure to it. To do so, a drug may be given by a constant-rate protocol, such as an intravenous infusion, or by repeated administration of single doses. The administration (dosage form, dosing rate, loading dose, maintenance dose, interval between doses, route of administration, and duration of therapy) used to achieve and maintain therapy is called a **dosage regimen**.

The rational design of safe and efficacious dosage regimens is now examined. In this section, fundamental aspects of dosage regimens are covered primarily from the point of view of treating a typical patient within the population, with a given disease or condition for which the drug is indicated. It is realized, of course, that individuals vary in their responses to drugs; later, in Section IV, focus is turned toward the individual patient.

A dosage regimen is basically derived from the kinds of information shown in Fig. 10-1 (next page). This scheme applies to essentially all drugs, but particularly to those intended to produce therapeutic effects systemically; for locally acting drugs, local exposure is critical, but systemic exposure remains a safety concern. There are several issues that determine a therapeutic dosage regimen. One consideration is how the body acts on the drug and its dosage form, the essence of pharmacokinetics. Another consideration is the relationship between systemic exposure and both efficacy

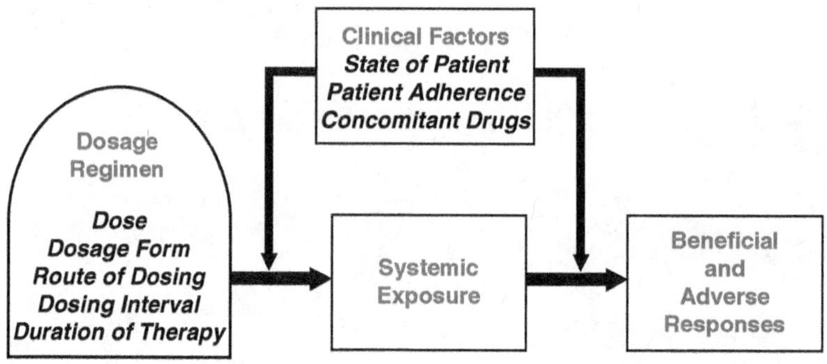

FIGURE 10-1 A dosage regimen of drug comprises dose, dosage form, dosing interval, route of administration, and duration of therapy. During drug development, these factors are adjusted to achieve an exposure profile that maximizes the benefits compared with adverse effects of the drug. Clinical factors that determine the optimal dosage regimen for an individual patient include the disease or condition being treated, the presence of other diseases and conditions, and other concomitantly administered drugs. These and other factors determine the optimal regimen for the individual by their effects on the drug's pharmacokinetics, pharmacodynamics, or both.

and safety of the drug, namely, pharmacodynamics. A third consideration, which can affect both the pharmacokinetics and the pharmacodynamics of a drug, is the clinical state of the patient. This includes the disease or condition being treated, other diseases or conditions that the patient may have, as well as associated additional drug therapy—that is, his or her *total* therapeutic regimen. A fourth set of issues includes all other factors such as genetics, age and weight, and the extent of adherence by the patient to the dosage regimen. Many of these determinants are, of course, interrelated and interdependent. For example, the requirement of frequent dosing can reduce the incidence of adherence to a regimen and thereby influence clinical outcome, whereas clinical outcome, particularly adverse effects without perceived benefit, can influence adherence even when maintenance of the regimen is critical to the ultimate therapeutic benefit.

Also critical to our understanding and to the optimal design and application of dosage regimen principles are changes in dosage requirements with time. The status of a patient is never static and, in addition to changes that occur soon after drug administration, there are often progressive changes in the disease or condition over the time span of treatment, particularly when the treatment extends over many months, years, or a lifetime. Such changes need to be taken into account when assessing the beneficial or adverse effects of a drug.

Dosage regimens are designed to achieve a therapeutic objective, namely, safe and effective therapy. This objective may be accomplished using various modalities of drug administration, extending from a single, or occasional, dose to continuous and constant input. An example of the former is the use of aspirin to treat an occasional headache; the continuous intravenous infusion of fentanyl, which is one option for the use of this opioid for the relief of pain after surgery, is an example of the latter. More commonly, drugs are administered repeatedly in discrete doses, a multiple-dosing regimen. The frequency and duration of a dosage regimen vary with the condition being treated. For many drugs, maintenance of a relatively constant systemic exposure is needed to maintain effect, which may, for example, be achieved by giving the drug three times daily for the duration of treatment. Other drugs do not require such a strict maintenance of systemic exposure and can be given relatively infrequently, which results in large fluctuations in the systemic exposure–time profile. Reasons for this latter approach being therapeutically desirable include the development of tolerance to the desired effect of the drug if exposure is maintained; the need to produce high exposure for short periods of time, as occurs in some antibiotic and anticancer chemotherapies; and persistence of drug effect even when the drug has been eliminated, as discussed in Chapter 9. To rapidly initiate therapy, the initial (or loading) dose of some drugs must be larger than the maintenance dose. In all cases, however, the general intent is to achieve and maintain effective therapy while minimizing harmful effects.

Evidence was presented in Chapter 3 that pharmacodynamic response is often better correlated with systemic exposure than with dose administered. Accordingly, it would seem to be most appropriate to apply pharmacokinetic principles to the design of dosage regimens to achieve desired systemic exposure–time profiles. Ultimately, however, the value of a dosage regimen must be assessed by the therapeutic and adverse responses produced when given to patients. Linking pharmacokinetics with pharmacodynamics, however, facilitates the achievement of an appropriate dosage regimen and serves as a useful means of evaluating existing dosage regimens.

In this chapter, various elements of the exposure–response relationship in the context of dosage regimens are explored; these build on principles developed in Chapters 3 and 9. Principles for achieving a desired exposure profile are discussed in the subsequent two chapters of this section, Chapters 11 and 12.

THERAPEUTIC WINDOW

Fig. 10-2 shows the probabilities of observing **beneficial** and **adverse effects** each as a function of the systemic exposure to a drug within its target patient population. In common with most drugs, the probability of each of a drug's effects increases progressively with increasing exposure. Also shown is the difference between the two probabilities, that is, the probability of achieving therapeutic benefit without harmful effects of the drug, a measure of its **therapeutic utility.** This difference plot is known

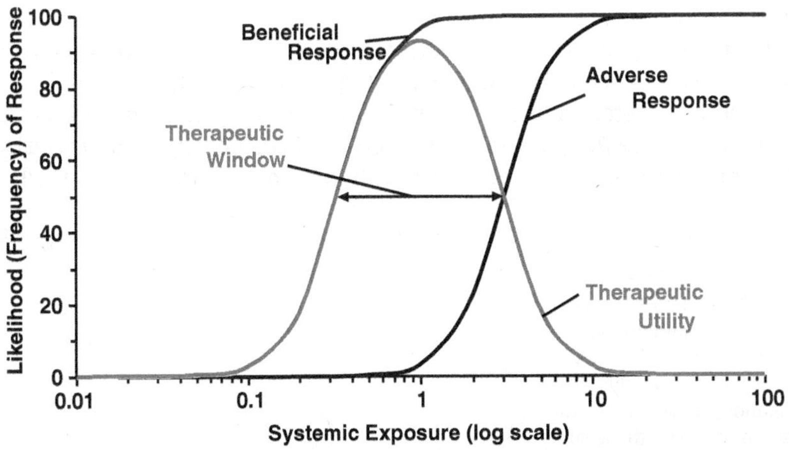

FIGURE 10-2 Schematic representation of the frequencies of effective therapy and adverse response within the target patient population as a function of systemic drug exposure. Also shown is the "therapeutic utility" (in *color*), or the curve of therapeutic success, given by the difference in frequencies of effective and adverse responses. The therapeutic window (*indicated by the width of the double-headed arrow*) is given by the range of exposures associated with frequencies of success in the patient population being equal to or greater than some preset value, in this case, 50%. In this example, the curves for both therapeutic and adverse responses are steep and well separated. The therapeutic window is therefore relatively wide (0.3 to 3) because there is little overlap between the exposure associated with attainment of total effective treatment within the patient population and the exposure associated with the likelihood of an adverse effect.

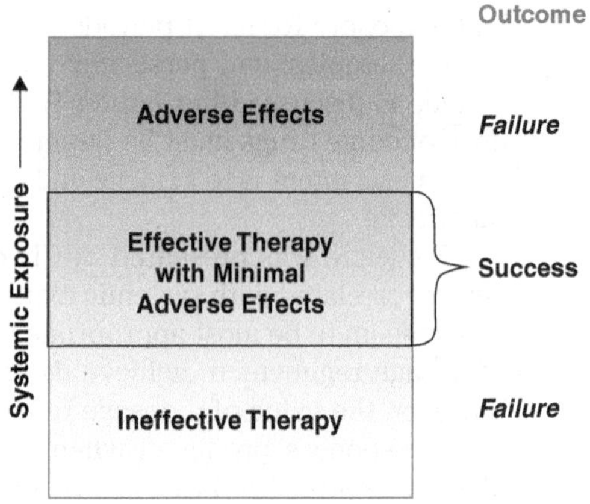

FIGURE 10-3 Schematic diagram depicting the therapeutic window of a drug, which lies between two regions of exposure associated with therapeutic failure. The lower region of failure is principally due to the absence of adequate efficacy, whereas the upper region is due to an inability to have adequate efficacy without an unacceptable adverse response.

as an unweighted **therapeutic utility curve** in that there is no particular significance, or weight, given to these two effects. They are treated equally. Here we see that the probability of achieving therapeutic utility increases with increasing exposure at low exposures, approaches a maximum, and then decreases at still higher exposures. Making the assumption that to be of therapeutic value the therapeutic utility should, for example, be in excess of 50%, we conclude that there is a range of exposures associated with successful therapy, the **therapeutic window** of the drug. This concept of a therapeutic window is depicted in Fig. 10-3.

At exposures below the window, therapy is deemed a failure because the probability of therapeutic benefit of the drug is too low despite the virtual absence of adverse effects. At exposures above the window, therapy is also deemed to fail; in this case, the probability of having a desired effect is high, but so too is the probability of being harmed. In other words, the risk of harm approaches and may even become greater than the likelihood of benefit.

In addition to the probability of desired and undesired effects, one should also consider the intensity or severity of these responses. In general, as discussed in Chapter 9, the frequency of more intense effects tends to increase with increasing exposure to the drug. This is seen, for example, in Fig. 10-4, by the greater incidence of severe central nervous system adverse effects with increasing exposure to the antiepileptic drug phenytoin. The first sign of adverse effects is usually nystagmus (jerky eye movement), which appears above a concentration of approximately 20 mg/L; gait ataxia

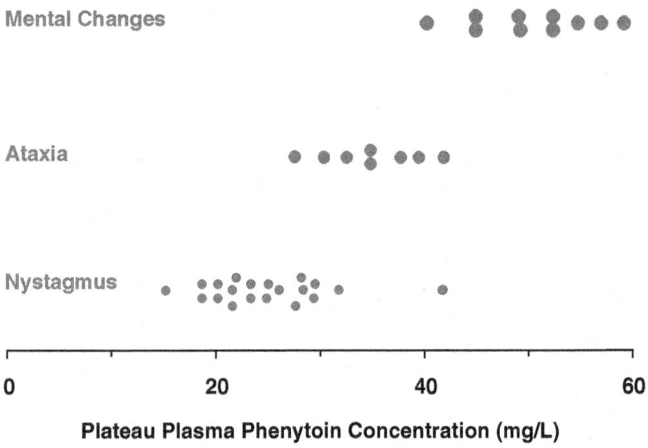

FIGURE 10-4 The occurrences of mild (nystagmus), moderate (ataxia), and severe (mental changes) untoward effects increase with the plasma concentration of the antiepileptic drug phenytoin (diphenylhydantoin). The values for nystagmus are for those subjects who have no more severe adverse effects. The values for ataxia are for those with no mental changes. (Modified from Kutt H, Winters W, Kokenge R, et al. Diphenylhydantoin metabolism, blood levels, and toxicity. *Arch Neurol* 1964;11:642-648. Copyright 1964, American Medical Association.)

(unsteadiness) usually appears with a concentration approaching 30 mg/L; and prolonged drowsiness and lethargy may be seen at concentrations greater than 40 mg/L.

In practice, then, desired and adverse effects need to be balanced with due consideration to their relative clinical importance. One must ask to what extent the beneficial effects of the drug outweigh its harmful effects. This relative weighting of effects requires judgment, which can vary depending on the drug, the condition being treated and the point of view of the evaluator. For example, appreciable gastrointestinal distress may be judged as a severe, and perhaps unacceptable, adverse effect for an analgesic drug, such as ibuprofen, being considered for relief of occasional headache. However, a more severe adverse effect, like constipation, may well be viewed as minor when a narcotic drug like morphine, a much stronger analgesic, is intended for the relief of severe pain in a patient suffering from the terminal stages of cancer. In addition, drugs may produce multiple adverse effects of different degrees of severity, judged as mild, moderate, and severe, as seen with phenytoin, with each requiring a different weighting. A therapeutic utility curve of greatest usefulness clinically is therefore one that takes into account all the above considerations. In reality, the utility curve cannot be very precise owing to the subjective nature of the weighting procedure. Also to be kept in mind is that such data are rarely, if ever, obtained in an individual. Rather, the data are the composite of limited data from many patients, each receiving a very small number of discrete dose strengths of the drug, such as 5 or 10 mg, with the spread of plasma concentrations, and responses, primarily resulting from the inherent pharmacokinetic and pharmacodynamic variabilities within the patient population.

Therapeutic windows, expressed in terms of the range of plasma, associated with successful therapy of the patient population with specific conditions, are listed in Table 10-1 (next three pages) for a select number of drugs. These are drugs taken by patients for relatively long periods of time, measured in months, years, and sometimes most of a lifetime. Several points are worth noting. First, for most of these drugs, the therapeutic concentration range is narrow in that the upper and lower limits differ by a factor of only 2 or 3. Of course, for many other drugs, this therapeutic window is much wider. This is certainly the case for amoxicillin and some other antibiotics. Second, some drugs are used to treat several diseases, and the therapeutic window may differ with the disease. For example, the dose, and associated systemic exposure, of aspirin needed to achieve an anticlotting effect is much lower than that needed to achieve an analgesic effect, and even higher doses are needed to relieve rheumatic symptoms. Next, the upper limit of the plasma concentration may be, like for the tricyclic antidepressant nortriptyline, a result of diminishing therapeutic efficacy at higher concentrations, producing a bell-shaped efficacy–concentration relationship. Or, it may be, like the immunosuppressant agent cyclosporine, used to prevent organ rejection after transplantation, a result of an increased likelihood of renal toxicity. The upper concentration limit may also be due to the drug being limited in its effectiveness, as with ibuprofen to relieve pain suffered by patients during severe trauma. Finally, an adverse effect may be either an extension of the pharmacologic property of the drug, or it may be totally distinct from its therapeutic effect. The hemorrhagic tendency associated with an excessive plasma concentration of the oral anticoagulant, warfarin, is an example of the former; the ototoxicity caused by the antibiotic gentamicin is an example of the latter.

A distinction also needs to be made between the steepness of a probability of response-versus-exposure curve and the width of a therapeutic window. In Fig. 10-2, the curves for the desired and adverse effects are both steep; yet because there is very little overlap between the two effects, the therapeutic window is relatively wide. For such a drug, the normal strategy would be to ensure that all patients receive a dosage

TABLE 10-1 | Selected Drugs and Their Plasma Concentrations Usually Associated With Successful Therapy

Drug	Disease/Condition	Therapeutic Window (mg/L)	Therapeutic Window (μmol/L)	Comments
Amikacin (aminoglycoside antibiotic)	Severe gram-negative infections	Every 8–12 hr:		Drug typically given in a 15–20 mg/kg/day dose as a single 30–60-min infusion daily or in divided doses every 8–12 hr. Peak (within 30 min of the end of the infusion) and trough (just before the next infusion) are used.
		Peak: 20–30	26–32	
		Trough: <10	<13	
		Once daily:		
		Peak: 60	77	
		Trough: undetectable		
Carbamazepine	Seizure disorders and used in psychiatric illnesses	4–12, although some prefer 4–8	17–51 17–34	The half-life of carbamazepine, 30–35 hr after a single dose, is about 15 hr during chronic therapy and about 10 hr in patients also receiving other antiepileptics (e.g., phenobarbital and phenytoin) due to autoinduction and induction of its metabolizing enzymes by these other drugs.
Cyclosporine	Immunosuppressive used in preventing and treating allograph rejection and in the treatment of various autoimmune diseases	Serum/plasma: 50–125	42–104	Absorption of cyclosporine has been a major problem that led to the development of a microemulsion dosage form that does not require the presence of bile and is less variable.
		Whole blood: 150–400	125–333	
Digoxin	Congestive heart failure (CHF) and atrial fibrillation	0.0008–0.002	0.001–0.0026	Blood samples should not be obtained within the first 6 hr after a dose no matter what the route of administration.
		0.0005–0.001 in CHF advocated by many	0.00064–0.00128	
Ethosuximide	Uncomplicated absence (petit mal) seizures	Trough: 40–100	284–710	
Gentamicin (aminoglycoside antibiotic)	Severe gram-negative infections	Every 8–12 hr:		Drug typically given in a 5–7 mg/kg/day dose as a single 30–60-min intravenous infusion daily or in divided doses every 8–12 hr. Peak (within 30 min of the end of the infusion) and trough (just before the next infusion) are used. Similar considerations apply to tobramycin and other aminoglycosides
		Peak: 5–8	10–17	
		Trough: <2	<4	
		Once daily:		
		Peak: 20	42	
		Trough: undetectable		

Lidocaine	Severe ventricular arrhythmias	1–5 mg/L	3.7–18	A loading dose is commonly given by a combination of several small bolus doses of 0.5–1.0 mg/kg or an infusion of 8 mg/min for 10–30 min (because of the distribution characteristics of the drug) followed by a maintenance rate of 1–4 mg/min.
Lithium	Treatment and prevention of various psychiatric conditions	–	0.6–0.8 mEq/L	Current practice is to obtain samples just before the morning dose and at least 12 hr after the last evening dose to minimize problems associated with the distribution kinetics of this drug.
Methotrexate	Used to treat several kinds of cancer. Also used to treat rheumatoid arthritis and psoriasis (a skin disease).	Variable	>0.1 for >48 hr >1 at 48 hr	Plasma concentrations exceeding 10^{-7} M for 48 hr are associated with methotrexate toxicity: myelosuppression, mucositis, and acute hepatic dysfunction. Leucovorin rescue may then be needed. Concentrations in excess of 10^{-6} M may require larger leucovorin doses.
Nortriptyline	Treatment of depression	0.05–0.15	0.17–0.5	Newer antidepressants (particularly serotonin uptake inhibitors) have replaced, in large part, the tricyclic antidepressants, but continue to be second-line agents.
Phenobarbital	Seizure disorders, insomnia, and anxiety	15–40	65–172	Because of its long half-life (4–5 d), it takes weeks to establish steady state when therapy is initiated or changed.
Phenytoin	Management of complex partial seizures and generalized tonic-clonic seizures and to treat cardiac arrhythmias when conventional options have failed or after cardiac glycoside intoxication.	10–20	40–80	Because of the drug's nonlinear kinetic behavior, adjustment of dosage must be carefully performed. Only a relatively small increase in daily dose may result in a large increase in the steady-state concentration.

(*continued*)

TABLE 10-1 | *(continued)*

Drug	Disease/Condition	Therapeutic Window (mg/L)	Therapeutic Window (μmol/L)	Comments
Procainamide	Ventricular and Atrial arrhythmias	4–8	15–30	Because procainamide has a short half-life (3 hr), steady-state concentrations are reached within 12 hr; however, sampling time is important for immediate-release dosage forms, less so for modified-release dosage forms. Usually, plasma samples are obtained just before the next dose.
Sirolimus	Macrolide antibiotic used as an immunosuppressive to prevent allograft rejection	0.005–0.015	0.0055–0.016	The typical loading dose of sirolimus is 6–15 mg (3 times the daily maintenance dose), because the half-life is 62 hr.
Tacrolimus	Macrolide antibiotic used as an immunosuppressive to prevent allograft rejection	0.005–0.02	0.0062–0.024	Tacrolimus blood samples are usually drawn just before the next dose (trough). As the half-life is 8–12 hr, the drug is usually given every 12 hr, and it is therefore reasonable to wait 36 hr or so after initiating or altering dosage to monitor plasma levels.
Theophylline	Bronchial asthma and certain other respiratory conditions	5–20	28–111	Currently is a third-line agent for treating asthma, but there is a large background of information for its safe use in those patients in whom its use is appropriate.
Valproic acid	Seizure disorders, prevention of migraines, and to treat a variety of psychiatric disorders such as bipolar disorder, anxiety, depression, psychosis, and substance-abuse withdrawal	50–100	350–700	Only trough concentrations are measured, because of the short half-life (6–8 hr in children, 10–12 hr in adults) of valproic acid. Modified-release products are typically used to treat migraines and monitoring of plasma concentrations is generally not recommended.

Abstracted from data in Winter ME. *Basic Clinical Pharmacokinetics*. 5th ed. Baltimore, MD: Lippincott Williams & Wilkins, 2010.

regimen that produces an exposure profile that achieves the therapeutic objective. Fig. 10-5 shows a drug with a narrow therapeutic window, despite the therapeutic curve being shallow. This narrowness arises because the curves overlap well below the point of maximal likelihood of therapeutic benefit, a result of the curve for adverse response being steep, so that it is difficult to find exposures that produce a high probability of efficacy without a high degree of a limiting adverse effect.

It is to be stressed that significant interindividual patient variability occurs in both therapeutic and adverse responses, leading to differences among individuals in the exposures where the desirable and undesirable effects occur. This should be kept in mind when considering the therapeutic windows listed in Table 10-1 for selective drugs for which concentration monitoring plays an important part in managing therapy. The values are derived from patient populations requiring the drugs, and they apply to the average patient within those populations. Also, one must keep in mind that the ultimate therapeutic objective is to treat each patient as efficaciously and safely as possible and not to keep his or her plasma concentrations within the recommended therapeutic window. This window can serve as a useful guide, however, particularly in the absence of additional information. When combined with pharmacokinetic information about the individual, as discussed further in Chapter 14, knowing the therapeutic window helps to define the dosage regimen to be used when initiating therapy. However, some patients fail to respond beneficially even when the plasma concentration lies within, or even considerably above, the normal therapeutic window. Such nonresponders may unknowingly lack or have a genetically different target receptor. Alternatively, the issue may be one of inaccurate diagnosis or misdiagnosis. For example, knowing that a patient suffers from cancer or an inflammatory disease does not guarantee that a particular anticancer or anti-inflammatory drug will be effective. The causes of such diseases are manifold, and no single drug is effective against all the causes of cancer or inflammation.

In many therapeutic situations several drugs are used in combination to treat a given condition or disease. An example is the use of a thiazide diuretic, a β-blocker, and an ACE (angiotensin-converting enzyme) inhibitor or angiotensin-receptor inhibitor in the treatment of hypertension. Each drug acts on a different part of the cardiovascular system to lower blood pressure. Another is the combination of acetaminophen with a nonsteroidal anti-inflammatory agent to relieve arthritic pain. Given that the adverse effects of drugs are often unrelated to their therapeutic effects, the

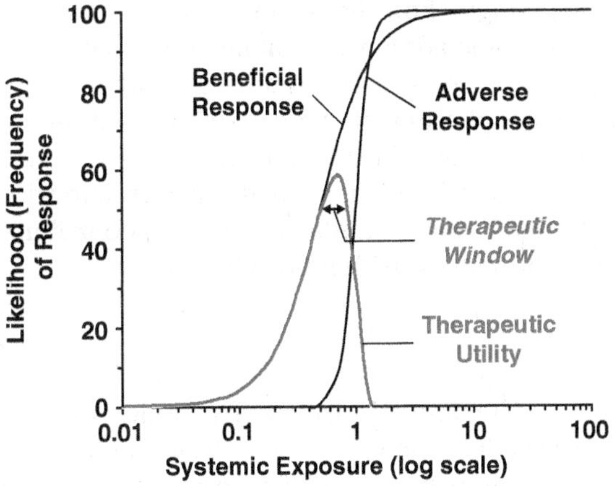

FIGURE 10-5 The width of a therapeutic window depends on the degree of overlap of the therapeutic and adverse exposure–response curves within the patient population. The therapeutic window (*indicated by the width of the double-headed arrow*) is narrow because of a high degree of overlap between efficacy and untoward effects caused by the adverse effect being the steeper of the two responses and making the utility curve (*color*) drop off sharply with increasing concentration. In this example, the therapeutic window is associated with exposures at which the frequency of success is greater than 50%. If a lower likelihood of success was clinically acceptable the therapeutic window would be wider.

advantage of such combinations is that the dose of each needed to produce a given therapeutic effect may be lower than if either is given alone, thereby reducing the likelihood of adverse effects. A combination of drugs is also often used in the treatment of infectious diseases, but for a somewhat different reason. For example, in the treatment of AIDS, patients are likely to receive a combination of one or two nucleoside/nucleotide reverse transcriptase inhibitors (faulty versions of the building block that the human immunodeficiency virus [HIV] needs to make more copies of itself so that reproduction of the virus is stalled), with either a nonnucleoside reverse transcriptase or a protease inhibitor (which disables protease, a protein that HIV needs to make more copies of itself). Each drug acts on a different critical pathway of the viral replication such that together they achieve a greater benefit than is possible with either drug alone, thereby reducing the chances of the emergence of resistant strains. Moreover, the combination allows the use of lower doses of each drug and again reduces the chances of associated adverse effects.

THERAPEUTIC CORRELATES

So far, plasma concentration has been assumed to be a better correlate of a drug's therapeutic response and harmful effects in a population of patients needing a drug than any other measure. However, because doses are administered and plasma concentration measurement requires invasive sampling and is costly, why not use dose as a therapeutic correlate? Certainly, in most cases, response and exposure both increase with increasing dose. Still, plasma concentration is expected to be a better correlate within the target patient population than dosage. This must be true after a single dose of drug, because with dose alone, no account is taken of time. It may also be true for continuous drug administration as well, but for different reasons.

The objective of much of drug therapy is to maintain a stable therapeutic response for the duration of treatment, usually by maintaining an effective plasma concentration. Recall, Fig. 1-7 (Chapter 1) shows the relationship between the steady-state plasma concentration and the rate of administration of the antiepileptic drug, phenytoin. Particularly noticeable are the large interindividual deviations in the plasma concentration at any specific dosing rate; in the patient cohort studied, the plasma concentration ranged from nearly 0 to 50 mg/L at a dosing rate of 6 mg/day/kg of body weight. Had no correction been made for body weight, the deviations may well have been even greater. In contrast, plasma concentration correlates reasonably well with effect. Thus, seizures are usually effectively controlled without undue adverse events at plasma concentrations between 10 and 20 mg/L. For phenytoin, plasma concentration is a better correlate than dose during chronic administration because pharmacokinetics is the major source of variability between dose and response. For other drugs, such as atenolol, used to lower blood pressure, pharmacokinetic variability within the patient population is relatively small, and variability in the concentration–response relationship is large. In such cases, plasma concentration is no better a correlate with response than dose, and indeed may be worse if, for example, metabolites contribute to therapeutic activity and toxicity (see Additional Considerations below).

THERAPEUTIC INDEX

A concept related to therapeutic window is **therapeutic index**. This index reflects how sensitive *an individual patient* is to the limiting effects of a drug on changing exposure, usually noticed in practice when dose is increased. The index is low when the dose required to elicit the desired therapeutic effect is very close to that producing the limiting adverse effect(s). Examples of low therapeutic index drugs are warfarin and digoxin. Minor increases in exposure with these drugs can tip a patient from having therapeutic benefit into experiencing unacceptable risk. In contrast to these drugs, most other drugs have a moderate to high therapeutic index; for them, patients are relatively insensitive to a moderate change in dose, although it is always good practice to use as low a dose as possible, commensurate with achieving adequate therapeutic effectiveness.

ADDITIONAL CONSIDERATIONS

Despite the appeal, measurement of plasma concentration, as an index of systemic exposure, to guide therapy is uncommon in clinical practice (see Chapter 14). One major reason is that for many drugs, there are direct and simple means of using therapeutic and adverse responses to guide therapy. Even then, appreciating the relationship among drug administration, exposure, and response over time aids in assuring rational use of such drugs. Another major reason for not monitoring plasma concentration is the wide margin of safety of many drugs, such as many antibiotics, so that high and effective doses may be given to virtually all patients, the exception being those with a known allergy to the drug or who have an idiosyncratic reaction (genetically related response peculiar to the individual) to the drug. Yet another is that plasma concentration often correlates poorly with measured response, especially when most of the variability in drug response is in its pharmacodynamics (subject of Chapter 13). Another reason for a poor correlation, discussed more fully in Chapter 12, is the development of tolerance to the drug whereby response diminishes with time, sometimes quite slowly and sometimes very rapidly, despite maintenance of a relatively constant plasma concentration. Some additional explanations for poor exposure–response correlations follow.

Multiple Active Species

Many drugs are converted to active metabolites in the body. Unless these metabolites are also measured, poor correlations with the parent drug may exist. For example, based on its plasma concentration, alprenolol is more active as a β-blocker when given as a single oral dose than when administered intravenously. This drug is highly cleared on its first passage through the liver; so in terms of the parent drug, the oral dose is poorly bioavailable. However, large amounts of metabolites, including an active species, 4-hydroxyalprenolol, are formed during the absorption process, which explains the above apparent discrepancy. The tricyclic antidepressant amitriptyline offers a second example. Its antidepressant activity correlates poorly with the plasma concentration of parent drug. Only when the contribution of its active desmethyl metabolite, nortriptyline, is also considered can more useful correlations be established. The analgesic activity after administration of codeine is thought to arise from its partial conversion to morphine; clearly, trying to correlate analgesic activity with codeine concentration alone is likely to be unsuccessful.

Single-Dose Therapy

One dose of aspirin often relieves a headache, which may not return even after the drug has been eliminated. Other examples of effective single-dose therapy include albuterol nebulizer to treat an acute asthmatic attack, nitroglycerin to relieve an acute episode of angina, and morphine to relieve acute severe pain. Although the specific mechanism of action may be poorly understood, the overall effect is known; the drug returns an out-of-balance physiologic system to within normal bounds. Thereafter, feedback control systems within the body maintain homeostasis. The need for drug has now ended. In these instances of single-dose therapy, a correlation between beneficial effect and peak exposure to drug may exist, but beyond the peak, any such correlation is unlikely.

Duration Versus Intensity of Exposure

Complexities can also exist in the relationships among effect, dose, and duration of therapy. For example, some chemotherapeutic agents, such as methotrexate, exhibit peculiar relationships between response and dose. The response observed relates more closely to the duration of dosing than to the actual dose used or the plasma concentrations produced. This behavior for methotrexate can be explained by its activity as an antimetabolite. It inhibits dihydrofolate reductase, an enzyme that plays a critical role in the building of DNA and other body constituents. This enzyme is involved in the synthesis of folic acid, a molecule that shuttles carbon atoms through methylation to enzymes that need them in their reactions. These reactions can be inhibited for short periods of time, such as a few days, without causing irreversible damage, but even smaller doses given over a prolonged period of time can become toxic. Although all attempts are made to minimize the effect of prolonged and excessive exposure, occasionally signs of inadvertent methotrexate toxicity are seen in patients. Then leucovorin, which is converted to folic acid within the body, is given as a rescue therapy to reverse the effect of methotrexate.

Another example is seen with corticosteroids. Massive doses can be administered acutely for the treatment of anaphylactic shock without significant adverse effects; yet even when relatively small doses are administered chronically for the treatment of some inflammatory conditions some patients develop a Cushingoid state, characterized by moonface and a buffalo hump associated with excessive deposits of fat on the face and back caused by a sustained state of higher-than-normal circulating corticosteroid.

Time Delays

As discussed in Chapter 9 (and again in Chapter 14), correlation between systemic exposure and response can be complicated owing to time delays, which are caused by time needed for drug to reach the active site, or because it takes time for the body to respond fully to a given systemic exposure. This type of complication often tends to diminish on chronic medication when exposure and response become relatively stable with time.

ACHIEVING THERAPEUTIC GOALS

We now need to integrate this information on the therapeutic window with basic principles for establishing and evaluating dosage regimens for those drugs that show reasonably valid and stable correlations of response with exposure and dose. Chapter 11 examines features of constant-rate input regimens, and Chapter 12 examines the principles underlying the administration of drug in discrete repetitive doses, to attain and maintain successful therapy.

SUMMARY

- A dosage regimen for the indicated patient population aims to achieve a desired therapeutic benefit while minimizing harm for the duration of therapy.
- A rational approach for many drugs toward achieving the therapeutic objective is to maintain the systemic exposure of the drug within a therapeutic window. Below the window, there is a higher likelihood of ineffective therapy; above the window, there is a higher likelihood that the adverse effects will outweigh the benefits.
- The difference between the likelihood of desired and adverse effects, weighted by their relative clinical importance, is a measure of the therapeutic utility of a drug.
- The width of the therapeutic window is a function of the degree of overlap and the steepness of the incidences of the beneficial and adverse response-versus-exposure curves. The greater the overlap, the narrower is the therapeutic window of a drug.
- The therapeutic index of a drug is a measure of the sensitivity in an individual patient to a change in exposure or dose. The index is low if only a minor increase in systemic exposure leads to unacceptable adverse effects, and is high if a relatively large increase in exposure is required to observe an unacceptable incidence of adverse effects.
- Situations exist in which the utility of using systemic exposure as a guide to the management of drug therapy is complicated, limited, or even misleading. These include the buildup of tolerance to a drug, the presence of active metabolites, single-dose therapy, time delays between drug administration and measured effects, and complex interplays among dose, duration of therapy, and effect.

KEY TERM REVIEW

Adverse effects	Therapeutic index
Beneficial effects	Therapeutic utility
Dosage regimen	Therapeutic utility curve
Therapeutic correlates	Therapeutic window

STUDY PROBLEMS

1. Which of the following statements is (are) correct?
   I. The method of administration of a drug (dosage form, dosing rate, loading dose, maintenance dose, interval between doses, route of administration, and duration of therapy) used to achieve and maintain therapy is called a dosage regimen.
   II. Dosage regimens are designed to achieve a therapeutic objective, namely, safe and effective therapy. This objective may be accomplished using various modalities of drug administration, extending from a single, or occasional, dose to continuous and constant input.
   III. The therapeutic window of a drug may be defined as the range of plasma concentrations that are associated with successful therapy in a patient population with a specific condition.

   A. I only **E.** I and III
   B. II only **F.** II and III
   C. III only **G.** All
   D. I and II **H.** None

2. Therapeutic window and therapeutic index are important concepts in drug therapy. Which *one* of the following statements about them is *incorrect*?
   a. The therapeutic index reflects how sensitive *an individual patient* is to the limiting effects of a drug on changing exposure, usually noticed in practice when dose is increased.
   b. Plasma drug concentration monitoring is potentially helpful as a supplemental piece of information for those drugs for which much, if not most, of the variability in their dose–response relationship is in their pharmacokinetics.
   c. One cannot have a wide therapeutic window if the therapeutic index is small.
   d. Many drugs are converted into active metabolites in the body. Poor correlations of efficacy or adverse events with the parent drug may be expected, unless these metabolites are also measured and taken into account.
3. Which *one* of the following statements about therapeutic window and therapeutic index is *correct*?
   a. Because of its appeal, measurement of plasma concentration, as an index of systemic exposure, to guide therapy is common in clinical practice. One major reason is that for most drugs, there are good, direct, and simple correlations of therapeutic and adverse responses with systemic exposure.
   b. One refers to the therapeutic index as being wide or narrow and the therapeutic window as being small or large.
   c. In common with most drugs, the probabilities of a drug's beneficial and adverse effects, each a function of the systemic exposure to a drug within its target patient population, increase progressively with increasing exposure on chronic administration. The difference between the two probabilities, that is, the probability of achieving therapeutic benefit without harmful effects of the drug in the target population, weighted for the benefits and risks involved, is a measure of its therapeutic utility.
   d. The therapeutic objective of pharmacotherapy cannot be met with a single dose of drug.
4. Briefly discuss why response is often better correlated with drug exposure than with dose.
5. Briefly discuss the statement: Drugs with steep adverse effect–exposure curves are ones with a narrow therapeutic window.
6. State why a combination of drugs may be beneficial in drug therapy to treat a specific disease or condition, and give two examples of such combinations.
7. Give three examples of situations in which a complexity arises in attempting to correlate response with drug exposure.

CHAPTER 11

Constant-Rate Regimens

OBJECTIVES

The reader will be able to:

- Define what is meant by a *plateau* plasma drug concentration and *plateau* amount of drug in the body following administration of a drug at a constant rate, and describe the factors controlling them.
- Describe the relationship between half-life of a drug and time required to approach steady state following a constant-rate input with or without a bolus dose.
- Estimate the values of half-life, volume of distribution, and clearance of a drug from plasma concentration data obtained during and following a short-term, constant-rate intravenous infusion.
- Determine the bolus dose needed to achieve the same amount in the body, or same plasma concentration, as that achieved at steady state on infusing a drug at a given constant rate.
- Determine the input rate needed to maintain the bolus amount in the body, or the initial plasma concentration, with time after giving an intravenous bolus dose.
- Using pharmacokinetic parameters, predict the plasma concentration and the amount in the body with time during and following constant-rate input with or without a bolus dose.
- Briefly discuss why short-term rapid infusions are often used when a single intravenous loading dose is called for.
- Briefly discuss pharmacokinetic and pharmacodynamic reasons for a delay in the onset of drug effect during a constant-rate intravenous infusion. Also discuss pharmacokinetic and pharmacodynamic reasons for the effect of a drug being sustained after stopping an infusion.

A single dose may rapidly produce a desired therapeutic concentration, but this mode of administration is unsuitable when careful maintenance of plasma or tissue concentrations and effect is desired. To maintain a constant plasma concentration, drug must be administered at a constant rate. This is most often accomplished by infusing drug intravenously. No other mode of administration provides such precise and readily controlled systemic drug input. One major advantage of this method of administration is that drug input can be stopped instantly if adverse effects occur. In contrast to extravascular administration, for which drug input continues, the drug concentration immediately begins to decrease when an intravenous infusion is stopped. A disadvantage of this form of administration is that it usually is restricted to institutional settings because it is invasive and requires special equipment and trained health care providers. Examples of drugs given by intravenous infusion are listed in

Table 11-1 | Examples of Drugs Given by Intravenous Infusion

Drug	Indication	Administration
Bivalirudin	Anticoagulation in patients with unstable angina undergoing percutaneous transluminal coronary angioplasty.	Bolus of 1 mg/kg followed by a 4-hr infusion at rate of 2.5 mg/kg/hr. An additional infusion of 0.2 mg/kg/hr for up to 20 hr may be given if needed.
Eptifibatide	Acute coronary syndrome and for patients undergoing percutaneous coronary intervention.	Bolus of 180 μg/kg followed by an infusion of 2.0 μg/kg/min until hospital discharge or initiation of coronary artery bypass graft for up to 96 hr.
Esmolol hydrochloride	For rapid control of supraventricular and intraoperative and postoperative tachycardia.	A loading dose of 0.5 mg/kg infused over 1 min, followed by 0.05 mg/kg/min for 4 min, then increased as necessary in steps of at least 4-min duration to a maximum of 0.2 mg/kg/min.
Nesiritide	Patients with acutely decompensated congestive heart failure who have dyspnea.	Bolus dose of 2 μg/kg followed by continuous infusion of 0.01 μg/kg/min.
Nicardipine hydrochloride	Short-term treatment of hypertension when oral therapy is not feasible or not desirable.	Therapy is initiated with 5 mg/hr. If desired blood pressure reduction is not achieved at this rate, the rate may be increased by 2.5 mg/hr every 5 min up to 15 mg/hr. Once the goal is achieved, the rate is adjusted to maintain the desired response.

Table 11-1. Many common drugs, approved for intravenous administration, are given by infusion under special circumstances, for example, when a patient is comatose or unable to take a drug orally, as sometimes occurs with patients who have undergone major small bowel resection.

A wider application of constant-rate therapy, beyond intravenous administration, has become possible with the development and use of constant-rate release devices and systems, which can be ingested or placed at a variety of body sites and which deliver drug for a period of time extending from hours to years. Some examples of these devices/systems and their applications are given in Table 11-2. Many of the transdermal systems previously discussed (see Table 8-10) fall into this category as well. When used to produce a systemic effect, absorption is a prerequisite to attain effective plasma concentrations for all methods that are extravascular in nature. For the purpose of understanding the principles in this chapter, drug delivery from these systems is assumed to be equivalent to a constant-rate intravenous infusion.

EXPOSURE–TIME RELATIONSHIPS

The salient features of the events following a constant-rate infusion are shown in Fig. 11-1 (p. 204) for tissue-type plasminogen activator (t-PA), a protein drug used to treat myocardial infarctions. The plasma concentration rises toward a constant value and drops off immediately after the infusion of 1.4 mg/min is stopped at 80 minutes.

Table 11-2 | Representative Constant-Rate Devices or Systems and Their Applications

Type of Therapeutic System	Drug	Rate Specifications	Application/Comment
Intramuscular injection	Haloperidol	Deep IM injection (50 and 100 mg/mL in sesame oil). Initial dose of 10–15 times dose of oral immediate-release product. Maintenance with once-monthly injection. Approximately 1/30 of the dose becomes systemically available daily, on average.	Used in treating schizophrenia patients who require prolonged parenteral therapy.
	Leuprolide	Dose depends on age of child (7.5, 11.25, or 15 mg/syringe). Starting dose is 0.3 mg/kg every 4 wk.	Used in the treatment of children with central precocious puberty.
Oral	Glipizide	2.5-, 5-, or 10-mg constant-rate release tablets administered once daily.	Oral blood glucose–lowering drug of sulfonylurea class with 24-hr constant-rate release.
	Nifedipine	30, 60, or 90 mg/day administered once daily.	Nondisintegrating system is designed to provide a constant rate of release for 24 hr. Used in treating vasospastic and chronic stable angina and hypertension.
Subcutaneous implant	Goserelin	Implanted subcutaneously. Continuous release of drug for a 12-wk period. Product is biodegradable.	Used in treating prostate carcinoma. Potent synthetic decapeptide agonist of luteinizing hormone-releasing hormone.
	Leuprolide acetate	Implant is nonbiodegradable. Implanted subcutaneously and removed and replaced once yearly. Contains 72-mg leuprolide acetate; delivers 120 μg/day.	Used as palliative treatment for advanced prostatic cancer.
Subcutaneous injection	Insulin glargine	Exhibits a relatively constant glucose-lowering effect over 24 hr, permitting once-a-day administration.	Treatment of adult and pediatric patients with type 1 diabetes mellitus or adults with type 2 diabetes mellitus who require long-acting insulin for control of hyperglycemia.
Vaginal ring	Etonogestrel/ ethinyl estradiol	On average, 0.12 mg of the progestin hormone and 0.05 mg of the estrogen are released per day.	Used to prevent pregnancy. Ring is inserted for 3 wk. After a 1-wk break, another is inserted.

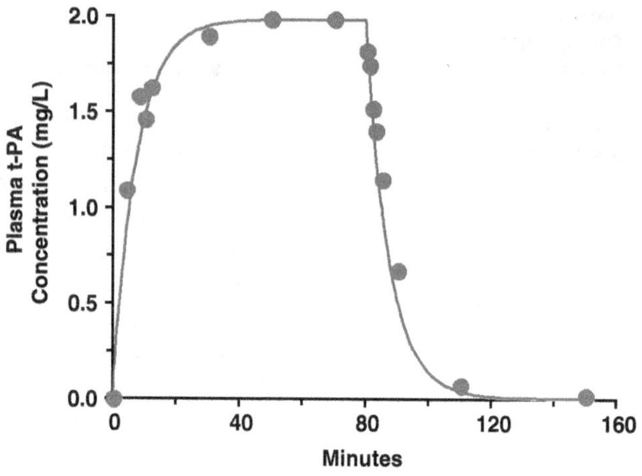

FIGURE 11-1 The plasma concentration of recombinant tissue-type plasminogen activator (t-PA) rapidly approaches a limiting value in a patient who receives 1.4 mg/min by constant-rate infusion for 80 minutes. On stopping the infusion, the plasma t-PA concentration drops rapidly toward 0 with a 5.2-minute half-life. The line from 0 to 80 minutes, during the infusion, is the function $C = 1.98\ (1 - e^{-0.133t})$, while $C = 1.98 \cdot e^{-0.133t}$ is the function postinfusion. The exponential value of 0.133/min corresponds to a half-life of 5.2 minutes. (Adapted from Koster RW, Cohen AF, Kluft C, et al. The pharmacokinetics of double-chain t-PA (duteplase): effects of bolus injection, infusions, and administration by weight in patients with myocardial infarction. *Clin Pharmacol Ther* 1991;50:267–277.)

The half-life of the compound in this patient is 5.2 minutes, so the drug has been infused for about 15 half-lives.

A drug is said to be given as a constant (rate) infusion when the intent is to maintain a stable plasma concentration or amount in the body. In contrast to the input of a bolus dose by a short-term infusion, the duration of a constant-rate infusion is usually much longer than the half-life of the drug. The essential features following a constant-rate infusion can be appreciated by considering the events depicted in Fig. 11-2, in which drug is introduced at a constant rate into the reservoir model previously presented (Fig. 5-3).

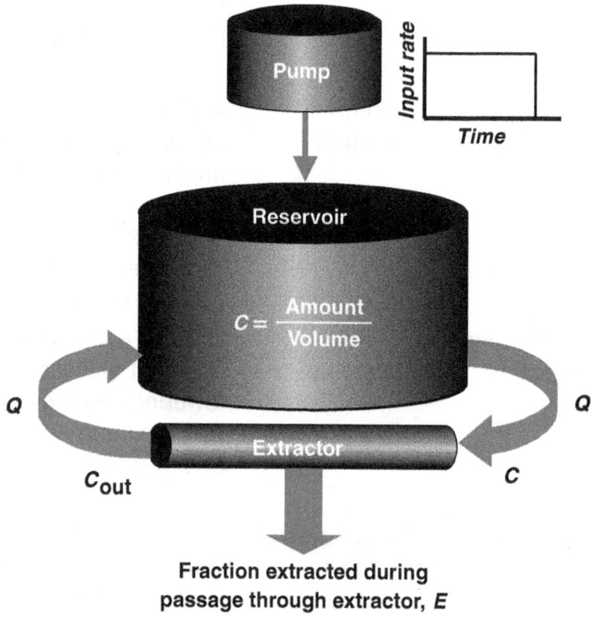

FIGURE 11-2 Drug is delivered at a constant rate (pump and rate of input shown) into a well-stirred reservoir (see Fig. 5-3). Fluid from the reservoir enters the extractor at flow rate Q. A fraction E of drug presented to the extractor is removed as the fluid passes through it; the remainder is returned to the reservoir. For modeling purposes, the volume of drug solution introduced by the pump and the amount of drug in the extractor are negligible compared with the volume of the reservoir and the amount of drug contained in it, respectively.

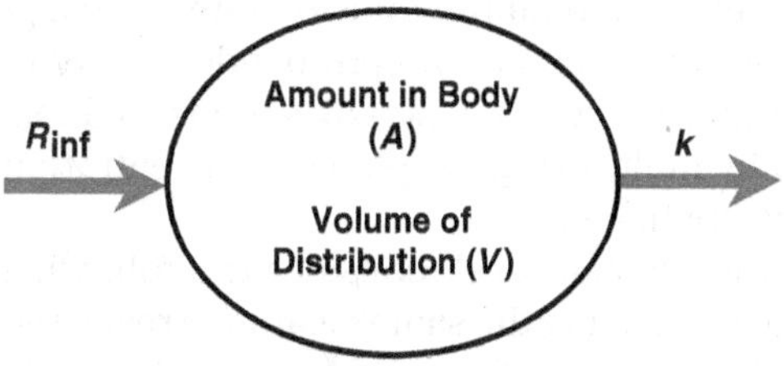

FIGURE 11-3 The time course of the amount of drug in the body during a constant-rate infusion depends on the rate of input and the rate of elimination. The simplest model for examining the time course is shown. The symbols are: R_{inf}, rate of infusion; A, amount in the body; V, volume of distribution; and k, the elimination rate constant. The rate of elimination is equal to $k \cdot A$: the plasma concentration is equal to A/V.

The Plateau Value

At any time during an infusion, the rate of change in the amount of drug in the body (or reservoir) is the difference between the rates of drug infusion and elimination. Using the model shown in Fig. 11-3,

$$\text{Rate of change of drug in the body} = \underset{\substack{\text{Constant rate}\\ \text{of infusion}}}{R_{inf}} - \underset{\substack{\text{Rate of}\\ \text{elimination}}}{k \cdot A} \quad \textbf{Eq. 11-1}$$

or expressing the equation in terms of the concentration of drug in plasma,

$$\text{Rate of change of drug in the body} = \underset{\substack{\text{Constant rate}\\ \text{of infusion}}}{R_{inf}} - \underset{\substack{\text{Rate of}\\ \text{elimination}}}{CL \cdot C} \quad \textbf{Eq. 11-2}$$

On starting a constant-rate infusion, the amount in the body (reservoir) is zero, and so there is no elimination. Therefore, the amount in the body initially rises at a rate equal to the infusion rate. The amount or plasma concentration continues to rise with time but at a diminishing rate because, as it does so, the rate of elimination increases. Eventually, the amount in the body is such that the rate of elimination matches the rate of infusion, at which time the amount in the body and plasma concentration are said to have reached a **steady state** or **plateau**, which continues as long as the same infusion rate is maintained. Since the net rate of change of amount in the body at plateau is zero, it follows that Equations 11-1 and 11-2 simplify to:

$$\underset{\substack{\text{Amount at}\\ \text{steady state}}}{A_{ss}} = \underset{\frac{\text{Infusion rate}}{\text{Elimination rate constant}}}{\frac{R_{inf}}{k}} \quad \textbf{Eq. 11-3}$$

$$\underset{\substack{\text{Concentration}\\ \text{at steady state}}}{C_{ss}} = \underset{\frac{\text{Infusion rate}}{\text{Clearance}}}{\frac{R_{inf}}{CL}} \quad \textbf{Eq. 11-4}$$

Clearly, the only factors governing amount at plateau are the rate of infusion and the elimination rate constant. Similarly, only infusion rate and clearance control the steady-state plasma concentration. For example, consider the case of eptifibatide (Integrilin), a cyclic heptapeptide derived from a protein found in the venom of the southeastern pygmy rattlesnake, used to treat acute coronary syndrome. Furthermore, suppose, for illustrative purposes, that a steady-state plasma eptifibatide concentration of 1 mg/L is desired in a 70-kg patient, whose clearance and volume of distribution are 4 L/hr (57 mL/hr/kg) and 14.3 L, respectively. The required infusion rate is 4.0 mg/hr (4 L/hr × 1 mg/L). Because the elimination rate constant of eptifibatide is 0.28/hr, the corresponding amount of drug in the body (reservoir) at steady state is 14.3 mg. Alternatively, the amount can be calculated by multiplying the plateau concentration (1 mg/L) by the volume of distribution of eptifibatide (14.3 L).

To emphasize the factors that control the plateau level, consider the following statement: "All drugs infused at the same rate and having the same clearance reach the same plateau concentration." This statement is true. The liver and kidneys clear only what is presented to them; the rate of elimination depends on clearance and plasma concentration. At plateau, rate of elimination equals rate of infusion and, therefore, the plasma concentration must be the same for all drugs with the same clearance if administered at the same rate. However, amount in the body also varies with volume of distribution. Only for drugs with the same clearance and volume of distribution are both plasma concentration *and* amount in the body at plateau the same when infused at the same rate. Now consider the next statement: "When infused at the same rate, the amount of drug in the body at steady state is the same for all drugs with the same half-life." This statement is also true, as seen from Equation 11-3. Drugs with the same half-life have the same elimination rate constant. As the elimination rate constant is the rate of elimination divided by the amount of drug in the body, and the rate of elimination equals the rate of infusion, the amount in the body at plateau must be the same. The corresponding plateau plasma concentration, however, varies inversely with the drug's volume of distribution, which can be different, but the ratio CL/V must be the same.

During therapy with a drug, it is not uncommon to adjust administration to observed clinical effects. This may require an increase or decrease in dosing rate. Knowledge of the plateau value at one particular infusion rate allows prediction of the infusion rate needed to achieve plateau values at other rates. Thus, provided that clearance is constant, a change in infusion rate produces a proportional change in plateau concentration. Returning to the eptifibatide example, one expects that a rate of 8 mg/hr is needed to produce a plateau concentration of 2 mg/L in our patient, because an infusion rate of 4 mg/hr resulted in a plateau concentration of 1 mg/L.

Time to Reach Plateau

A delay always exists between the start of an infusion and the establishment of plateau. *The sole factor controlling the approach to plateau is the half-life of the drug.* To appreciate this point, consider a situation in which a bolus dose is given at the start of a constant-rate infusion to immediately attain the amount achieved at plateau; clearly, the size of the bolus dose must be A_{ss}. Thereafter, the amount in the body is maintained at the plateau value by the constant-rate infusion. Imagine that a way exists to monitor separately drug remaining in the body from the bolus and that accumulating due to the infusion. The events are depicted in Fig. 11-4. Drug in the body associated with each mode of administration is eliminated as if the other were not present. The amount associated with the bolus dose declines exponentially, and at any time,

$$\text{Amount remaining in the body from bolus dose} = A_{SS} \cdot e^{-k \cdot t} \quad \textbf{Eq. 11-5}$$

However, as long as the infusion is maintained, this decline is exactly matched by the gain resulting from the infusion. This must be so because the sum always equals the

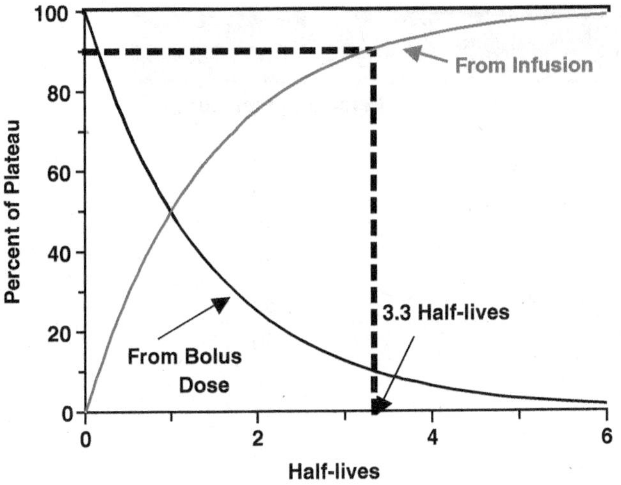

FIGURE 11-4 The time to approach plateau is controlled only by the half-life of the drug. Depicted is a situation in which a bolus dose immediately attains and a constant infusion rate thereafter maintains a constant amount in the body (*solid horizontal line at top*). As the amount of the bolus dose remaining in the body (*black line*) falls, there must be a complementary rise resulting from the infusion (*colored line*). Therefore, by 3.3 half-lives, the amount in the body associated with the bolus is 10% of the initial value, and that associated with the infusion has reached 90% of the plateau value.

amount at plateau, A_{ss}. It therefore follows that the amount in the body associated with a constant-rate infusion (A_{inf}) is always the difference between the amount at plateau (A_{ss}) and the amount remaining from the bolus dose, namely,

$$A_{inf} = A_{ss} - A_{ss} \cdot e^{-kt} = A_{ss}\,(1 - e^{-kt}) \qquad \text{Eq. 11-6}$$

or, upon dividing through by the volume of distribution,

$$C_{inf} = C_{ss}\,(1 - e^{-kt}) \qquad \text{Eq. 11-7}$$

Thus, both the amount in the body and the plasma concentration (C_{inf}) rise toward their respective plateau values after constant-rate drug infusion without a bolus dose.

The amount of drug in the body, or plasma concentration, expressed as a percent of the plateau value at different times after initiation of an infusion, is shown in Table 11-3 (next page). In 1 half-life, the value in the body is 50% of the plateau value. In 2 half-lives, it is 75% of the plateau value. Theoretically, a plateau is reached only when the drug has been infused for an infinite number of half-lives. *Practically, however, the plateau may be considered to be reached in 3.3 half-lives (when the amount or concentration has reached 90% of the steady-state value)*, because the 10% difference is only of marginal significance both experimentally and clinically. Thus, the shorter the half-life, the sooner the concentration approaches its plateau. For example, t-PA (half-life of 5 minutes) reaches a plateau within minutes (3.3 half-lives is 17 minutes), whereas it takes more than 8 hours of constant eptifibatide administration (half-life of 2.5 hours) before the plateau is reached (3.3 half-lives is 8.25 hours). The important point to remember is that the approach to plateau depends *solely* on the half-life of the drug. This is so whether 8 mg/hr of eptifibatide is infused to attain a plateau concentration of 2 mg/L or the infusion rate is 4 mg/hr to maintain a plateau concentration of 1 mg/L. In the former case, the eptifibatide plasma concentration at 1 half-life is half the corresponding plateau value of 2 mg/L or 1 mg/L. So a plateau concentration of 2 mg/L can be achieved more quickly by first infusing at a rate of 16 mg/hr for 1 half-life (2.5 hours) and then maintaining the resulting 2 mg/L by halving the initial rate, that is, by infusing at a rate of 8 mg/hr.

Table 11-3 | Approach to Plateau with Time Following a Constant-Rate Drug Infusion

Time (in Half-lives)	Percent of Plateau[a] (%)
0.25	16
0.5	29
1	50
2	75
3	88
3.3	90
4	94
5	97
6	98
7	99

[a]Values are rounded off to the nearest percent.

Postinfusion

After stopping an infusion, the amount in the body or the plasma concentration falls by one-half each half-life. Indeed, given only the declining values of a drug, one cannot conclude whether a bolus or an infusion had been given. In the example of eptifibatide, 28.6 mg (2 mg/L × 14.3 L) are in the body (reservoir) at plateau after an infusion rate of 8 mg/hr. At 8.25 hours (3.3 half-lives) after stopping the infusion, only one-tenth of the plateau value, or 2.86 mg, remains in the body. The same amount of drug would be found in the body 8.25 hours after an IV bolus dose of 28.6 mg.

A comment should be made about removing constant-rate transdermal devices or systems. After removing some of them, drug continues to be released from storage sites in skin for appreciable periods of time. In this instance, as a result of continued systemic input, the plasma drug concentration falls more slowly than what would be seen when stopping an intravenous infusion.

Changing Infusion Rates

The rate of infusion of a drug is sometimes changed during therapy because of excessive toxicity or an inadequate therapeutic response. If the object of the change is to produce a new plateau, then the time to go from one plateau to another—whether higher or lower—depends *solely* on the half-life of the drug.

Consider, for illustrative purposes, our patient stabilized on a 4-mg/hr infusion rate of eptifibatide, which, with a clearance of 4 L/hr, should produce a plateau plasma concentration of 1.0 mg/L. Suppose that the clinical situation now demands a plateau concentration of 2.0 mg/L. This new plateau value is achieved by doubling the infusion rate to 8 mg/hr. Imagine that, instead of increasing the infusion rate, the additional 4 mg/hr is administered at a different site and that a way exists to monitor drug in the body from the two infusions separately. The events illustrated in Fig. 11-5 show that the eptifibatide concentration associated with the supplementary infusion is expected to rise to its steady-state concentration of 1 mg/L in exactly the same time as in the first infusion. The concentration half-way toward the new plateau (2.0 mg/L), namely

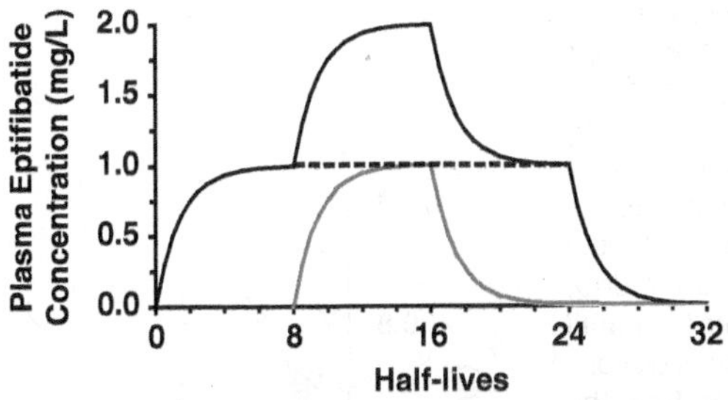

FIGURE 11-5 Situation illustrating that the time to reach a new plateau, whether higher or lower than the previous value, depends only on the half-life of a drug. A plateau concentration of 1 mg/L is reached in approximately 3.3 half-lives after starting a constant infusion of 4 mg/hr of eptifibatide in the patient under consideration. Doubling the infusion rate is like maintaining 4 mg/hr (which would maintain the plateau concentration of 1 mg/L; dotted line) and starting another constant infusion of 4 mg/hr (*colored line*). In approximately 3.3 half-lives, the total eptifibatide concentration rises from 1 mg/L to close to 2 mg/L. Halving an infusion rate of 8 mg/hr is analogous to stopping the supplementary 4 mg/hr infusion. The plasma concentration of eptifibatide returns to the previous plateau concentration of 1 mg/L in approximately 3.3 half-lives. When drug infusion is completely stopped, the concentration falls exponentially toward zero at a rate, again, depending on its half-life. The half-life of eptifibatide is about 2.5 hours. The total time span, 32 half-lives, is then about 80 hours and 3.3 half-lives is 8.25 hours.

1.5 mg/L (comprising 1 mg/L from the first infusion plus 0.5 mg/L from the second one), is achieved in one elimination half-life (2.5 hours), and so on. Clearly, half-life is the sole determinant of the time to go from 1.0 to 2.0 mg/L or from any initial value to a new steady-state value during constant-rate input.

The decline from a high plateau to a low one is likewise related to the half-life. Consider, for example, the events after stopping the supplementary 4-mg/hr infusion rate discussed above. The eptifibatide concentration associated with this supplementary infusion falls to half of the initial value in 1 half-life. In 3.3 half-lives, the total concentration has almost returned to the 1.0-mg/L concentration. In addition, it will take another 3.3 half-lives for most of the eptifibatide to be removed from the body if the original 4-mg/hr infusion is also stopped.

An example of the change in plasma concentration on changing from one infusion rate to another is again demonstrated by data on tissue plasminogen activator in Fig. 11-6 (next page). The half-life is the determinant of the speed of attaining the new steady state. Clearance determines the steady-state concentration.

Bolus Plus Infusion

It takes 8.25 hours of constant infusion of eptifibatide before the plateau concentration is reached in the patient with a 2.5-hour half-life. An even longer time is required for drugs with half-lives greater than that of eptifibatide. Situations sometimes demand that the plateau be reached more rapidly, as is the case clinically for eptifibatide. One solution, as previously stated, is to double the infusion rate for the first half-life. Fig. 11-4 suggests another solution. That is, at the start of an infusion, give a bolus dose equal to the amount desired in the body at plateau. Usually, the bolus dose is a therapeutic dose, and the infusion rate is adjusted to maintain the therapeutic level. When the bolus dose and infusion rate are exactly matched, as in Fig. 11-4, the amounts of drug in the body associated with the two modes of administration are complementary; the gain from the infusion offsets the loss of drug from the bolus.

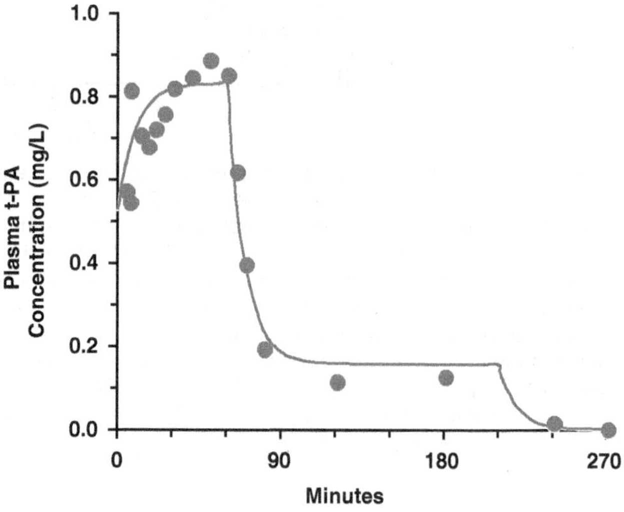

FIGURE 11-6 The plasma concentration of tissue plasminogen activator (t-PA) starts at about 0.6 mg/L and approaches a plateau of 0.8 mg/L following an IV bolus of 10 mg and a constant-rate infusion of 1.6 mg/min for 60 minutes to an individual subject. Subsequently, the plasma concentration drops as the drug infusion is decreased to 0.3 mg/min until 210 minutes when the infusion is discontinued. The time required to go from the first steady state to the second one (0.16 mg/L) depends on the half-life of the drug—6.6 minutes in this subject—as does the time to decline after drug administration is stopped. The line is the best fit of the parameters of an infusion model to the observations (circles). (Adapted from Koster RW, Cohen AF, Kluft C, et al. The pharmacokinetics of double-chain t-PA (duteplase): effects of bolus injection, infusions, and administration by weight in patients with myocardial infarction. *Clin Pharmacol Ther* 1991;50:267–277.)

Now consider two additional situations: The first, shown in Fig. 11-7, is one in which different bolus doses are given at the start of a constant-rate infusion. In case A, drug is infused at a rate of 4 mg/min, following which the plasma concentration rises and reaches a plateau of 1 mg/L in approximately 4 half-lives. In case B, a bolus dose of 15 mg immediately attains, and the infusion rate thereafter maintains the initial concentration. In case C, the bolus dose of 30 mg is excessive, because the rate of loss is initially greater than the rate of infusion; consequently, the concentration falls. This fall continues until the same plateau as in case B is reached. It should be noticed that the time to reach the plateau depends solely on the half-life of the drug. Thus, in case C at 1 half-life, the concentration of 1.5 mg/L, composed of 1 mg/L remaining from the bolus and 0.5 mg/L arising from the infusion, lies midway between the values immediately after the bolus dose and the plateau concentration achieved by the infusion. By 2 half-lives, the concentration of 1.25 mg/L lies 75% of the way toward the plateau. By 3.3 half-lives, only 10% of the initial concentration resulting from the bolus remains (0.2 mg/L) and the concentration from the infused drug is 0.9 mg/L. We are now (1.1 mg/L) within 10% of the plateau. In case D, the bolus dose of 7.5 mg is below the plateau amount. Because the rate of infusion now exceeds the rate of drug elimination, the plasma concentration continuously rises until the same plateau, as in the previous cases, is reached. Once again, the time to approach the plateau is controlled solely by the half-life of the drug.

Case D is demonstrated by t-PA in Fig. 11-6. The bolus dose of 10 mg was insufficient to immediately attain the steady state achieved on infusing 1.6 mg/min. This result is expected from the 6.6-minute half-life in this patient, as the amount in the body at plateau (R_{inf}/k) is 15 mg.

In the second and more common situation, depicted in Fig. 11-8 (p. 212), the same bolus dose and infusion rate of eptifibatide are administered to three patients, A, B, and C, with different clearance and associated half-life values, but with the same volume of distribution. The half-lives in these patients are 2.5, 5, and 7.5 hours, respectively. All patients start with the same amount of drug in the body, and therefore the same

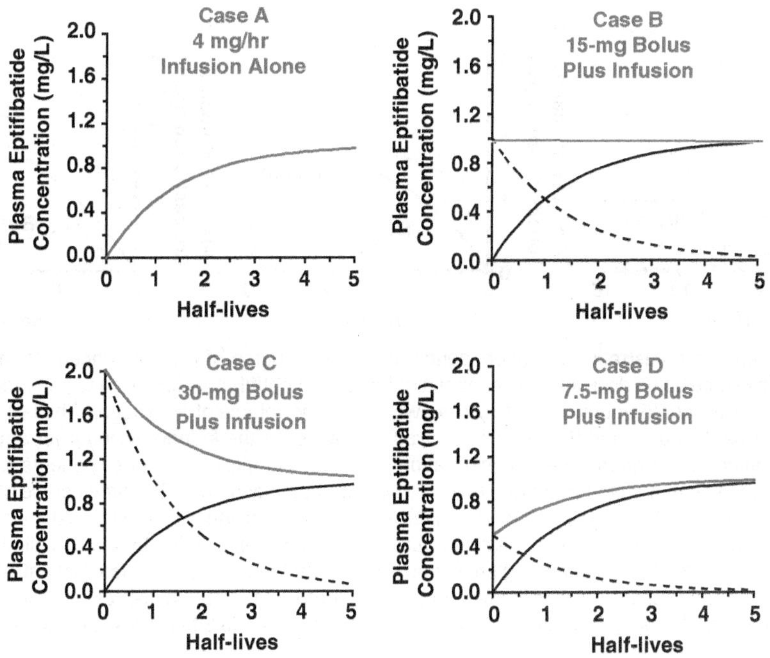

FIGURE 11-7 Situations illustrating that the plateau depends on the infusion rate and not on the initial bolus dose. Whether a bolus dose of eptifibatide is given (cases B–D) or not (case A), at the start of the infusion, the plasma concentrations at the plateau are the same when a given infusion rate is used. The plasma concentration associated with the bolus dose declines exponentially (*dashed line*), whereas the concentration associated with the infusion in all cases rises asymptotically toward plateau (*solid line*), as portrayed by case A. In cases B–D, the observed concentration (*colored line*) is the sum of the two. When not initially achieved by the bolus, it takes approximately 3.3 half-lives to reach 90% of the way between the initial and the plateau value (cases A, C, and D), regardless of whether the initial value is greater or less than the plateau. This is reflected in cases A, C, and D by the observation that at 1 half-life, the plasma concentration lies midway between initial and plateau values. The simulation is based on an 83-kg patient given bolus doses of 15 mg (case B), 30 mg (case C), and 7.5 mg (case D) and an infusion rate of 4 mg/hr.

plasma concentration. In patient A, the initial concentration is maintained because rate of infusion is exactly matched by rate of elimination. Since elimination is slower, the concentration in patient B rises until rate of elimination equals infusion rate. The time to reach this higher plateau value is governed solely by the half-life of the drug in this patient. Thus, by 1 half-life (5 hours), the plasma concentration in patient B is midway between that from the bolus dose and that at plateau. By the time the plateau is reached, the entire bolus dose has been eliminated. Also, it follows from Equation 11-4 that for a given infusion rate, concentration at plateau is inversely proportional to the clearance. This is seen in Fig. 11-8C, where the concentration in patient C at plateau is 50% higher than that in patient B. Patient C eliminates the drug even more slowly than does patient B, resulting in a longer time to reach plateau. Clearly, the time to reach plateau is governed solely by the half-life.

SHORT-TERM INFUSIONS

In many therapeutic settings, drugs are said to be given by intravenous infusion when, in fact, they are intended to be given as intravenous bolus doses. Short-term infusions are used because the incidence of adverse events associated with the sudden and high

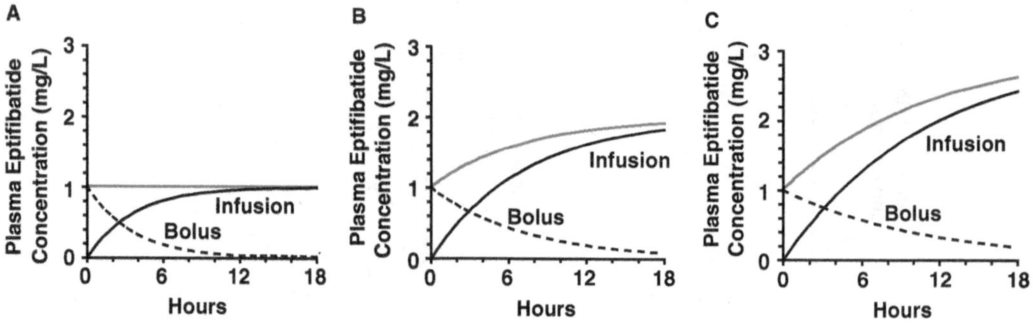

FIGURE 11-8 Situations illustrating the dependence of the time course of plasma concentration on half-life and clearance. The same bolus dose and rate of constant infusion of eptifibatide are given to patients A, B, and C, with half-lives of 2.5, 5, and 7.5 hours, respectively, but with the same volume of distribution. The last two patients have decreased renal function, and therefore decreased clearance, as the kidneys account for a major part of this drug's elimination. Although the initial concentration is the same (1 mg/L) in all three patients (same volume of distribution), the plateau concentration differs inversely with their clearances. The time course of the plasma concentration associated with the bolus (*dotted line*) depends on the individual's half-life, as does the rise in the plasma concentration associated with the constant infusion (*black solid line*). Only when rate of elimination is immediately matched by rate of infusion is the plateau immediately attained and maintained (patient A). Otherwise, the plasma concentration (*colored line*) changes, until after approximately 3.3 half-lives, a plateau is reached (patients B and C). Note for patient C that it would take at least 25 hours (3.3 half-lives) to reach a plateau.

spike concentrations may occur when the rate of administration is too rapid. The antiepileptic drug phenytoin is one example. This poorly soluble drug, with a pK_a of 8.8, is dissolved using a high pH (12) and a high concentration of propylene glycol (40%) in the intravenous dosage form. Slow administration is required to avoid precipitation of the drug in the vein, producing phlebitis, and systemic toxicity produced by high plasma concentrations of propylene glycol. Sometimes, it is an effect of the drug itself that limits the rate of input. An example here is propofol, an intravenous anesthetic agent. When given as a true bolus dose, followed immediately by a maintenance infusion, the very high concentration initially reaching the well-perfused brain, without time to be diluted by distribution to other tissues of the body, produces excessive anesthesia. If the size of the bolus dose is reduced, then the anesthesia is not adequately maintained with time, because the drug moves quickly from brain out into other tissues. To overcome this problem, the loading dose must be given over at least 40 seconds. Trastuzumab, used to treat metastatic breast cancer in patients whose tumors overexpress the epidermal growth factor receptor 2 (HER2) protein, is an example of an antibody (MW = 185,000 g/mol) that produces fever and chills if injected too rapidly. The loading dose of 4 mg/kg is given over a minimum of 90 minutes, and the weekly maintenance dose of 3 mg/kg is given over 30 minutes if the loading dose is tolerated in the 90-minute period of infusion.

PARAMETER VALUES

Clearance is readily determined when both the rate of infusion and the plateau concentration are available, as previously stated. Half-life can be obtained from the terminal decline after an infusion is stopped. Volume of distribution can be estimated from the clearance and the half-life values. These values can also be obtained from data following a short-term infusion even when the plateau is not achieved. As with an intravenous bolus, all that is needed is the total amount infused (dose) and the total area under the curve (AUC), from the start of the infusion until the drug has been completely eliminated from the body. Recall that

$$\text{Rate of elimination} = CL \cdot C \quad \text{Eq. 11-8}$$

On integrating this equation,

$$\text{Amount eliminated} = \text{Dose} = CL \cdot \text{AUC} \quad \text{Eq. 11-9}$$

$$CL = \frac{\text{Dose}}{\text{AUC}} \quad \text{Eq. 11-10}$$

CONSEQUENCE OF SLOW TISSUE DISTRIBUTION

As discussed for an intravenous bolus dose in Chapter 5, the body is more complex than the reservoir portrayed in Fig. 11-2. The approach of the plasma concentration toward steady state during a constant-rate infusion, the time course of the decline after discontinuing an infusion, and the time course of the concentration after a combined bolus dose and constant-rate infusion are often not simple functions of the terminal half-life of the drug, because of slow distribution to and from the tissues.

The intravenous anesthetic agent, propofol, a lipophilic (n-octanol:water partition coefficient of 6760:1) phenol (pK_a of 11), exemplifies what happens when tissue distribution is relatively slow. When infused at a constant rate, the blood concentration rises quickly within the first 20 minutes, and then continues to rise at a slower rate (Fig. 11-9). A model, in which the drug distributes into three pools (Fig. 11-10), helps to explain the following events: the rapid induction of anesthesia even without a bolus

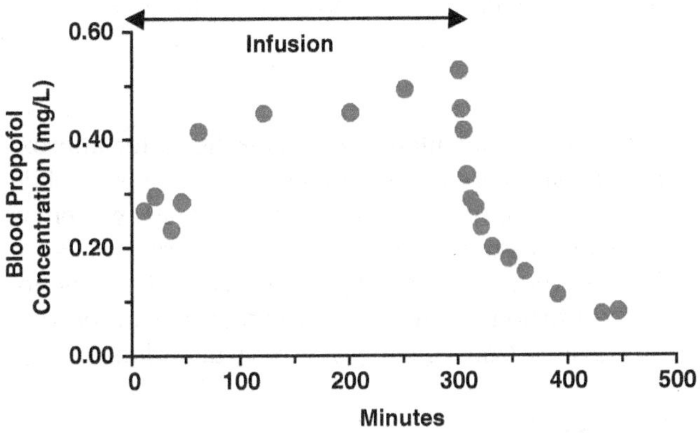

FIGURE 11-9 Blood concentration-time profile of propofol, an intravenous anesthetic agent, following a constant-rate infusion of 1.0 mg/hr/kg for 5 hours (300 minutes) in a patient after coronary artery bypass surgery. Data (*circles*) for a specific intravenous formulation (Diprivan 10) are shown. (Data from Knibbe CAJ, Aarts LP, Kuks PF, et al. Pharmacokinetics and pharmacodynamics of propofol 6% SAZN versus propofol 1% SAZN and Diprivan-10 for short-term sedation following coronary artery bypass surgery. *Eur J Clin Pharmacol* 2000;56:89–95.)

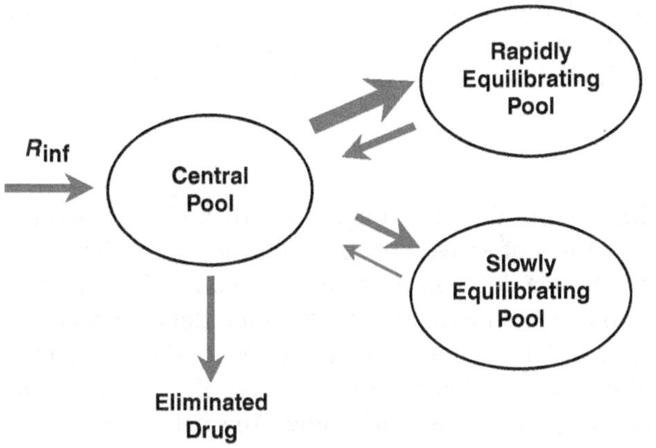

FIGURE 11-10 Model simulating the effect of distribution to tissues on the approach of the plasma concentration of propofol toward steady state following a constant-rate infusion and its decline when the infusion is stopped. Drug distribution in the body is represented by three body pools (or compartments). Drug in the central pool, which includes blood and brain, distributes to and from a rapidly equilibrating pool and a slowly equilibrating pool, which includes fat. The size of the arrows indicates the relative rapidity of the processes: the larger and heavier the arrow, the more rapid the process.

dose and in spite of a 2-day terminal half-life; the need to decrease the input rate when the drug is infused for long periods of time to avoid oversedation; and the increase in recovery time after discontinuance when infused for long periods of time. Each of these events is now considered.

Rapid Induction of Anesthesia

After an intravenous bolus dose, there is very rapid equilibration of propofol (1–3 minutes) between the blood and the very highly perfused brain. Even without a bolus dose, anesthesia develops rapidly because of this rapid equilibration.

Decrease in Infusion Rate on Chronic Administration

The time for equilibration between blood and the rapidly equilibrating pool, including muscle tissue, takes more time than does equilibration of propofol between brain and blood; this explains the slow rise in the concentration observed in Fig. 11-9. Equilibration of drug in the slowly equilibrating tissue, which includes fat, with that in blood takes much longer and is not shown in Fig. 11-9. As a consequence of the gradual buildup in this slowly equilibrating large pool in fat when the infusion is maintained, there is a decreased long-term net rate of movement of drug out of blood into the tissues, which in turn results in a slow but continuous rise in the blood concentration on approach to the plateau. Accordingly, when the drug is used for long periods of time, the rate of infusion needs to be reduced at later times. Failure to do so may result in excessive depth of anesthesia due to very high blood, and hence brain, concentrations of the drug.

Recovery From Anesthesia

Discontinuation of the infusion rate after the maintenance of anesthesia for approximately 1 hour, or for sedation in an intensive care unit for 1 day, results in a prompt decrease (within a few minutes) in the blood propofol concentration and rapid awakening. Longer infusions (e.g., 10 days of sedation within an intensive care unit) result in accumulation of significant tissue stores of propofol, particularly in fat, so that the reduction in circulating propofol on stopping the infusion is slowed by the greater rate of return of drug from these slowly equilibrating tissues. Consequently, recovery takes longer.

PHARMACODYNAMIC CONSIDERATIONS

Although an intravenous infusion provides a highly controlled means of delivering drug to the systemic circulation, drug response depends on exposure–response relationships as well. Let us examine a few of these additional considerations.

Onset of Response

Onset or time course of the development of drug response depends on both the pharmacokinetics and the pharmacodynamics of a given drug. As discussed in Chapter 9, there are many reasons why drugs show a delay in response, including slow specific distribution to the site of action (pharmacokinetic in nature) and a delayed relationship between the measured response and the actual measured effect of the drug (pharmacodynamic in nature). Under these circumstances, the addition of an intravenous bolus dose to constant-rate therapy may be of marginal value. An example is that of leuprolide acetate implant, used in treating advanced prostatic cancer. The drug inhibits the formation of both follicle-stimulating hormone and luteinizing hormone, which subsequently reduce the levels of testosterone and dihydrotestosterone to below castration values. However, because of the relatively slow kinetics of these physiologic systems, it takes 2–4 weeks for the pharmacodynamic effect to fully develop. Giving a bolus to start therapy quickly is consequently of little value. Furthermore, treatment often continues for years; there is no urgency for immediately obtaining the response.

Response on Stopping an Infusion

The expected time course of response after stopping an infusion depends on both the pharmacokinetics and the pharmacodynamics of a drug as well. Recall that a prolongation of effect occurs, relative to the disappearance of the drug, when the drug has a delayed effect (e.g., warfarin, Fig. 9-4); the initial response is in Region 3 of the concentration–response relationship (e.g., succinylcholine, Fig. 9-7); or the drug reacts irreversibly with a receptor aspirin, (Fig. 9-9), so that the effect continues until new receptor is formed, a period of time much longer than that required for removal of drug from the body.

This chapter has been devoted to constant-rate input. In the next chapter, we turn to the much more common situation of regimens involving the administration of fixed doses given at regular intervals.

SUMMARY

- On administering a drug at a constant rate, the amount in the body and the plasma concentration rise until the rate of elimination equals the rate of input and a plateau (steady state) is reached.
- The steady-state plasma drug concentration depends on the rate of input and clearance. By definition, the rate of elimination is the product of clearance and concentration.
- The steady-state amount of drug in the body depends on the rate of input and the elimination rate constant (or half-life as $t_{1/2} = 0.693/k$).
- The approach to steady state is a function of the half-life of the drug, as is the decline after input is stopped.
- The infusion rate needed to maintain the amount in the body from an intravenous bolus dose is the product of the elimination rate constant and the bolus dose ($k \cdot$ Dose).
- The intravenous bolus dose needed at the start of a given rate of infusion to achieve the steady-state amount in the body is equal to the infusion rate divided by the elimination rate constant (R_{inf}/k). It can also be calculated knowing the steady-state plasma concentration and the volume of distribution ($V \cdot C_{ss}$).
- Slow distribution to tissues can affect the onset of action, the infusion rate needed to maintain drug effect chronically, and the recovery from drug effects when the infusion is discontinued, as illustrated by the intravenous anesthetic agent propofol.
- Many drugs are given by short-term infusions with the intent to give a bolus dose, but avoid or reduce the adverse events associated with too rapid administration.
- A delayed onset of action during an infusion or a prolonged response, relative to its systemic exposure, after stopping an infusion may be explained by the kinetics either of the drug (pharmacokinetics) or of the systems within the body that the drug affects (pharmacodynamics), whichever is the rate-limiting step.

KEY TERM REVIEW

Bolus dose
Bolus plus infusion
Constant-rate release device
Duration of infusion
Intravenous infusion
Onset of response
Plateau
Plateau plasma concentration
Rate of infusion
Rate of input
Steady state
Steady-state amount in the body
Steady-state plasma concentration
Time to reach plateau

KEY RELATIONSHIPS

$$A_{ss} = \frac{R_{inf}}{k}$$

$$C_{ss} = \frac{R_{inf}}{CL}$$

$$A_{inf} = A_{ss} - A_{ss} \cdot e^{-kt} = A_{ss}\,(1 - e^{-kt})$$

$$C_{inf} = C_{ss}\,(1 - e^{-kt})$$

STUDY PROBLEMS

1. Which *one* of the following statements is *incorrect*?
   a. At any time during an intravenous infusion, the rate of change in the amount of drug in the body is the difference between the rates of drug infusion and elimination.
   b. The time to reach 75% of the plateau concentration depends on the rate at which a drug is infused.
   c. All drugs having the same clearance reach the same plateau concentration when administered at the same infusion rate.
   d. All drugs having the same volume of distribution and clearance values have the same amount in the body at plateau when administered at the same infusion rate.
   e. The time required to go from one plateau concentration to another when the infusion rate is abruptly changed to another value depends solely on the half-life of the drug.
2. Which of the following statements is (are) *correct* for a drug with a clearance of 10 L/hr and a 5-hour half-life?
   I. When given by intravenous infusion at a rate of 5 mg/hr, the plateau concentration expected is 1.0 mg/L.
   II. The time required to reach 50% of the plateau value when given by a constant-rate intravenous infusion is 2.5 hours.
   III. The plasma concentration expected after distribution equilibrium is established (assume less than 15 minutes and that virtually no drug is eliminated during this time) after a 40-mg intravenous bolus dose is 0.80 mg/L.

   A. I only
   B. II only
   C. III only
   D. I and II
   E. I and III
   F. II and III
   G. All
   H. None

3. An anesthetic drug has a high affinity for, but a slow distribution to, fat and exhibits rapid distribution to the tissue (brain) where the site of action is located. The concentration in the brain producing a given level of anesthesia does not change with time. Which *one* of the response characteristics below would you expect this anesthetic to definitely *not* exhibit when infused at a fixed constant rate that generally produces anesthesia?
   a. A rapid induction of anesthesia.
   b. A prolonged recovery time when the drug is discontinued when it has been infused for long periods of time. The longer the infusion time, the longer is the recovery time.
   c. The need for a decrease in the infusion rate with time if the same level of anesthesia is to be maintained.
   d. All other factors remaining the same, the greater the affinity of fat for the drug, the shorter will be the recovery time after a 24-hour infusion.
4. Briefly answer each of the following questions that apply to *constant-rate infusion conditions*.
   a. Does the time to reach a given fraction of the plateau concentration depend on the rate of infusion?
   b. For a given infusion rate will a decrease in clearance of a drug in a patient increase the plateau concentration but not the time to reach it?
   c. Do drugs with the same clearance generally reach their respective plateau concentrations at the same time?
   d. Can the amount of drug in the body at plateau be the same when drugs with different clearance values are infused at the same rate?
   e. Does the time to go from one plateau concentration to another depend solely on the half-life of the drug?
5. In the graphs in Fig. 11-11 (next page), on the left are three multiple infusion rate regimens of a drug, with time expressed in half-lives. Sketch in the anticipated plasma drug concentration–time profiles (concentration at each half-life) on the respective graphs on the right. Appropriately scale the concentration axes of the three graphs. The total clearance of the drug is 0.1 L/min. Hint: Had any particular infusion rate been continued, it would ultimately reach a steady-state concentration given by Infusion Rate/*CL*.
6. Fig. 11-12 (p. 219) was published in the literature for the concentration–time profile of a drug in a patient during a period of time when the drug was infused intravenously at one constant rate, then at a second lower constant rate until the infusion was discontinued altogether.
   a. Knowing published values for clearance (20 L/hr) and volume of distribution (28.8 L), do you agree with the time scale used? To help with your analysis of the graph, the specific data points in the graph are listed in Table 11-4 (p. 219).
   b. Determine the most likely rates (mg/hr) of the two constant-rate infusions.
   c. Determine the intravenous bolus dose (in mg) that would be needed to achieve a concentration of 50 μg/L immediately.
7. A drug is administered intravenously as a bolus of 500 mg followed immediately by a constant infusion of 120 mg/hr for 16 hours. Estimate the values of volume of distribution, half-life, and clearance from the data in Table 11-5 (p. 219) and in Fig. 11-13 (p. 220). The AUC is 202.28 mg-hr/L.
8. Nifedipine is administered for management of hypertension and angina. The drug, which has a half-life of 2 hours, is available in several oral modified-release products. One of these dosage forms is Nifedipine GITS (Gastrointestinal Therapeutic System, Procardia XL Extended Release Tablet). This modified-release dosage form

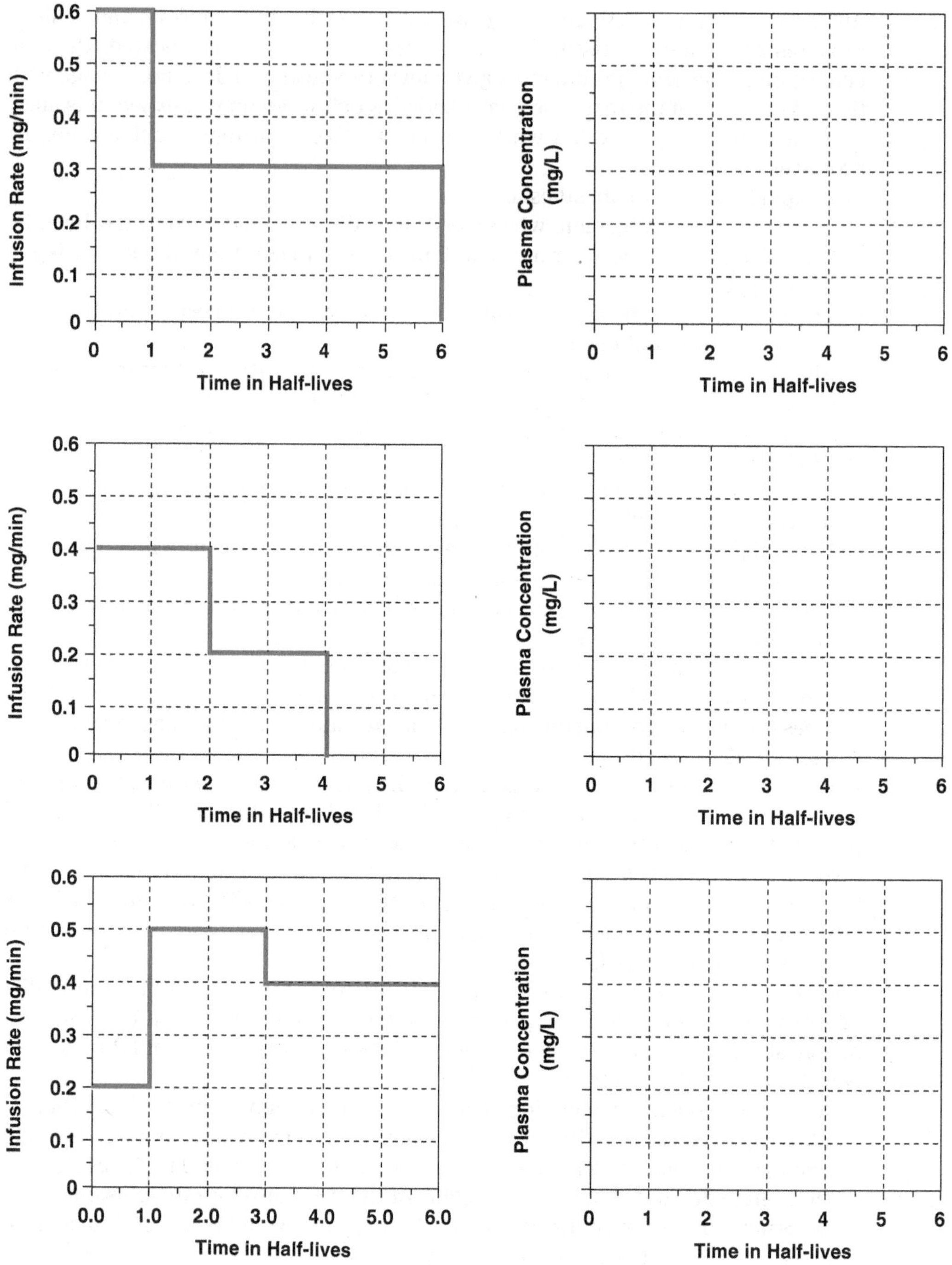
Infusion Rate (mg/min)
0.6
0.5
0.4
0.3
0.2
0.1
0
0 1 2 3 4 5 6
Time in Half-lives
Plasma Concentration (mg/L)
0 1 2 3 4 5 6
Time in Half-lives
Infusion Rate (mg/min)
0.6
0.5
0.4
0.3
0.2
0.1
0
0 1 2 3 4 5 6
Time in Half-lives
Plasma Concentration (mg/L)
0 1 2 3 4 5 6
Time in Half-lives
Infusion Rate (mg/min)
0.6
0.5
0.4
0.3
0.2
0.1
0
0.0 1.0 2.0 3.0 4.0 5.0 6.0
Time in Half-lives
Plasma Concentration (mg/L)
0 1 2 3 4 5 6
Time in Half-lives

FIGURE 11–11

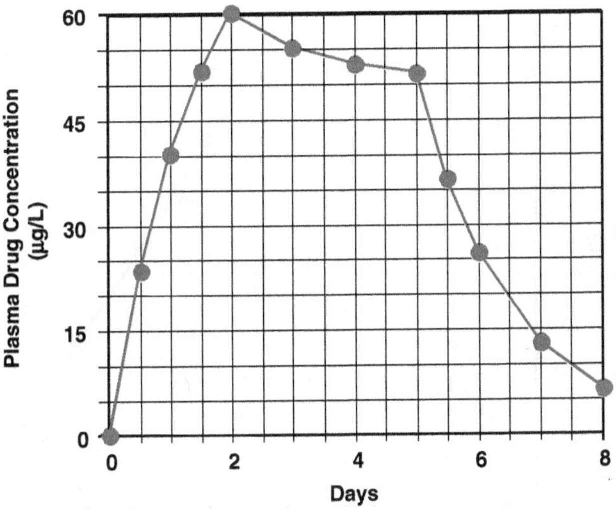

FIGURE 11-12

TABLE 11-4 | Plasma Concentration During and Following Constant Rate Infusion of the Drug (Data Shown in Fig. 11-12)

Time (days)	0	0.5	1	1.5	2	3	4	5	5.5	6	7	8
Plasma drug concentration (μg/L)	0	23.4	40	51.7	60	55	52.5	51.3	36.2	25.7	12.8	6.4

Table 11-5 | Plasma Concentration of a Drug During and After a Constant-Rate Infusion (120 mg/hr) for 16 Hours

Time (hr)	Plasma Concentration (mg/L)
During Drug Infusion	
0.083	5.0
2	6.1
4	6.9
6	7.6
8	8.1
12	8.8
16	9.3
Postinfusion	
2	7.3
4	5.7
6	4.5
8	3.5
12	2.2
16	1.4

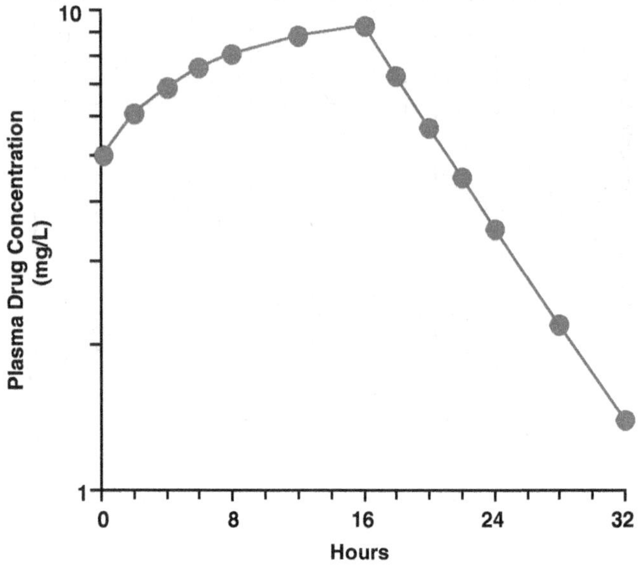

FIGURE 11-13

is taken once daily and releases drug at an essentially constant rate over 24 hours. The difference between single doses of the conventional immediate-release capsule (two 10-mg capsules) and the 60-mg modified-release tablet (*colored line*) is demonstrated by the plasma concentration–time profiles in Fig. 11-14.

a. Given that the clearance of nifedipine is 7 mL/min/kg, estimate the rate of input of nifedipine into the systemic circulation from the apparent plateau observations for the modified-release product (*in color*) in Fig. 11-14. Use a steady-state concentration of 40 μg/L and a 70-kg body weight.
b. Determine the total amount delivered systemically from the GITS formulation over a period of 24 hours of delivery at the rate calculated in part a.
c. The oral bioavailability of an immediate-release dosage form (*black curve*) is about 50%. Is the bioavailability from the oral modified-release dosage form in approximate agreement with this number?

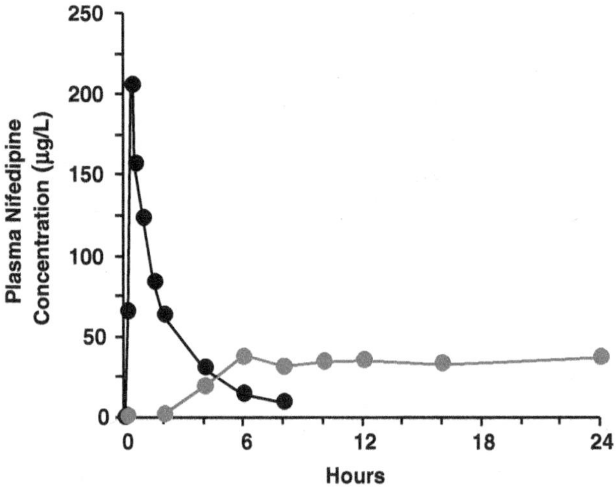

FIGURE 11-14

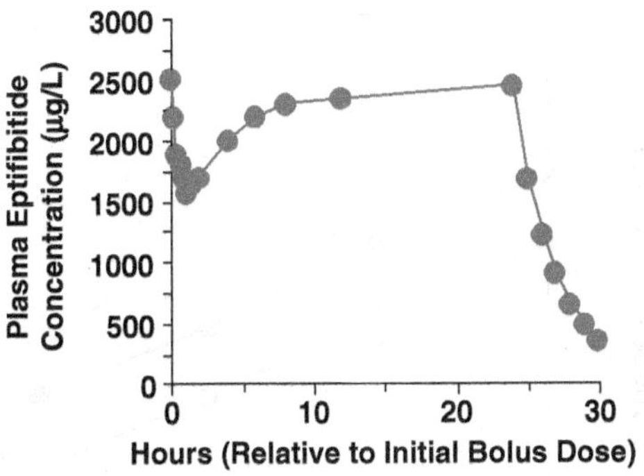

FIGURE 11-15 Plasma eptifibitide concentration in an 80-kg patient receiving a 250 µg/kg intravenous bolus dose, immediately followed by a 3 µg/kg/min constant-rate infusion of the drug for 24 hours. (Adapted from data in Gilchrist IC, O'Shea JC, Kosoglou T, et al. Pharmacodynamics and pharmacokinetics of higher-dose, double-dose eptifibitide in percutaneous coronary intervention. *Circulation* 2001;104:406–411.)

d. Briefly discuss your findings with respect to where nifedipine is released along the gastrointestinal tract, and whether you think the gastrointestinal tract is highly permeable to this drug.

9. Fig. 11-15 above shows the plasma eptifibitide concentration resulting from an intravenous 250-µg/kg bolus dose, followed immediately by an intravenous infusion of 3 µg/kg/min to an 80-kg patient. The half-life of the terminal phase is 2.2 hours.
   a. What is the approximate value of clearance of this drug?
   b. Determine the volume of distribution (V) for this drug.
   c. What would the steady-state concentration of the drug be if the infusion rate were halved?
   d. Eptifibatide shows two-compartment distribution characteristics. How can one explain the dip in the plasma concentration–time curve at about 0.5–8 hours when the drug is given as stated above?

10. Droperidol, a butyrophenone derivative, has been used for the prevention and treatment of nausea and vomiting in postoperative patients and in patients undergoing chemotherapy. Droperidol is currently administered intravenously and intramuscularly, both invasive procedures. The oral route creates a problem for patients who are nauseous or vomiting, a common occurrence with chemotherapy. To overcome this problem, Gupta et al. (1992) evaluated a continuous-release rectal drug-delivery system as a means of achieving therapy for an extended period. Table 11-6 lists the mean plasma concentrations of droperidol obtained following use of this device, designed to deliver drug at a constant rate for 15 hours. Fig. 11-16A (next page) shows the data (colored line) in graphical form. Fig. 11-16B shows the data after 24 hours on a semilogarithmic plot. The results are compared with those following a 24-hr constant-rate (0.125 mg/hr) intravenous infusion (black line). The rectal device contained a total of 3-mg droperidol. No drug was found in the recovered device.

Table 11-6 | Mean Plasma Droperidol Concentrations (mg/L) following an Intravenous Infusion and the Use of a Rectal Device in Eight Subjects

Time (hr)	0	0.5	2	4	6	8	10	14	18	24	26	28	30
IV Infusion	0	0.90	1.80	2.60	2.50	2.50	2.70	2.70	2.90	2.90	1.40	0.61	0.30
Rectal Device	0	0	0.49	0.99	1.83	1.84	1.93	1.52	1.43	1.41	0.65	0.29	0.14

Adapted from data in Gupta SK, Southam M, Hwang S. Pharmacokinetics of droperidol in healthy volunteers following intravenous infusion and rectal administration from an osmotic drug delivery module. *Pharm Res* 1992;9:694–696.

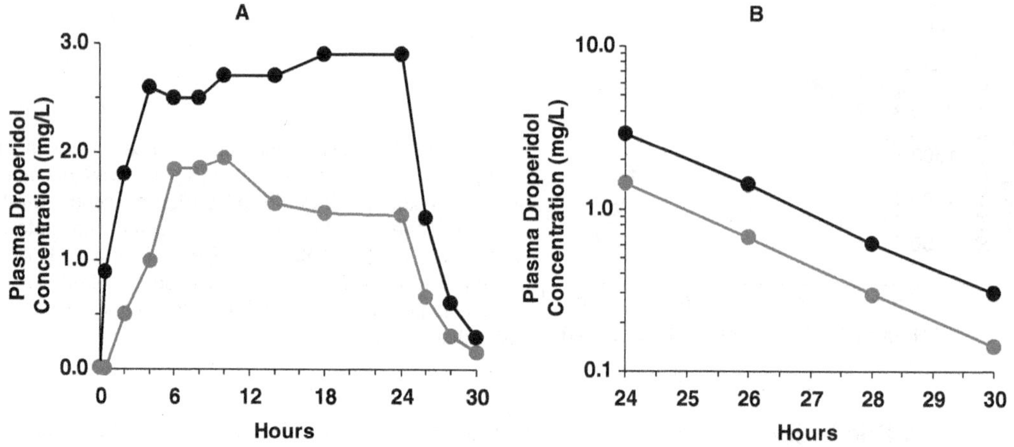

FIGURE 11-16

a. From the plasma concentration data after stopping the IV infusion at 24 hours, estimate the elimination half-life of droperidol. Also comment on whether you think a one-compartment or 2-compartment model best describes this drug's distribution characteristics.
b. Calculate the AUC up to the last time point for both routes of administration using the data in Table 11-6 and the trapezoidal approximation (Appendix D).
c. Calculate the clearance of droperidol.
d. What is the volume of distribution of droperidol?
e. The plasma to blood concentration ratio of droperidol is 1.0. Using a hepatic blood flow of 1.35 L/hr, can the decreased bioavailability (F) of the rectal device be solely explained by the hepatic first-pass effect? Much of the rectal blood supply is drained into the portal system.
f. Comment on the delivery of droperidol by the rectal device. Do you think it was pharmacokinetically successful?

CHAPTER 12

Multiple-Dose Regimens

OBJECTIVES

The reader will be able to:

- Define the meaning of the following words and phrases: accumulation index, acquired resistance, average level at plateau, dose dumping, drug accumulation, fluctuation, loading dose, maintenance dose, modified-release product, multiple-dose regimen, plateau, priming dose, relative fluctuation, trough concentration.
- Predict the plasma concentration–time profile following a fixed dose and dosing interval regimen of a drug when given its plasma concentration–time profile after a single dose.
- Predict the extent of drug accumulation for a given regimen of fixed dose and dosing interval.
- Explain why the time for the amount in the body to reach plateau on a multiple-dose regimen depends only on the half-life for a drug showing linear kinetics and rapid distribution.
- Discuss the rationale behind a loading dose, and calculate the maintenance dose needed to maintain the same peak amount in the body, knowing the half-life, the loading dose, and the dosing interval.
- Calculate the loading dose when the maintenance dose, half-life, and dosing interval are given.
- Offer examples of drugs for which the oral dosage regimen is primarily determined by its half-life and therapeutic index.
- Discuss the use of modified-release products to develop more convenient dosage regimens.
- Explain why the time for the response to a drug to stabilize when the patient is on a multiple-dose regimen is sometimes governed more by its pharmacodynamics than by its pharmacokinetics. Give two examples illustrating this situation.
- Discuss how tolerance to either the desired or adverse effects of a drug can impact the optimal design and use of multiple-dose regimens.
- Give an example of a situation that requires intermittent, rather than continual, drug administration for optimal therapy.

The previous chapter dealt with constant-rate regimens. Although these regimens possess many desirable features, they are not the most common ones. The more common approach to the attainment and maintenance of chronic drug therapy is to give multiple discrete doses. This chapter covers the pharmacokinetic and, to some degree, pharmacodynamic principles associated with the establishment of appropriate multiple-dose regimens. Emphasis is on oral administration, the commonest route for many small molecular weight drugs, although the principles apply equally to other extravascular routes of administration and to large molecular weight protein drugs. Also covered is the design and application of regimens using modified-release dosage forms.

PRINCIPLES OF DRUG ACCUMULATION

Drugs are most commonly prescribed to be taken on a fixed dose, fixed time interval basis, such as 20 mg once daily or 50 mg three times a day (every 8 hours). Associated with this kind of repetitive administration, the plasma concentration and amount in the body fluctuate and, similar to an infusion, generally rise toward a plateau.

To appreciate what happens when such regimens are taken, consider the plasma concentration–time data over 120 hours (5 days) in Table 12-1, also displayed in Fig. 12-1, following the oral administration of a single 200-mg dose of a drug. This drug is relatively slowly eliminated and is completely absorbed. Because it is very rapidly absorbed, the peak concentration occurs at the first time of measurement—1 hour after administration. The intention is to give the same dose of this drug once daily, and we wish to predict the anticipated concentration–time profile over the first 5 days. To do this, we expect the profile associated with each dose to be the same as that following the first dose, except that each profile is displaced in time by the number of days since the first dose was given, as listed in Table 12-1 and shown as black dashed lines

Table 12-1 | Plasma Concentrations of a Drug Following a Regimen of 200 mg Once Daily for 5 Days

Time After First Dose (hr)	Plasma Concentration Associated With Each Dose (mg/L)					Total Concentration (mg/L)
	1st Dose	2nd Dose	3rd Dose	4th Dose	5th Dose	
0	0					0
1	9.6					9.6
12	6.1					6.1
24	3.7	0				3.7
25	3.5	9.6				13.1
36	2.2	6.1				8.3
48	1.35	3.7	0			5.05
49	1.30	3.5	9.6			14.4
60	0.82	2.2	6.1			9.12
72	0.50	1.35	3.7	0		5.55
73	0.47	1.30	3.5	9.6		14.87
84	0.30	0.82	2.2	6.1		9.42
96	0.18	0.50	1.35	3.7	0	5.73
97	0.17	0.47	1.30	3.5	9.6	15.04
108	0.11	0.30	0.82	2.2	6.1	9.53
120	0.07	0.18	0.50	1.35	3.7	5.80

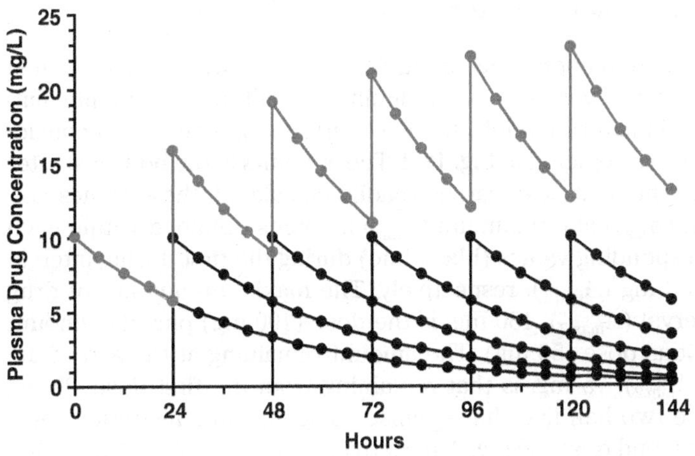

FIGURE 12-1 Accumulation on approach to plateau. When the plasma concentration–time profile following a single dose of drug is known, the anticipated profile following repetitive administration of a fixed dose of drug at regular intervals can be estimated by replicating the single-dose profile after each new dose (*black curves*) and summing at each time the resultant concentrations associated with each dose. The result (*colored curve*) is a typical saw-tooth profile rising toward a plateau. The data used to generate these profiles are given in Table 12-1.

in Fig. 12-1. The expected plasma concentration at each time (colored solid line) is the sum of the concentrations then associated with each of the doses. These total concentrations are listed in the last column of Table 12-1. For example, the concentration at 1 hour after the second dose (25 hours since the first dose) is the sum of that remaining from the first dose at 25 hours (3.5 mg/L) plus that associated with the second dose at 1 hour after dosing (9.6 mg/L), or 13.1 mg/L. Similarly, the concentration at 12 hours after the fifth dose, or 108 hours (4 × 24 + 12) after the first dose, is given by:

$$\text{Total } C_5(12\text{ hr}) = \begin{matrix} C_5(12\text{ hr}) + & C_4(36\text{ hr}) + & C_3(60\text{ hr}) + & C_2(84\text{ hr}) + & C_1(108\text{ hr}) \\ 6.1 \quad + & 2.2 \quad + & 0.82 \quad + & 0.30 \quad + & 0.11 \end{matrix}$$

$$= 9.53 \text{ mg / L}$$

where the subscript denotes the dose number and the time in parentheses denotes the time since that dose was administered.

Several points are worth noting. First, clear evidence of **accumulation** in the plasma concentration is seen resulting in a characteristic rising saw-tooth profile, showing **fluctuation** in concentration within each dosing interval. This accumulation occurs because there is some drug left in the body from previous doses. Second, accumulation continues until a **plateau** concentration is reached, after which time there is no further increase in it from one dosing interval to the next. Analysis of the data in Table 12-1 shows that the lack of further increase occurs because by that time—about 4 days in the current example—virtually nothing is left in the body from the first dose. Indeed, appreciable amounts remain from only the last 3–4 doses. This pattern repeats itself for each subsequent dosing interval no matter how long the drug might be given. Lastly, this calculation requires no knowledge of any pharmacokinetic parameter. All that is needed is the profile after a single dose, regardless of its shape or complexity as long as the drug exhibits linear kinetics. Generally speaking, linear kinetics occurs *when the rate of a process is directly proportional to the level of the variable driving the process.* For example, metabolism is linear when the rate of formation of a metabolite varies in direct proportion to the concentration of the drug being metabolized. Sometimes, the kinetics of a drug changes with dose and the duration of therapy, a topic that is beyond the scope of this book.

We now consider a model for calculating the level of a drug in the body *at any time after any number of intravenous bolus doses.*

Maxima and Minima on Accumulation to the Plateau

To appreciate further the phenomenon of accumulation, consider what happens when a 100-mg bolus dose is given intravenously every elimination half-life. To simplify matters, we again start with administration into the well-stirred reservoir model considered in Fig. 5-3. The events are depicted in Fig. 12-2. The amounts in the body just after each dose and just before the next dose can be readily calculated; these values correspond to the maximum (A_{max}) and minimum (A_{min}) amounts obtained within each dosing interval. The corresponding values (black line) during the first dosing interval are 100 mg ($A_{max,1}$) and 50 mg ($A_{min,1}$), respectively. The maximum amount of drug in the second dosing interval ($A_{max,2}$), 150 mg, is the dose (100 mg) plus the amount remaining from the previous dose (50 mg). The amount remaining at the end of the second dosing interval ($A_{min,2}$), 75 mg, is that remaining from the first dose, 25 mg (100 mg × ½ × ½, because two half-lives have elapsed since its administration) plus that remaining from the second dose, 50 mg. Alternatively, the value, 75 mg, may simply be calculated by recognizing that one-half of the amount just after the second dose, 150 mg, remains at the end of that dosing interval. Upon repeating this procedure, it is readily seen that drug accumulation, viewed in terms of either maximum or minimum amounts in the body, continues until a limit is reached. At the limit, in each dosing interval, the amount lost equals the amount gained, the dose. In this example, the maximum and the minimum amounts in the body at steady state are 200 and 100 mg, respectively. This must be so because the difference between the maximum and minimum amounts is the dose, 100 mg, and because at the end of the interval, 1 half-life, the amount remaining must be one-half that at the beginning of the interval.

Recall, following a constant-rate input, a *plateau* is reached when rate of elimination matches rate of input. Then the level of drug in the body is constant as long as the input rate is maintained. With discrete dosing, the level is not constant within a dosing interval, but the values at a given time within the interval are the same from one dosing interval to another, that is, *at that given time between consecutive intervals, the amount lost equals the amount gained.* The term **plateau** is also applied to this interdosing steady-state condition.

The foregoing considerations can be expanded for the more general situation in which a drug is given at a dosing interval, τ, not equal to the half-life. The general

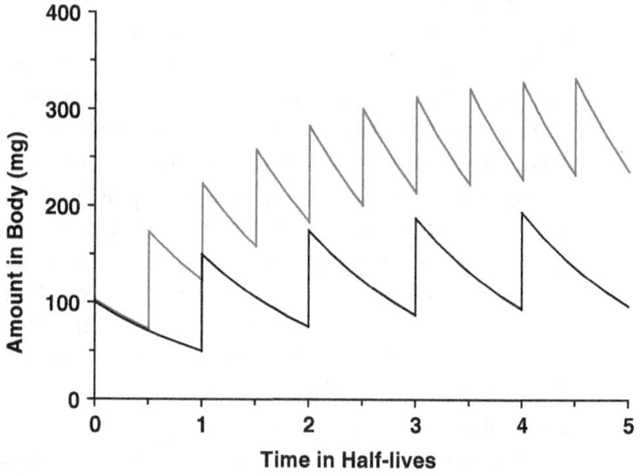

FIGURE 12-2 Dosing frequency controls the degree of drug accumulation. When an intravenous bolus dose (100 mg) is administered once every half of a half-life (*colored line*), the accumulation is much greater than when the same bolus dose is administered once every half-life (*black line*). Note that time is expressed in half-life units.

equations are derived in Appendix E for the maximum and minimum amounts in the body after the Nth dose ($A_{max,N}$; $A_{min,N}$) and at steady state ($A_{max,ss}$; $A_{min,ss}$). These are

$$\text{Maximum amount in body after the } N\text{th dose, } A_{max,N} = \text{Dose}\left[\frac{1-e^{-N\cdot k\cdot\tau}}{1-e^{-k\cdot\tau}}\right] = \text{Dose}\left[\frac{1-e^{-N\cdot k\cdot\tau}}{\text{Fraction lost in interval}}\right] \qquad \textbf{Eq. 12-1}$$

$$\text{Minimum amount in body after the } N\text{th dose, } A_{min,N} = A_{max,N}\cdot e^{-k\cdot\tau} \qquad \textbf{Eq. 12-2}$$

$$\text{Maximum amount in body at steady state, } A_{max,ss} = \frac{\text{Dose}}{(1-e^{-k\cdot\tau})} = \frac{\text{Dose}}{\text{Fraction lost in interval}} \qquad \textbf{Eq. 12-3}$$

$$\text{Minimum amount in body at steady state, } A_{min,ss} = A_{max,ss}\cdot e^{-k\cdot\tau} = A_{max,ss} - \text{Dose} \qquad \textbf{Eq. 12-4}$$

Recall from Chapter 5 that the function $e^{-k\cdot t}$ is the fraction of the initial amount remaining in the body at time t. So that $e^{-k\cdot\tau}$ is the fraction of drug remaining at the end of the dosing interval τ, and therefore $1 - e^{-k\cdot\tau}$ is the fraction of drug lost during that interval. Similarly, the amount in the body at the end of a dosing interval τ of a multiple-dose regimen ($A_{min,N}$), frequently called the **trough** value, is obtained by multiplying the corresponding maximum amount by $e^{-k\cdot\tau}$, that is, $A_{min,N} = A_{max,N} \cdot e^{-k\cdot\tau}$ and $A_{min,ss} = A_{max,ss} \cdot e^{-k\cdot\tau}$.

The corresponding values for the plasma concentration are obtained by dividing the equations above by the volume of distribution of the drug. Returning to the example in Table 12-1, which approximates an IV bolus situation, the half-life of this drug, gained from a semilogarithmic plot of the plasma concentration after the single dose, is 16.7 hours, and its volume of distribution is 20 L. Given this information, it is readily seen that the maximum and minimum concentrations anticipated at plateau, $C_{max,ss}$ and $C_{min,ss}$, when a 200-mg dose is given once daily (every 24 hours) are, by substitution

$$C_{max,ss} = \frac{A_{max,ss}}{V} = \frac{200\text{ mg}}{20L\times 1-e^{-(0.693/16.7\text{hr})\times 24\text{hr}}} = 15.82\text{ mg/L}$$

$$C_{min,ss} = \frac{A_{min,ss}}{V} = \frac{200\text{ mg}\times e^{-(0.693/16.7\text{hr})\times 24\text{hr}}}{20L\times 1-e^{-(0.693/16.7\text{hr})\times 24\text{hr}}} = 5.82\text{ mg/L}$$

Notice that the previously calculated maximum and minimum values after the fifth dose (15.0 and 5.8 mg/L, Table 12-1) are very close to the correspondingly predicted maximum and minimum plateau concentrations, indicating that for all practical purposes (≥90%, as with constant-rate input) a plateau is anticipated to be reached by day 5 of dosing for this drug. Also, it is apparent that Equation 12-3, upon dividing by V, offers a rapid way of calculating the maximum exposure, and often the maximum response (desired or adverse) likely to occur with a given dosage regimen when response tracks plasma concentration, once the half-life (or value of k) and volume of distribution of a drug following a single dose are known.

Equations 12-1 to 12-4 apply only to intravascular bolus administration. They are reasonable approximations following extravascular administration when, as in the above example, absorption is complete and rapid relative to elimination. The next discussion deals with a less restrictive view of accumulation, which applies to all routes of administration.

Average Level at Plateau

In many respects, the accumulation of drugs administered in multiple doses is the same as that observed following a constant-rate IV infusion. The average amount in the body at plateau is readily calculated using the steady-state concept: Average *rate in* must equal average *rate out.* The average rate in is $F \cdot \text{Dose}/\tau$, where F is the bioavailability of the drug. The average rate out is $k \cdot A_{av,ss}$, where $A_{av,ss}$ is the average amount of drug in the body over the dosing interval, τ, at plateau. Therefore,

$$\frac{F \cdot \text{Dose}}{\tau} = k \cdot A_{av,ss} \qquad \textbf{Eq. 12-5}$$

or

$$\frac{F \cdot \text{Dose}}{\tau} = CL \cdot C_{av,ss} \qquad \textbf{Eq. 12-6}$$

where $C_{av,ss}$ is the average plasma concentration at plateau. Since $k = 0.693/t_{1/2}$, it also follows from Equation 12-5 that

$$A_{av,ss} = 1.44 \cdot F \cdot \text{Dose} \cdot \left(\frac{t_{1/2}}{\tau} \right) \qquad \textbf{Eq. 12-7}$$

while rearranging Equation 12-6 yields

$$C_{av,ss} = \frac{F \cdot \text{Dose}}{CL \cdot \tau} \qquad \textbf{Eq. 12-8}$$

These are fundamental relationships; they show how the average amount in the body at steady state depends on rate of administration (Dose/τ), bioavailability, and half-life, and how the corresponding average concentration depends on the first two factors and clearance. Returning to the first example, with a half-life of 16.7 hours (or 0.693 day) and $\tau = 1$ day, the average amount in the body at plateau is 200 mg. This amount lies approximately midway between the maximum and minimum amounts of 316 and 116 mg (calculated by multiplying the respective concentrations by the volume of distribution, 20 L). Notice also that, as expected, the difference between the maximum and minimum amounts is the dose, in this case 200 mg. That $A_{av,ss}$ = Dose in this example is because the half-life is 0.693 of the dosing interval. If, for example, $F = 0.5$, or the dosing interval had been changed from 1 day to 12 hours, thereby doubling the frequency of administration, then clearly $A_{av,ss}$ would no longer equal the Dose.

Drug accumulation is not a phenomenon that implicitly depends on the property of a drug, nor are there drugs that are cumulative and others that are not. *Accumulation, particularly the extent of it, is a result of the frequency of administration relative to half-life of the drug* ($t_{1/2}/\tau$ or $1/k\tau$), as shown in Fig. 12-2. Here, we see that by halving the dosing interval from 1 half-life to one-half of a half-life, the extent of accumulation has doubled. Notice, however, that the time for the trough concentrations to approach the plateau has not changed.

For convenience and to assure adherence to a regimen, drugs (except for many protein drugs) are commonly given once or twice a day, with three and four times daily being less desirable. As a consequence, extensive drug accumulation is more common for those drugs with half-lives greater than 1 day and is particularly noticeable when the half-life of the drug is 1 week or longer. Conversely, drugs with half-lives less than 2 hours hardly accumulate at all even when given three or four times daily.

Rate of Accumulation to Plateau

The amount in the body rises on multiple dosing just as it does following a constant-rate IV infusion (Chapter 11). That is, *the approach to the plateau depends solely on the drug's half-life.* The simulation for the antiepileptic drug phenobarbital in Table 12-2, which shows the ratio of the minimum amount during various dosing intervals to the minimum amount at plateau, illustrates this point. This drug has a half-life of 4 days and is given at a dose of 1–3 mg/kg daily (a dose of 100 mg given daily is used in the calculations below) for the treatment of partial and generalized seizures (especially those formerly known as grand mal). It is a first-line treatment in large part because of its cheapness. In more affluent countries, it is no longer recommended as a first- or second-line choice anticonvulsant for most seizure types, although it is still commonly used to treat neonatal seizures. Observe that it takes 1 half-life (4 days), or 4 doses, to be at 50% of the value at plateau; 2 half-lives (8 days), or 8 doses, to be at 75% of the plateau value; and so on.

Accumulation of phenobarbital takes a long time because of its long half-life. Although once a day appears to be infrequent, relative to the regimens of many drugs, it is frequent relative to phenobarbital's half-life of 4 days. The degree of accumulation is extensive because of relatively frequent administration. The frequent administration also determines the small **relative fluctuation** in the plasma concentration (and amount in the body) of drug at plateau, defined as the difference between the maximum and minimum values relative to the average.

$$\text{Relative fluctuation} = \frac{C_{\text{max,ss}} - C_{\text{min,ss}}}{C_{\text{av,ss}}} \qquad \textbf{Eq. 12-9}$$

At plateau, 100 mg of phenobarbital is lost every dosing interval, the dose, which is small compared with the maximum and minimum amounts (from Equations 12-3 and 12-4) in the body at plateau, namely 630 and 530 mg.

The approach to steady state, observed for the minimum amounts of phenobarbital in the body, also holds true for the maximum amounts (proof in Appendix E), that is, on dividing Equation 12-1 by Equation 12-3, and Equation 12-2 by Equation 12-4:

$$\frac{A_{\text{max,N}}}{A_{\text{max,ss}}} = \frac{A_{\text{min,N}}}{A_{\text{min,ss}}} = 1 - e^{-k \cdot N \cdot \tau} \qquad \textbf{Eq. 12-10}$$

Table 12-2 | Approach to Plateau on Daily Administration of Phenobarbital

Time (days)[a]	0	1	2	3	4	8	12	16	20	24	∞
Number of doses (N)	0	1	2	3	4	8	12	16	20	24	∞
$\left[\frac{\text{Minimum Amount}}{\text{Minimum Amount at Plateau}}\right]^b$	0	0.16	0.29	0.40	0.50	0.75	0.875	0.94	0.97	0.98	1.00

[a]Time after first dose.
[b]$A_{\text{min,N}}/A_{\text{min,ss}} = 1 - e^{-0.173N}$

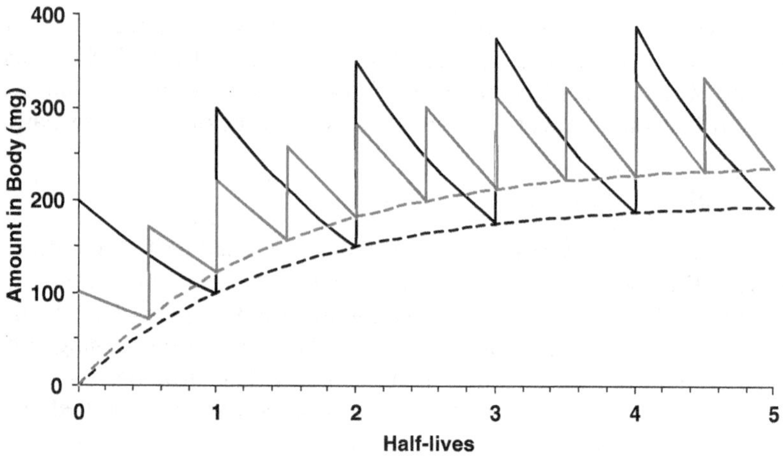

FIGURE 12-3 Plot showing that the general approach of amount of drug in the body to the plateau on giving the daily dose in multiple doses is independent of the dosing interval. Here, the same average dosing rate was administered with increasing frequency (100 mg at onehalf of a half-life [*colored line*] vs. 200 mg every half-life [*black line*]). Although the relative fluctuation around the average value within a dosing interval varies with the dosing interval, the time to reach the plateau, as reflected by the trough values (*dashed lines*), does not.

By recognizing that $N \cdot \tau$ is the total time elapsed since starting administration, expressed in multiples of the dosing interval, the similarity of Equation 12-10 to the equation describing the rise of drug in the body to plateau, relative to the plateau amount, with time following a constant-rate infusion ($1 - e^{-k \cdot \tau}$; Equation 11-6) becomes apparent. This point is further illustrated by the events depicted in Fig. 12-3. Here, the average dosing rate is maintained at 100 mg a day, but the drug is given with increasing frequency, which, in the limiting case of the dosing interval becoming infinitesimally small, is a constant-rate input. It is seen that the time course of average amount in the body is the same in all cases, but the less frequent the administration the greater is the fluctuation.

Accumulation Index

When the amounts at steady state are compared with the corresponding values after the first dose, a measure of the extent of accumulation is obtained. This value can be thought of as an **accumulation index (R_{ac})**,

$$\text{Accumulation index } (R_{ac}) = \frac{A_{max,ss}}{A_{max,1}} = \frac{A_{min,ss}}{A_{min,1}} = \frac{1}{1 - e^{-k \cdot \tau}}$$
$$= \frac{1}{\text{Fraction lost in interval}} \qquad \text{Eq. 12-11}$$

Thus, the quantity $1/(1 - e^{-k \cdot \tau})$ is an accumulation index. When phenobarbital is given once daily ($k = 0.173$/day, $\tau = 1$ day), the accumulation index is 5.8. Thus, the maximum and minimum amounts (and, for that matter, the amount at any given time within the dosing interval at plateau) are 5.8 times the corresponding values after a single dose. Recall that our model assumes that absorption and distribution of the drug are very fast and that the kinetics of the drug is linear. These are reasonable approximations for phenobarbital.

Change in Regimen

Sometimes, the dose of drug has to be changed because the body's response to it is either too low or excessive. Suppose, for example, that the decision is made to double the amount of phenobarbital in the body at plateau because of an insufficient control of seizures. The need for a twofold increase in the rate of administration—from 100 to 200 mg/day—follows from Equation 12-7. However, due consideration has to be given to the time needed to achieve a new plateau on changing the dosing rate. This often guides how long one needs to wait to ensure the achievement of the full response associated with the change in dosage, before deciding whether any further adjustments in drug therapy are needed. As with IV infusion, it takes 1 half-life to go one-half the way from the original plateau to the new one, 2 half-lives to go three-quarters of the way, and 3.3 half-lives to reach plateau. For phenobarbital, it would take about 14 days (3.3 half-lives) to go from the original plateau ($A_{max,ss}$ = 630 mg; $A_{min,ss}$ = 530 mg) to the new one ($A_{max,ss}$ = 1260 mg; $A_{min,ss}$ = 1060 mg) on doubling the daily dose. Hence, we would not expect to see the full benefits associated with this increase in dose for at least 2 weeks.

RELATIONSHIP BETWEEN INITIAL AND MAINTENANCE DOSES

It is sometimes therapeutically desirable to establish the required amount of drug in the body as soon as possible, rather than wait for the full therapeutic effect to be achieved by repeatedly giving the same dose at a regular interval. When a larger first or initial dose is given to quickly achieve a therapeutic level, it is referred to as a **loading (or priming) dose**. A case in point is sirolimus, an immunosuppressive drug used as part of therapy to prevent rejection following organ transplantation. Sirolimus has a half-life of about 2.5 days, and the usual oral maintenance dose is 2 mg once a day. Given in this manner, it would take approximately 1 week to reach the plateau, which is much too long to prevent the increased risk of organ rejection. Instead, patients first receive a loading dose of 6 mg followed by 2 mg daily. Another example is digoxin used in the treatment of chronic atrial fibrillation; it has a half-life of about 2 days, and the usual oral maintenance dose is 0.25 mg taken once a day. Taken in this manner, it would take approximately 1 week to reach the plateau. In some patients, it is important to reach effective levels in the body relatively rapidly. In this case, digoxin is given as a larger initial dose, followed by the regular daily doses. For digoxin, a low therapeutic index drug, the initial oral dose up to 1 mg is often administered in divided doses to minimize the risk of overdosing. Several procedures are followed, but a divided initial dose of 0.25 mg is often given every 6 hours until the desired therapeutic response is obtained. In this way, each patient is titrated to his or her required initial therapeutic dose, and a full therapeutic effect is achieved relatively rapidly, within 18–36 hours.

Instead of determining the loading dose when the maintenance dose is given, it is more common to determine the maintenance dose required to sustain a therapeutic amount in the body. The initial dose rapidly achieves the therapeutic response; subsequent doses maintain the response by replacing drug lost during the dosing interval. The **maintenance dose,** therefore, is the difference between the loading dose and the amount remaining at the end of the dosing interval, Loading dose $\cdot\, e^{-k\cdot\tau}$, that is,

$$\begin{aligned}\text{Maintenance Dose} &= \text{Loading Dose}\cdot(1-e^{-k\cdot\tau}) \\ &= \text{Loading Dose}\cdot[\text{Fraction lost in interval}]\end{aligned} \qquad \textbf{Eq. 12-12}$$

Likewise, if the maintenance dose is known, the initial dose can be estimated:

$$\text{Loading Dose} = \frac{\text{Maintenance Dose}}{(1-e^{-k\cdot\tau})} = \frac{\text{Maintenance Dose}}{[\text{Fraction lost in interval}]}$$
$$= R_{ac} \cdot \text{Maintenance Dose} \qquad \textbf{Eq. 12-13}$$

The relationship between loading dose and accumulation index, R_{ac}, follows from Equation 12-10. For sirolimus, Equation 12-13 predicts that a daily maintenance dose of 2 mg requires a loading dose of 8 mg. As noted previously, clinical experience indicates that a slightly lower initial dose (6 mg) safely suffices.

The similarity between Equations 12-3 and 12-12 should be noted. From the viewpoint of accumulation, Equation 12-3 relates to the maximum amount at plateau on administering a given dose repetitively. If the maximum amount were put into the body initially, then Equation 12-12 indicates the dose needed to maintain that amount. The relationships are the same, although they were derived starting from different viewpoints. These equations form the heart of multiple-dose administration.

The ratio of loading to maintenance doses depends on the dosing interval and the half-life, and is equal to the accumulation index, R_{ac} (Equation 12-13). For example, the antibiotic doxycycline has approximately a 1-day half-life, and a dose in the range of 200 mg is considered to provide effective antimicrobial drug concentrations. Therefore, a reasonable schedule is 200 mg (two 100-mg capsules) initially, followed by 100 mg once a day (a half-life), as shown in Fig. 12-4. (In practice, it is recommended that the initial amount be divided into two 100-mg doses taken 12 hours apart.) A dosage regimen, such as that for doxycycline, consisting of a priming dose equal to twice the maintenance dose and a dosing interval of one half-life is convenient for drugs with half-lives between 8 and 24 hours. The frequency of administration for such drugs varies from three times a day to once daily, respectively. For drugs with half-lives less than 3 hours, or with half-lives longer than 24 hours, this regimen is often impractical.

Although a loading or priming dose greater than the maintenance dose seems appropriate for drugs with half-lives longer than 24 hours, such is often not the case. There are various reasons why this is so, which are discussed at greater length later in this chapter and also in Chapter 14. Here, we note a few examples. For piroxicam, an analgesic/antipyretic drug with a half-life of 2 days, the most common adverse effects are gastrointestinal reactions. Such reactions may be increased if a loading dose, which would be three to four times the maintenance dose (Equation 12-12, $\tau = 1$ day), were to be given. Another example is that of protriptyline (an antidepressant with a

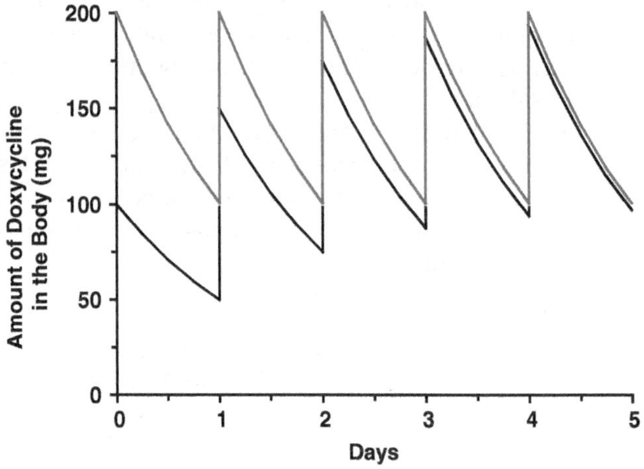

FIGURE 12-4 Sketch of the amount of doxycycline in the body with time in an individual with a 24-hour half-life after intravenous administration of 200 mg initially and 100 mg once daily thereafter (*colored line*). When the initial and maintenance doses are the same, one can conclude that the plateau has been reached by the fifth dose (4 days, 4 half-lives, *black line*). Thereafter, the two lines are essentially the same.

half-life of 3 days), for which larger doses slow gastric emptying and gastrointestinal activity (anticholinergic effect), resulting in slower and more erratic absorption of this and other coadministered drugs.

MAINTENANCE OF DRUG IN THE THERAPEUTIC RANGE

Dosage regimens that achieve effective therapy for drugs with both high and medium-to-low therapeutic indices and with various half-lives are listed in Table 12-3.

TABLE 12-3 | Oral Dosage Regimens for Continuous Maintenance of Therapy

Therapeutic Index	Half-life	Ratio of Initial Dose to Maintenance Dose	Ratio of Dosing Interval to Half-life	General Comments	Drug Examples
High	<30 min	–	–	Candidate for constant-rate administration and/or short-term therapy.	Nitroglycerin[a]
	30 min–3 hr	1	3–6	To be given any less often than every 3 half-lives, drug must have very high therapeutic index.	Cephalosporins
					Ibuprofen
	3–8 hr	1–2	1–3		Clopidogrel
	8–24 hr	2	1	Very common and desirable regimen.	Doxycycline
	>24 hr	>2	<1	Once daily is practical.	Azithromycin
					Piroxicam
Medium-to-low	<30 min	–	–	Not a candidate except under very closely controlled infusion.	Esmolol[b]
	30 min–3 hr	–	–	By infusion or frequent administration; less frequently with modified-release formulation.	Morphine
	3–8 hr	1–2	~1	Requires 3–4 doses/day, but less frequently with modified-release formulation.	Oxycodone
	8–24 hr	2–3	0.5–1	Very common and desirable regimen.	Flecanide[c]
	>24 hr	>2	<1	Daily dosing is the norm.	Sirolimus[d]

[a]Tolerance to drug prevents its continuous administration throughout the day.
[b]Despite a half-life of 9 minutes with rapid attainment of steady state, an intravenous bolus loading dose is given due to the use of the drug in emergency settings.
[c]As with many other drugs in this category, rather than administering a loading dose, dosage is progressively elevated until the desired response is achieved.
[d]Loading dose often not given for drugs with these pharmacokinetic characteristics, or given as smaller divided doses over several days, to avoid acute exposure to high concentrations and excessive adverse effects.

Half-Lives Less Than 30 Minutes

Great difficulty is encountered in trying to maintain therapeutic levels of such drugs. This is particularly true for a drug with a low therapeutic index, such as heparin and esmolol, which have half-lives of approximately 30 and 10 minutes, respectively. Such drugs must be either infused or discarded unless intermittent systemic exposures are permissible. Drugs with a high therapeutic index may be given less frequently, but the longer the dosing interval, the greater is the maintenance dose required to ensure that drug in the body stays above a minimum effective value, and the greater is the degree of fluctuation. Penicillin is a notable example of a drug for which the dosing interval (4–6 hours) is many times longer than its half-life (approximately 30 minutes). This is possible because the dose given greatly exceeds that required to yield plasma concentrations of antibiotic equivalent to the minimum inhibitory concentration for most penicillin-sensitive microorganisms. With the dosing interval some 8–12 times longer than the half-life, there is negligible accumulation of this drug.

Half-Lives Between 30 Minutes and 8 Hours

For drugs in this category, the major considerations are therapeutic index and convenience of dosing. A drug with a high therapeutic index need only be administered once every 1–3 half-lives or even less frequently. An example is the nonsteroidal anti-inflammatory drug ibuprofen; it has a half-life of about 2 hours, but dosing once every 6 hours, or even 8 hours, is adequate for effective treatment of various inflammatory conditions. A drug with a relatively low therapeutic index must be given approximately every half-life or more frequently, or be given by infusion. Theophylline, now relegated to a third-line bronchodilator after inhaled anticholinergics and β_2 agonists, but still recognized as a useful treatment in patients with severe chronic obstructive pulmonary disease (COPD), is an example. It has a half-life of 6–8 hours and needs to be given 3–4 times a day in its immediate-release dosage form; more convenient dosing is achieved by slowing the release of the drug (see Modified-Release Dosage Forms later in this chapter).

Half-Lives Between 8 and 24 Hours

Here, the most convenient and desirable regimen is one in which a dose is given every half-life. If immediate achievement of steady state is desired, then, as previously mentioned, the initial dose must be twice the maintenance dose; the minimum and maximum amounts in the body are equivalent to one and two maintenance doses, respectively. We have already discussed the example of doxycycline (see Table 12-3); naproxen is another (see below).

Half-Lives Greater Than 24 Hours

For drugs with half-lives longer than 1 day, administration once daily is common and convenient, and promotes patient adherence to the prescribed regimen. For some drugs with very long half-lives, in the order of weeks or more, and with a moderate to relatively high therapeutic index, once-weekly, biweekly, or monthly administration is adequate. Examples are mefloquine (half-life 3 weeks), used as a prophylaxis against malaria; alendronate, a bisphosphonate (retained and very slowly released from bone) used in the treatment of osteoporosis, both given once weekly; and adalimumab, an antibody drug used to treat autoimmune inflammatory disorders, given once every other week. Indeed, most antibody drugs are given in this manner or even once monthly and even less frequently.

If an immediate therapeutic effect is desired, a loading dose may need to be given initially. Otherwise, the initial and maintenance doses are the same, in which case several doses may be necessary before the drug accumulates to therapeutic levels. The decision whether or not to give larger initial doses is often a practical matter. Side effects to large oral doses (gastrointestinal side effects) or to acutely high concentrations of drug in the body may dictate against the use of a loading dose. This is particularly so when, as in many situations, tolerance develops to the adverse effects of a drug (see Tolerance, later in this chapter, for further discussion of this topic).

Reinforcing the Principles

To summarize the foregoing discussion, consider the recommended maintenance dosage regimens given in Table 12-4 for three drugs, namely, the antibiotic amoxicillin, used to treat several bacterial infections; the anti-inflammatory agent naproxen, when used to treat an acute attack of gout; and piroxicam, another anti-inflammatory agent, when used to treat arthritic joint pain. Listed in Table 12-5 are: the corresponding fractions of the initial amounts remaining at the end of a dosing interval, and the average, maximum, and minimum values. Absorption is assumed to be instantaneous and complete, which are reasonable approximations for these drugs.

The maintenance regimens of amoxicillin and naproxen are the same, but the amounts of them in the body with time are not. Also, despite the difference in maintenance regimens, the average amount in the body at plateau is not that different for amoxicillin and piroxicam. The explanation is readily visualized with a sketch.

For naproxen, the amount in the body immediately after the first dose is 250 mg. At the end of the 8-hour dosing interval, with a half-life of 14 hours, the fraction

TABLE 12-4 | Dosage Regimens and Half-lives of Three Drugs

Drug	Loading Dose (mg)	Maintenance Dose (mg)	Dosing Interval (hr)	Half-Life (hr)
Amoxicillin	–	250	8	1
Naproxen	750	250	8	14
Piroxicam	20	20	24	50

TABLE 12-5 | Amount of Drug in Body (mg) on Regimens Given in Table 12-4

Drug[a]	Fraction Remaining at End of Interval[b]	Average at Steady State[c]	Maximum at Steady State[d]	Minimum at Steady State[e]
Amoxicillin	0.004	45	251	0.98
Naproxen	0.67	630	765	515
Piroxicam	0.71	60	70.7	50.7

[a]Bioavailability of all three drugs is 100% ($F = 1$).
[b]Given by $e^{-k\tau}$
[c]$1.44 \cdot F \cdot$ Maintenance dose $\cdot t_{1/2}/\tau$.
[d]$F \cdot$ Maintenance dose$/(1 - e^{-k\tau})$.
[e]$A_{ss,max} - F \cdot$ Maintenance dose.

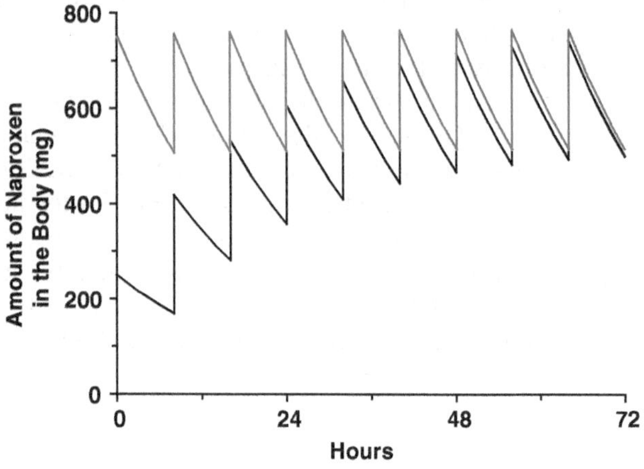

FIGURE 12-5 Sketch of the amount of naproxen in the body with time; simulation of 250 mg given intravenously every 8 hours (*black line*). Because the half-life, 14 hours, is somewhat longer than the dosing interval, the degree of accumulation and the relative fluctuation at plateau are both modest. Notice that a loading dose of 750 mg immediately achieves steady-state conditions (*colored line*).

remaining is 0.67, and the amount remaining is therefore 168 mg. The second maintenance dose of 250 mg raises the amount to 418 mg, and so on. Fig. 12-5, black line, is thus readily drawn, from which it is clear that it takes approximately 2 to 3 days to reach steady state. At steady state, the average amount in the body is 630 mg (Equation 12-7), and that the accumulation index is 3.06 (Equation 12-10). Sometimes, a full therapeutic effect needs to be established faster, in which case a loading dose of 750 mg (3 × 250 mg) is administered. As can readily be seen, following the loading dose, the amount remaining at the end of the first dosing interval is 505 mg (0.67 × 750 mg), and the amount lost is 245 mg. The maintenance dose of 250 mg then essentially replaces that lost within this first dosing interval, thereby ensuring that steady-state conditions are essentially achieved and maintained throughout the regimen (colored line of Fig. 12-5).

For amoxicillin with a half-life of 1 hour, when 250 mg is given every 8 hours, virtually none remains at the end of the dosing interval (8 half-lives), such that a steady state is reached by the time the second dose is administered. Events in each subsequent dosing interval essentially repeat that observed following the first dose; fluctuation between maximum and minimum amounts is very large. In contrast to naproxen for the same dosage regimen, the average amount of drug within a dosing interval at plateau is only 45 mg (average amount/dose = 2.5 for naproxen and 0.18 for amoxicillin; Equation 12-7). Fig. 12-6 is a sketch of the amounts of amoxycillin in the body with time.

The results are markedly different for piroxicam than for amoxicillin. At the end of each 1-day dosing interval, with a half-life of 50 hours, the fraction remaining for piroxicam is 0.712. Accumulation then occurs until the 29% lost in each interval is equal to the dose, and the maximum amount in the body at steady state is therefore about 3.53 times the 20-mg maintenance dose, that is, 71 mg. The minimum amount at steady state is 51 mg. From the calculated value of the maximum amount at plateau and the half-life, it is apparent that a sketch must be scaled to at least 71 mg on the y-axis and to about 7 days on the x-axis (Fig. 12-7). The amount in the body at its half-life, 50 hours, is one-half of that at steady state; at 100 hours, the level is 75% of the plateau amount, and so on. Practically, fluctuations are relatively minor, and the average amount at plateau of 60 mg is now comparable to that obtained with amoxicillin, despite the 12-fold difference in the maintenance dose. Clearly, maintenance dose alone does not convey what the amount of drug will be in the body at plateau.

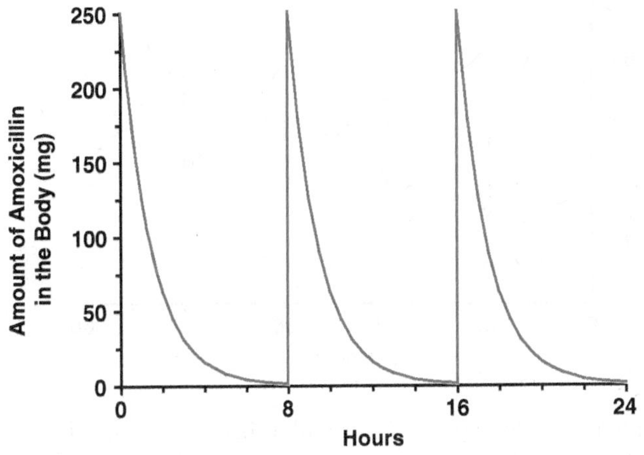

FIGURE 12-6 Sketch of the amount of amoxicillin in the body with time when 250 mg is given intravenously every 8 hours. Because the half-life, 1 hour, is very short relative to the dosing interval, the degree of accumulation is negligible, and the relative fluctuation is extremely large, as the average is only 45 mg (0.18 of a dose, not shown).

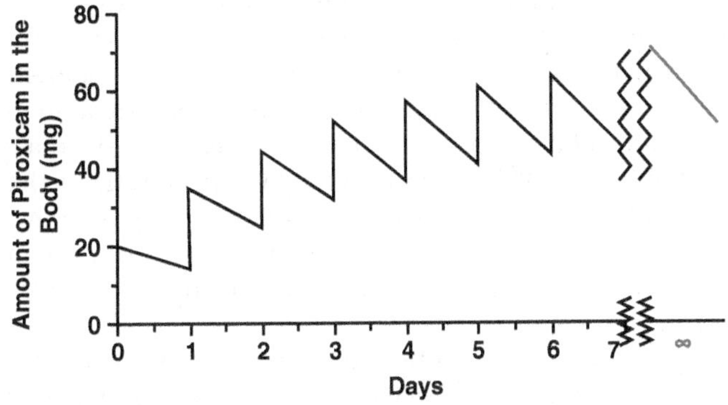

FIGURE 12-7 Sketch of the amount of piroxicam in the body with time; simulation of 20 mg given intravenously once daily. Because the half-life, 50 hours, is long relative to the dosing interval, the degree of accumulation is large, and the relative fluctuation at plateau is low. The maximum and minimum values during a dosing interval at steady state, 71 and 51 mg, are shown by the colored line. The difference between these two amounts at plateau is the dose, and the average amount is 60 mg.

ADDITIONAL CONSIDERATIONS

So far, consideration has been given primarily to the amount of drug in the body after multiple IV bolus injections or their equivalent, at equally spaced intervals. In practice, chronic administration is usually by the oral route. Furthermore, only drug concentration in plasma or in blood can be measured and not amount of drug in the body. These aspects are now considered. Issues related to unequal doses and dosing intervals and to missed doses, which arise when adherence to the dosage regimen is poor, are covered in Chapter 14.

Extravascular Administration

The oral (also intramuscular, buccal, subcutaneous, and rectal) administration of drugs requires an added step, systemic absorption. Equations 12-1 to 12-4 also apply to extravascular administration, provided that absorption has essentially ended within a small fraction of a dosing interval, a condition similar to IV bolus administration. Even so, a correction must be made if bioavailability is less than 1. For example, the maximum amount of drug in the body at plateau, $A_{max,ss}$, is then

$$A_{max,ss} = \frac{F \cdot \text{Dose}}{(1 - e^{-k \cdot \tau})} \quad \text{Eq. 12-14}$$

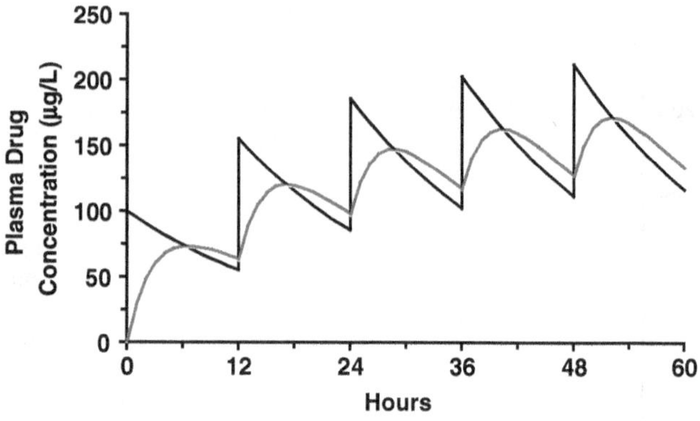

FIGURE 12-8 Compared with an intravenous bolus regimen (*black line*), when given orally the peak is lower and the trough (*colored line*) is higher. In this example of the impact of prolonged input, the average amount of drug in the body at steady state remains the same because the extent of absorption (bioavailability) of the drug is unchanged.

Equations 12-10 through 12-13 also still apply even if bioavailability is less than 1, provided that absorption is much faster than elimination, so that the bolus assumption holds.

When absorption becomes slower, within each dosing interval the peak concentration becomes lower and the trough (minimum) value higher than after rapid absorption. This decreases the **relative fluctuation** around the average value, as is apparent when extravascular administration is contrasted with intravenous bolus dose administration, Fig. 12-8. Notice that the impact of absorption kinetics is greater on decreasing the peak than on increasing the trough. This occurs because the peak reflects the condition when rate of input matches the rate of output, and hence is very sensitive to changes in input rate. In contrast, the trough better reflects the amount of drug in the body once absorption is over, and, as such, is relatively less sensitive to changes in absorption kinetics.

The therapeutic impact of differences in absorption kinetics, but not in bioavailability, of extravascularly administered drug products given continuously also depends on the frequency of their administration. As illustrated in Fig. 12-9, major differences in absorption kinetics seen following a single dose only persist and are of potential therapeutic concern at plateau when the drug products are given infrequently relative to the half-life of the drug. The differences between them almost disappear at plateau when the products are given frequently. In the latter case, with extensive accumulation of drug, the concentration at plateau is relatively insensitive to variations in the absorption rate-time profile.

When absorption continues throughout a dosing interval or longer, then Equations 12-1 through 12-4 do not strictly apply, but the steady-state relationships of Equations 12-7 and 12-8 still hold. These latter relationships allow estimation of the average plateau amount in the body and the average plateau concentration, respectively. The slowness of drug absorption affects the degree of fluctuation around, but not the value of, the average level. The exception is when absorption becomes so slow that there is insufficient time for complete absorption, such as when limited by the transit time within the gastrointestinal tract, in which case bioavailability becomes dependent on absorption kinetics.

Plasma Concentration Versus Amount in Body

During multiple dosing, the plasma concentration can be calculated at any time by dividing the corresponding equations defining amount by volume of distribution. However, distribution equilibrium between drug in the tissues and that in plasma takes

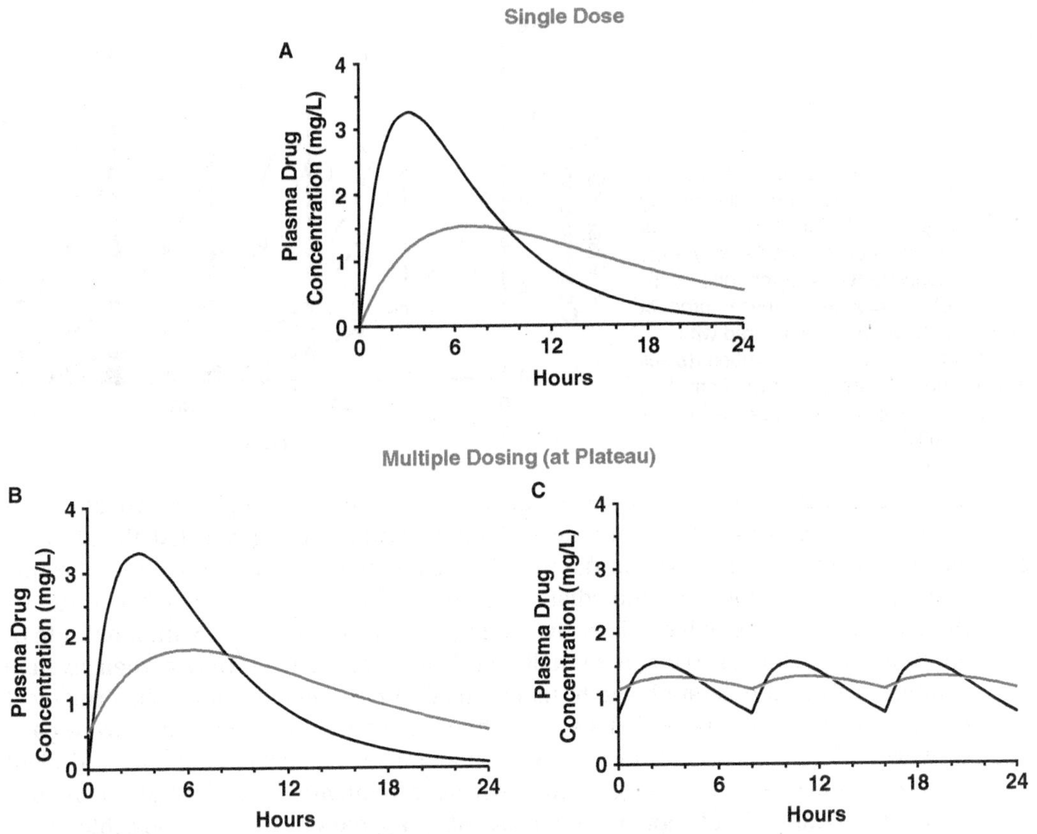

FIGURE 12-9 Differences in the absorption kinetics between two dosage forms following a single extravascular dose (*top panel*) may have a major therapeutic impact at plateau during multiple dosing, depending on the relative frequency of administration. The impact is greater when the products are given relatively infrequently (*lower left*) than when the total daily dose is given in divided doses and more frequently, i.e., with a shorter dosing interval (lower *right panel*). The colored line is the plasma concentration associated with the dosage form showing the slower absorption.

time. Thus, observed maximum concentrations may be appreciably greater than those calculated by dividing Equations 12-1 and 12-3 by *V*, which assume distribution equilibrium applies at all times.

The average plateau concentration may be calculated using Equation 12-8. This equation is applicable to any route, method of administration, or dosage form as long as bioavailability and clearance remain constant with both time and dose.

MODIFIED-RELEASE PRODUCTS

One way of maintaining a relatively constant response is by constant-rate administration. Although some constant-rate release systems have been developed (Chapter 11), other dosage forms exist from which drug release is not constant but is much slower than from conventional immediate-release dosage forms. Such **modified-release products** reduce considerably the relative fluctuation in the plasma concentration at plateau when compared with that following immediate-release products, when evaluated over the same dosing interval. They are particularly useful for oral administration when maintenance of a therapeutic level requires frequent dosing of the immediate-release dosage form, such as three or four times a day. The dosing interval may then

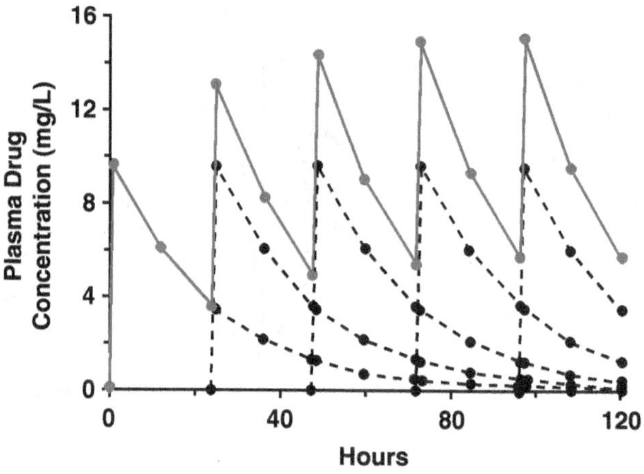

FIGURE 12-10 An oral modified-release dosage form allows for once-daily dosing of morphine, despite its short half-life of approximately 2 hours. Mean steady-state plasma concentrations after once-daily dosing of a modified-release product (Avinza, *colored circle*) compared with administration of morphine solution (*black circle*) every 4 hours. (Redrawn from data provided in *Physicians' Desk Reference*. 58th Ed. 2004).

be increased to give a more convenient once- or twice-daily regimen provided that the drug is well absorbed from much of the intestinal tract, given that the slow release is likely to lead to drug in the product being moved further along the intestine than experienced with the immediate-release product. This is readily illustrated by the data in Fig. 12-10, which show events at plateau for morphine, with a half-life of approximately 2 hours. With an immediate-release oral dosage form, or when given in solution, absorption is rapid, and to maintain effective concentrations, the drug must be taken very frequently, perhaps every 4 hours for the relief of chronic severe pain. However, effective concentrations can be maintained throughout the day and night with a modified-release dosage form given as infrequently as once daily. This long dosing interval, without reducing bioavailability, appears to be made possible in the particular case of morphine for most patients because this drug slows gastrointestinal motility, thereby retaining the product in the gastrointestinal tract for longer than normal. Other examples of useful oral modified-release dosage forms are those developed for theophylline, oxycodone, and lithium, all drugs with short half-lives and that are well absorbed throughout the gastrointestinal tract.

To maintain the same exposure at plateau for the 24-hour interval, because it is given less frequently, the maintenance dose contained in a modified-release product must be proportionally larger than that of the conventional immediate-release product. Obviously, modified-release products must perform reliably and, in particular, should not be sensitive to food that, through increased gastric retention and contraction, may markedly modify the release of drug. If the entire dose were released immediately, as when a modified-released product is chewed, unacceptably high plasma concentrations would result. This may also occur with some products taken concurrently with high alcohol-content drinks, in which the alcohol dissolves and destroys the matrix that normally retards the release of drug. This process is called **dose dumping** and can lead to excessive adverse effects.

For oral administration, once or twice daily is desirable. Accordingly, for drugs with half-lives longer than 12 hours, oral modified-release products may be of little value, not only because the usual regimen is already convenient but because protracted release may put drug into the large intestine or perhaps out of the alimentary canal before release is complete. Decreased bioavailability then becomes a major concern, especially in patients with conditions, for example, ulcerative colitis, in which gastrointestinal transit time is shortened.

For a drug that is usually given intramuscularly, or subcutaneously, multiple injections are inconvenient and painful, and a modified-release (or depot) injectable dosage form may be advantageous. Depending on the total dose required and on the local effects of the injection mixture, it may only be necessary to administer the injection weekly, monthly, or perhaps even as a single dose. For example, leuprolide (a synthetic nonapeptide analog of naturally occurring gonadotropin-releasing hormone), with a half-life of approximately 3 hours, is available in depot preparations (Table 11-2 in Chapter 11) for subcutaneous or intramuscular administration every 1, 3, 4, or 6 months for the treatment of advanced prostate cancer, endometriosis, uterine leiomyomata, and breast cancer.

PHARMACODYNAMIC CONSIDERATIONS

In the examples of dosage regimens for continuous maintenance of therapy listed in Table 12-3, the main driving force for defining appropriate multiple-dose regimens, particularly the dosing interval and time to achieve full therapeutic effect, is pharmacokinetics. This is because response tracks plasma concentration with relatively little time delay for the drugs listed. However, even then, the dosing interval is also determined by what part of the exposure–response relationship is needed for therapeutic efficacy, commensurate with being within the therapeutic window. This is illustrated in Fig. 12-11 (next page) during maintenance therapy at steady state for a drug with a half-life of 8 hours. Based on pharmacokinetic considerations alone, a reasonable dosing interval might be 8 hours, which would maintain the level within a twofold range. This may well be appropriate if the required response lies at or below 50% of the maximum response, E_{max}, as then for the most part, response is in the range in which it varies in direct proportion to the logarithm of the level (Fig. 12-11A). However, if the peak response is closer to E_{max} then, as large changes in systemic exposure produce minimal changes in response, the 8-hour dosing interval will maintain essentially the same response throughout the interval (Fig. 12-11B). Alternatively, it may well be possible to extend the dosing interval to 24 hours, permitting once-daily administration and still maintain response within an acceptable range (Fig. 12-11C). For example, although the elimination half-life of atenolol is approximately 6 hours, a dose of 50 or 100 mg can be administered once daily because the plasma concentrations remain sufficiently high so that the therapeutic effects (β-blockade and antihypertensive effect) persist throughout the 24-hour interval and the drug has a relatively wide therapeutic index.

Sometimes, response declines more slowly than the plasma concentration, which also allows for a longer dosing interval than one based on pharmacokinetic principles. For example, as discussed in Chapter 9, although both omeprazole and aspirin have half-lives of 1 hour or less, the decline in their responses is very sluggish. For these drugs, once-daily administration for the sustained reduction in secretion of gastric acidity and in platelet adhesion, respectively, is adequate. In addition, there are aspects of the pharmacokinetic–pharmacodynamic relationship of drugs and drug classes that influence the ultimate therapeutic regimen. These may argue for the need for a fluctuating or even an intermittent exposure profile rather than constant exposure, and for the need to wait for many days or even weeks or months before the full therapeutic effect of the drug, despite a relatively short half-life of a drug. We now consider some examples.

Time to Achieve Therapeutic Effect

Statins are widely used to reduce the risk of coronary heart disease and cardiovascular events, which is attributable to their lowering of the concentration of cholesterol and inhibiting its synthesis in the liver. One such statin is atorvastatin, which has

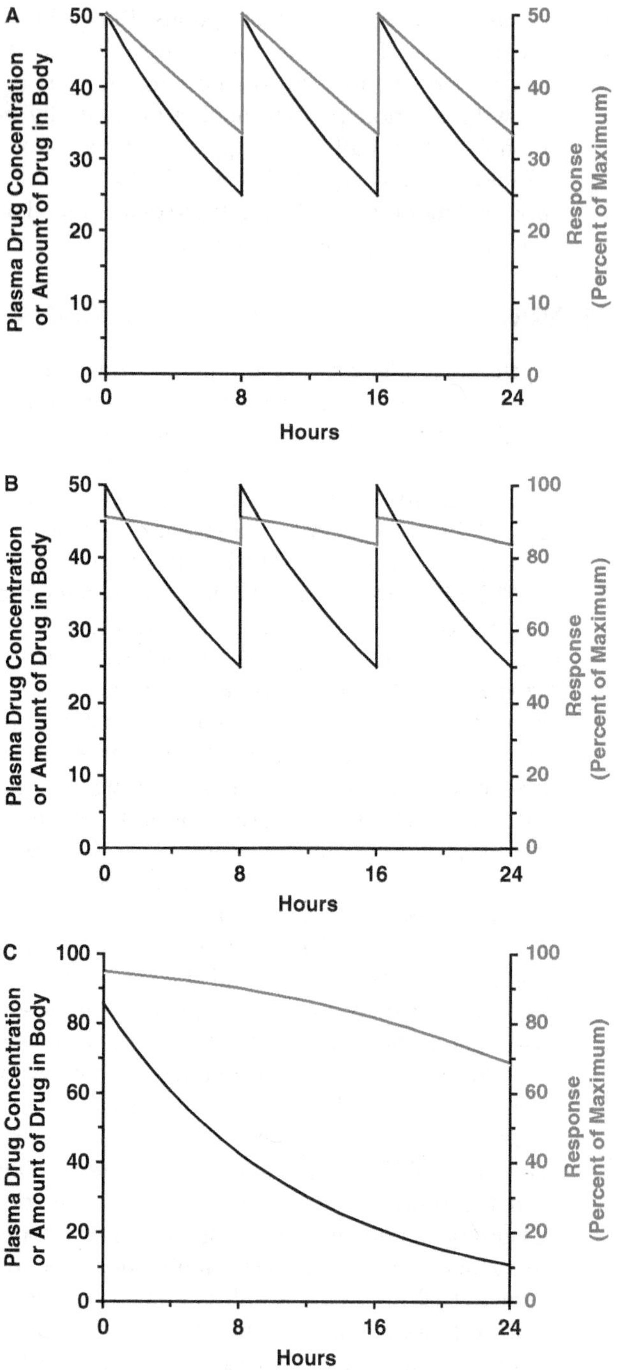

FIGURE 12-11 The dosing interval on maintenance therapy depends not only on the pharmacokinetics of a drug (*black lines*), but also on its pharmacodynamics (*colored lines*), even when response tracks the plasma concentration or amount of drug in the body, as shown here at plateau (using an arbitrary scale) for a drug with a half-life of 8 hours. **(A)** When the therapeutic response corresponding to the maximum plasma concentration lies at or below 50% of the maximum response, response declines similarly to that of the plasma concentration, although less so, as response is proportional to the logarithm of plasma concentration (see Fig. 3-5). Here, a dosing interval of 8 hours may well be reasonable. **(B)** When the therapeutic response corresponding to the maximum plasma concentration now lies close to the maximum response, then because response changes little with plasma concentration over the range of concentrations during the dosing interval, response remains relatively constant within the 8-hour dosing interval. Furthermore, it may well be possible to triple the dose of this drug and lengthen the dosing interval three fold to 24 hours, thereby maintaining the same total daily dose, yet still maintain adequate response during the entire interval **(C)**. Even though the fluctuation of the plasma concentration is large, the response remains quite constant because during the entire interval, the plasma concentration exceeds the C_{50}. In these simulations, while the pharmacokinetics of the drug is unchanged, the C_{50} value is 50 units in case A, and 5 units in cases B and C.

rather a relatively short half-life, about 12 hours; yet it is given once daily. One needs to wait for at least 3–4 weeks before considering a dose adjustment rather than the 2 days that might be expected based solely on its pharmacokinetics. The reason lies in the sluggish response of cholesterol to a decrease in its rate of synthesis, as seen in Fig. 12-12. This is due to the slow removal of cholesterol from the body in much the

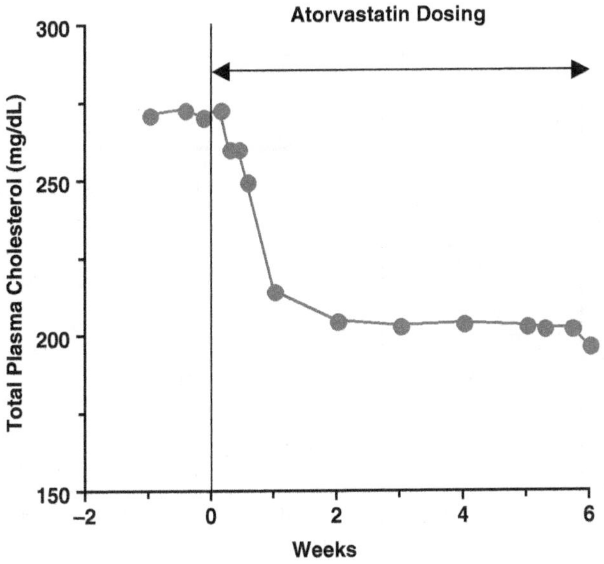

FIGURE 12-12 Plot of total plasma cholesterol against time , a week before and following oral administration of 5-mg atorvastatin once daily for 6 weeks. Atorvastatin is a selective, competitive inhibitor of HMG-CoA reductase, the rate-limiting enzyme that converts 3-hydroxy-3-methylglutaryl-coenzyme A to mevalonate, a precursor of sterols, including cholesterol. Note that despite the relatively short half-life of atorvastatin (14 hours, not shown), it takes almost 2 weeks to see the full effect of inhibition of cholesterol synthesis. (Redrawn from Stern RH, Yang BB, Hounslow NJ, et al. Pharmacodynamics and pharmacokinetic-pharmacodynamic relationship of atorvastatin, an HMG-CoA reductase inhibitor. *J Clin Pharmacol* 2000;40:616–623.)

same way that the plasma concentrations of drugs with long half-lives change slowly in response to a change in the rate of input during chronic administration.

The second example is erythropoietin, an antianemic agent given to patients with end-stage renal disease, who have developed anemia because the kidney is the source of synthesis of endogenous erythropoietin, which stimulates red cell production. Erythropoietin has a short half-life of only 9 hours and reaches steady state on chronic administration within 2 days. Yet it is commonly given twice to three times weekly, but even then, as the data in Fig. 12-13 (next page) show, following chronic administration of the drug, the hematocrit rises for about 70 days and sometimes longer before it levels off. Accordingly, adjustment in dosage is generally no more frequent than once a month.

One might be tempted to conclude that the effect of erythropoietin takes time to develop. In fact, the drug increases the rate of production of red blood cells throughout the entire course of its administration. What is observed is the accumulation of newly formed cells until they have reached their lifetime potential of around 70 days, after which they begin to die. The rates of production and death of the cells subsequently come into balance; the hematocrit now fully reflects the increased production of cells induced by the drug.

Intermittent Administration

Intermittent administration is relatively common in cancer chemotherapy. The gap between administrations is often 2–3 weeks, essentially independent of the pharmacokinetics of the drug, whose half-lives are often in the order of hours. Many of these agents act by irreversibly binding to DNA, resulting in death of proliferating cells, especially the most rapidly proliferating cancerous cells. However, there is also unavoidable death of rapidly proliferating healthy cells, including those of the erythropoietic system, such as leukocytes, neutrophils, and platelets. The gap between administrations is to allow healthy cells to recover. The recovery can be sluggish, occurring in weeks rather than days, as seen with red cells following administration of erythropoietin.

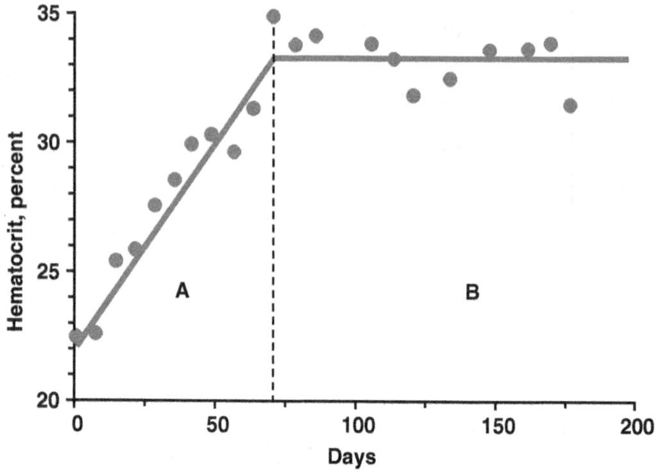

FIGURE 12-13 The hematocrit (*circles*) in a uremic patient undergoing dialysis and receiving erythropoietin after dialysis three times a week continuously throughout the study increases for 70 days (*dotted line*) and then levels off. (A) The drug increases erythrocyte production rate; hematocrit increases because the newly produced erythrocytes do not die at this early stage. (B) Erythropoietin continues to stimulate production of erythrocytes. However, after reaching 1 life span of 70 days, erythrocytes die at the current higher production rate, and a new steady state is reached. (Redrawn from Uehlinger DE, Gotch FA, Sheiner LB. A pharmacodynamic model of erythropoietin therapy for uremic anemia. *Clin Pharmacol Ther* 1992;51:76–89.)

Development of Tolerance

The effectiveness of a drug can diminish with continual use. **Acquired resistance** denotes the diminished sensitivity of a population of cells (microorganisms, viruses, neoplasms) to a chemotherapeutic agent; **tolerance** denotes a diminished pharmacologic responsiveness to a drug. The degree of acquired resistance through mutation varies; it may be complete, thereby rendering the agent, such as an antibiotic or antiviral agent, ineffective against a microorganism or virus. The degree of tolerance also varies, but is never complete. For example, within days or weeks of its repeated use, subjects can develop a profound tolerance but not total unresponsiveness to the pharmacologic effects (euphoria, sedation, respiratory depression) of morphine. Tolerance can develop slowly; for example, tolerance to the central nervous system effects of ethanol takes weeks. Tolerance can also occur acutely; it is then called **tachyphylaxis**. For example, tolerance, expressed by a diminished cardiovascular responsiveness, seen as a decrease in the degree of tachycardia, develops within minutes after repetitive intake (through smoking) of nicotine. At any moment, a correlation might be found between the intensity of response and the plasma concentration of the drug, but the relationship varies with time.

The therapeutic implication of tolerance depends on whether it involves the beneficial or harmful effects of the drug. The development of tolerance to desired responses may require adjustment in the manner of delivery of a drug. For example, nitroglycerin, a drug used in treating or preventing angina, has an elimination half-life of just minutes and is very quickly absorbed when given sublingually. This produces an effective pulse in its systemic response. When placed in a transdermal constant-rate release patch, a normally therapeutic systemic concentration of nitroglycerin can be maintained for 24 hours or more. Such products, however, are no longer used in this manner. They were shown to be ineffective long-term because of the development of tolerance to the prophylactic effects of the drug. The current recommendation is to remove the patch overnight to allow the concentration of nitroglycerin to fall and thereby reduce the development of tolerance.

Tolerance to the harmful effects of drugs, such as a side effect of headache or a sense of nausea, can be an advantage. Although a loading dose may seem appropriate for a drug with a long half-life, acutely high concentrations can produce excessive adverse effects, which may limit the tolerability of an otherwise useful drug. Such adverse effects are less frequently encountered when drug is allowed to slowly accumulate in the body with a regimen that comprises only the maintenance dose. This is certainly the case with the antidepressant protriptyline. Recall that this drug has a long half-life (3 days); yet no loading dose is given. There are several reasons for this. In addition to the previously mentioned adverse gastrointestinal effects experienced with large doses, many of the adverse central nervous system effects are mitigated against owing to tolerance to these effects as drug builds up slowly on maintenance therapy. Also, in common with many other antidepressants, independent of the pharmacokinetics of the drug, the development of the full benefit of the therapeutic effect is delayed usually for 2–4 or even more weeks for pharmacodynamic reasons related to the kinetics of the underlying affected system within the brain.

Modality of Administration

Fig. 12-14 (next page) illustrates another situation—this time with antimicrobial agents—for which modality of administration can influence therapeutic outcome. Shown are major differences in the effect of dosing frequency on the daily dose of ceftazidime and gentamicin required to produce 50% of maximal efficacy in treating pneumonia that is due to *Klebsiella pneumoniae* in neutropenic mice. Whereas decreasing the frequency of administration and hence increasing the degree of fluctuation in plasma concentration drastically diminished the effectiveness of ceftazidime, it had minimal effect on gentamicin. The explanation lies in the different pharmacodynamic profiles of these two drugs.

Ceftazidime, like other β-lactam antibiotics, exhibits only minimal concentration-dependent bactericidal activity, so that bacterial killing is more dependent on time above the minimal inhibitory concentration (MIC) than on the magnitude of the drug concentration. Greater benefit is therefore achieved with more frequent administration that minimizes the possibility of the plasma concentration falling too low. An additional reason for frequent administration is that the duration of the postantibiotic effect—whereby bacterial growth is suppressed for some time after intermittent exposure of bacteria to the antimicrobial agent—is very short with the β-lactam antibiotics.

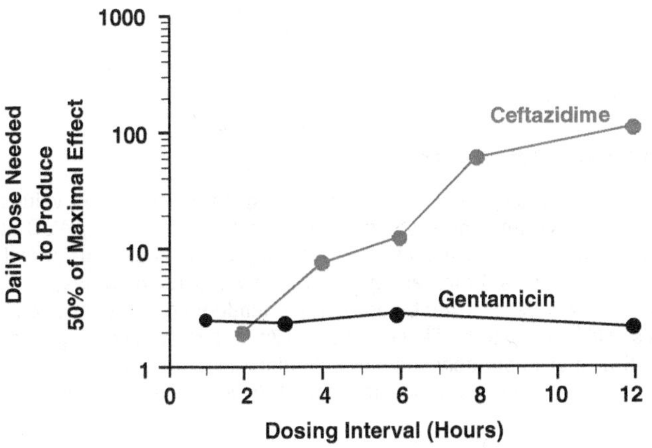

FIGURE 12-14 The influence of lengthening the dosing interval on the daily dose needed to produce 50% of maximal efficacy in treating pneumonia due to *Klebsiella pneumoniae* in neutropenic mice varies with the antimicrobial agent. Whereas no change in daily dose is needed with gentamicin (*black curve*), much larger daily doses of ceftazidime (*colored curve*) are needed when administered less frequently. (From Leggett JE, Fantin B, Ebert SC, et al. Comparative antibiotic dose-effect relationships of several dosing intervals in murine pneumonitis and thigh-infection models. *J Infect Dis* 1989;159:281–292.)

In contrast to ceftazidime, gentamicin, and other aminoglycosides produce a prolonged postantibiotic effect. They also exhibit marked concentration-dependent killing over a wide range of concentrations, with higher values having a more pronounced effect on the rate and extent of bactericidal activity. Accordingly, for the same daily dose, large infrequent doses of gentamicin are as effective as smaller more frequent ones.

Although data in patients with infections are of necessity more variable than those obtained in the experimental mouse model, they do tend to bear out the findings in Fig. 12-14. First, for the antibiotics exhibiting a minimal concentration dependence, a long half-life has proved to be a distinct advantage in allowing longer dosing intervals while maintaining efficacy. Second, studies indicate that for the same daily dose, once-daily regimens of aminoglycosides are as effective as more frequent ones, despite the short (about 2- to 3-hour) half-lives of these compounds. This explains the increasing move from a previous thrice-daily administration, which was based almost solely on half-life considerations, to once-daily administration of gentamicin. However, regardless of the mode of action of the antibiotic, if treatment is to be effective in eradicating the infection and increasing the probability of the microorganism remaining susceptible to the antibiotic, evidence such as that shown in Fig. 12-15 indicates that the ratio of 24-hour AUC of antibiotic to the corresponding AUC at the MIC (minimum inhibitory concentration) of the microorganism (commonly referred to as the area under the inhibitor curve [AUIC]) needs to be in excess of 100 throughout treatment.

This section has dealt with the principles surrounding the design and application of dosage regimens intended for the treatment or amelioration of a condition or disease in a typical patient. However, patients vary in their response to drugs, and the final section of the book deals with the issue of individualization of drug therapy. It starts with a chapter on evidence and expressions of interindividual variability in pharmacokinetics and response, and finishes with a chapter dealing with how this information is used in the initiation and management of drug therapy.

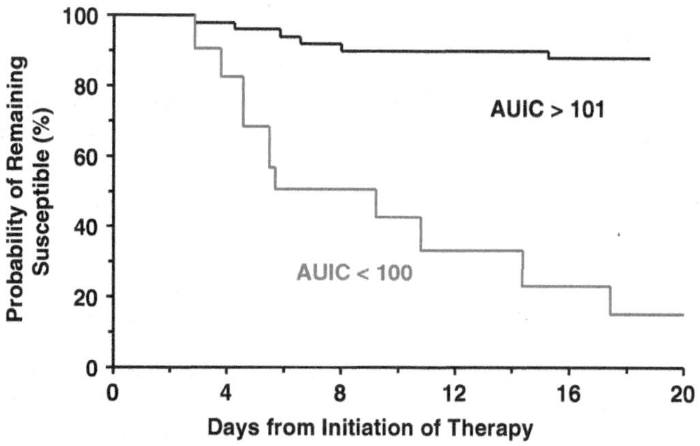

FIGURE 12-15 Area under the microbiological inhibitory curve (AUIC) and organism resistance. At values of AUIC (ratio of AUC of antibiotic during the dosing interval at steady state to the corresponding AUC at the minimal inhibitory concentration [MIC] of the antibiotic against the microorganism) above 101 (*black line*), only 9% of patients developed resistant organisms. Whereas, at AUIC below 100 (*colored line*), only 50% of the organisms remained susceptible after 5 days of antibiotic therapy. Inadequate concentrations, particularly if they fall below the organism's MIC, increase the likelihood of resistant strains emerging. (Redrawn from Thomas JK, Forrest A, Bhavnani SM, et al. Pharmacodynamic evaluation of factors associated with the development of bacterial resistance in acutely ill patients during therapy. *Antimicrob Agents Chemother* 1998;42:521–527.)

SUMMARY

- The plasma concentration–time profile following a fixed-dose and dosing-interval extravascular regimen of a drug can be predicted from the plasma concentration–time profile after a single dose. The same applies to repeated short-term infusions and intravenous doses.
- The rate and extent of accumulation of a drug given on a regimen of fixed dose and interval can be predicted when the pharmacokinetic parameters from a single dose are known.
- On repetitive dosing, drug accumulates until a plateau or steady state is achieved, when, within a dosing interval, amount eliminated from the body equals the amount absorbed.
- The extent of accumulation depends on the frequency of administration relative to the elimination half-life of the drug.
- Because the dosing interval of orally administered drugs is usually restricted to 6–24 hours, drugs with long half-lives (greater than 1 day) tend to accumulate more extensively than short half-life drugs (less than 3 hours) on repetitive dosing.
- How quickly drug in the body accumulates to steady state on repetitive dosing depends on its half-life.
- A loading dose, if needed, allows the rapid attainment of a therapeutic level for drugs given frequently relative to their half-lives. The ratio of loading to maintenance doses is determined by the fraction of drug initially present that is lost within a dosing interval.
- Modified-release dosage forms can reduce fluctuation in systemic exposure or allow regimens of longer dosing intervals than with regular rapidly releasing dosage forms, or both.
- Pharmacodynamic considerations that influence a multiple-dose regimen of a drug include:
  - The speed of decline in response following single-dose administration.
  - The need to sometimes administer a drug intermittently, regardless of its pharmacokinetics, to allow the body to recover from unavoidable adverse effects.
  - Development of tolerance to desired and harmful effects.
  - Impact of modality of administration on efficacy and safety.

KEY TERM REVIEW

Accumulation
Accumulation index
Acquired resistance
Dose dumping
Drug accumulation
Fluctuation
Loading dose
Maintenance dose
Modified-release product
Plateau
Priming dose
Relative fluctuation
Tachyphylaxis
Tolerance
Trough concentration

KEY RELATIONSHIPS

$$\text{Maximum amount in body at steady state, } A_{max,ss} = \frac{\text{Dose}}{(1 - e^{-k \cdot \tau})} = \frac{\text{Dose}}{\text{Fraction lost in interval}}$$

$$\text{Minimum amount in body at steady state, } A_{min,ss} = A_{max,ss} \cdot e^{-k \cdot \tau} = A_{max,ss} - \text{Dose}$$

$$C_{av,ss} = \frac{F \cdot \text{Dose}}{CL \cdot \tau}$$

$$\text{Accumulation index } (R_{ac}) = \frac{A_{max,ss}}{A_{max,1}} = \frac{A_{min,ss}}{A_{min,1}} = \frac{1}{1 - e^{-k \cdot \tau}}$$

$$= \frac{1}{\text{Fraction lost in interval}}$$

$$\text{Maintenance Dose} = \text{Loading Dose} \cdot (1 - e^{-k \cdot \tau})$$
$$= \text{Loading Dose} \cdot [\text{Fraction lost in interval}]$$

$$\text{Loading Dose} = \frac{\text{Maintenance Dose}}{(1 - e^{-k \cdot \tau})} = \frac{\text{Maintenance Dose}}{[\text{Fraction lost in interval}]}$$
$$= R_{ac} \cdot \text{Maintenance Dose}$$

STUDY PROBLEMS

1. Administration of a fixed oral dose of a drug repetitively every approximately fixed time interval is the most common manner of giving drugs. Which of the following statements accurately reflects this manner of drug administration?
   I. The amount eliminated in the first dosing interval is greater than the amount systemically absorbed from the first dose.
   II. The accumulation index at plateau depends only on the dosing frequency.
   III. At plateau, the amount of drug lost within a dosing interval equals the oral maintenance dose.
   A. I only **E.** I and III
   B. II only **F.** II and III
   C. III only **G.** All
   D. I and II **H.** None
2. A drug is given in a dose of 100 mg intravenously once every half-life ($\tau = 12$ hours) for 10 doses. Which of the following quantities are correct?
   I. The maximum amount in the body just after the third dose is 175 mg.
   II. The minimum amount at steady state is 100 mg.
   III. The amount in the body 24 hours just after the 10th dose is 50 mg.
   A. I only **E.** I and III
   B. II only **F.** II and III
   C. III only **G.** All
   D. I and II **H.** None
3. The half-life of a drug is 48 hours. It is commonly given in a regimen of 60 mg once daily with no loading dose. A patient has an acute problem for which the decision is made to give a loading dose. Using a model of multiple intravenous doses, which *one* of the loading doses listed below comes the closest to achieving initially the steady-state maximum amount in the body?
   a. 25 mg
   b. 50 mg
   c. 100 mg
   d. 200 mg
   e. 400 mg

4. There are many pharmacodynamic considerations to defining appropriate dosage regimens of drugs. Which of the following statements is (are) correct?
   I. The effectiveness of a drug can diminish with continual use. Acquired resistance denotes the diminished sensitivity of a population of cells (microorganisms, viruses, neoplasms) to a chemotherapeutic agent; tolerance denotes a diminished pharmacologic responsiveness to a drug.
   II. Sometimes a response declines more slowly with time than the plasma concentration, that is, the response is pharmacodynamically rate limited. Such a condition would require a much shorter dosing interval to be used than what one would predict on the basis of pharmacokinetic principles alone.
   III. If the peak response to a drug during a dosing interval is close to E_{max}, then large changes in systemic exposure might produce minimal changes in response throughout the dosing interval.

   A. I only **E.** I and III
   B. II only **F.** II and III
   C. III only **G.** All
   D. I and II **H.** None
5. Comment on the accuracy of the following statements with regard to drugs given in an oral multiple-dose regimen.
   a. The process of accumulation always occurs.
   b. The accumulation index at plateau depends only on the dosing frequency for a drug with a given half-life.
   c. The time to reach plateau occurs sooner, the more frequently drug is administered.
   d. The smaller the volume of distribution, the higher is the average plateau plasma concentration.
6. It has been said that maintenance of an effect is best achieved by maintaining a constant systemic exposure (plasma concentration) to a drug. Would you support this view? Discuss briefly.
7. A dose of 10 mg of a drug is taken orally twice daily (every 12 hours) by a patient for 2 weeks. The drug is very rapidly absorbed, is fully bioavailable, and has a half-life of 18 hours. Assuming that this regimen approximates intravenous dosing:
   a. Is the 2-week period of time long enough for a plateau to have been practically ($C = 0.9 \times C_{ss}$) reached?
   b. Determine the maximum amount of drug in the body just after the sixth dose from:
      (1) Adding up the amounts of drug remaining in the body from previous doses to the one just given at plateau.
      (2) Direct calculation using the appropriate equation.
   c. What is the minimum amount of drug in the body at plateau?
8. Table 12-6 lists typical pharmacokinetic parameter values and dosage regimens frequently used for acetaminophen, ibuprofen, and naproxen, three nonprescription analgesic/antipyretic agents.
   a. Calculate the average plateau plasma concentrations of these three drugs when subjects are on the regimens given in Table 12-6.
   b. For which of the three drugs is the plateau reached the fastest?
   c. For which of the three drugs is the degree of accumulation the greatest on the common regimens given in Table 12-6.
   d. Assuming instantaneous absorption, calculate the maximum plateau plasma concentration for ibuprofen and naproxen on the regimens given in Table 12-6.

TABLE 12-6 | Pharmacokinetic Parameters and Regimens of Three Drugs

Drug	*F*	*V* (L)	*CL* (L/hr)	Common Oral Dosage Regimen
Acetaminophen	0.9	67	21	1000 mg/6 hr
Ibuprofen	0.7	10	3.5	400 mg/6 hr
Naproxen	0.95	11	0.55	500 mg/12 hr

e. Assuming instantaneous absorption, calculate the minimum plateau plasma concentration for ibuprofen and naproxen on the regimens given in Table 12-6.

f. Assuming instantaneous absorption, calculate the relative fluctuations of ibuprofen and naproxen on the regimens given in Table 12-6. Relative fluctuation is defined as $(C_{max,ss} - C_{min,ss})/C_{av,ss}$. How do you rationalize the difference between these two drugs?

9. Fig. 12-16 shows the mean concentration of albuterol, a β_2-adrenergic agonist bronchodilator, within a 12-hour period at steady state, following oral administration of one 4-mg immediate-release tablet every 6 hours (*black curve*) and one 8-mg extended-release tablet every 12 hours (*colored line*). The areas under the curve within the 12-hour period are 134 μg-hr/L for the immediate-release product and 132 μg-hr/L for the extended-release product.

a. From the data in Fig. 12-16, calculate the relative fluctuation of the plasma concentration at steady state after administration of the two dosage forms, given that the average plasma albuterol concentrations associated with the 6- and 12-hour regimens are 11.2 and 11.0 μg/L, respectively. Relative fluctuation is defined as $(C_{max,ss} - C_{min,ss})/C_{av,ss}$.

b. Is the bioavailability of the drug altered in the extended-release dosage form?

c. Is the increase in the time of occurrence of the peak concentration with the extended-release dosage form expected?

d. Albuterol given in the immediate-release dosage form was found to have a mean half-life of 7.2 hours. Does this alone make the drug a candidate for extended

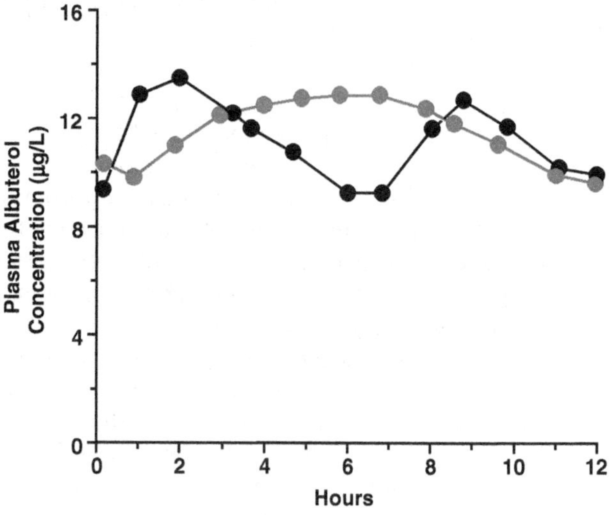

FIGURE 12-16 Mean plasma albuterol concentration with time plots within a 12-hour dosing interval at plateau following a regimen of 4 mg orally of an immediate-release tablet taken every 6 hours (*black circle*) and one 8-mg extended-release tablet taken every 12 hours (*colored circle*). (Taken from *Physician Desk Reference*. 58th Ed. 2004.)

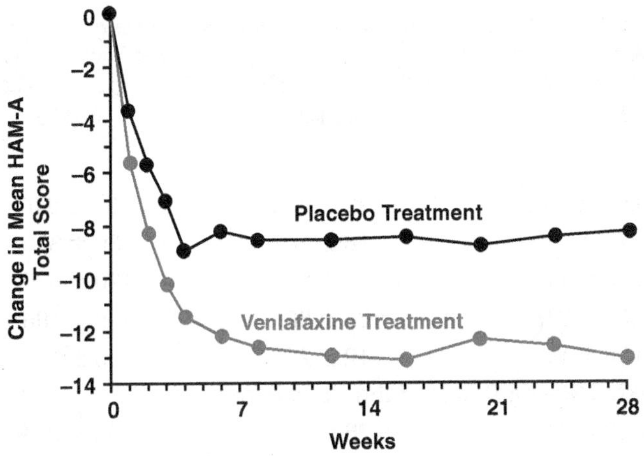

FIGURE 12-17 Changes from baseline in the Hamilton Rating Scale for Anxiety (HAM-A) score in patients receiving either a placebo (*black curve*) or venlafaxine (*colored curve*) (either 75, 150, or 225 mg/day) for 6 months. (From Greenberg AJ, Lydiard RB, Rudolph RL, et al. Efficacy of venlafaxine extended-release capsules in nondepressed outpatients with generalized anxiety disorder. *JAMA* 2000;283:3082–3088.)

release? Discuss other factors that determine the therapeutic usefulness of developing a modified-release dosage form.

10. Venlafaxine is used in the treatment of generalized anxiety disorders. Displayed in Fig. 12-17 are the changes from baseline in the Hamilton Rating Scale for Anxiety (HAM-A) score, an interviewer based measure. A reduction in the HAM-A score is taken as a measure of clinical benefit. The study involved patients receiving either a placebo or venlafaxine (either 75, 150, or 225 mg/day) for 6 months. Venlafaxine, itself active, is extensively metabolized to a major active metabolite, *O*-desmethylvenlafaxine.

    Given that the mean half-lives of venlafaxine and *O*-desmethylvenlafaxine are 5 and 11 hours, respectively, comment on the relationship between the pharmacokinetics of venlafaxine and the clinical response with time.

11. Table 12-7 lists key pharmacokinetic parameters and measures of mefloquine (MQ), an antimalarial agent effective against many strains of multidrug-resistant plasmodium vivax and plasmodium falciparum. The drug is administered as a racemate. The values given in the table are for the racemate and each of the enantiomers after oral administration of the racemate.

    Answer the following questions, given that the drug follows first-order kinetics and a one-compartment model. Use mean values only, except for Part d.

    a. Is the drug rapidly absorbed? Justify your answer.
    b. Does a difference in clearance or volume of distribution, or both, explain the observed kinetic differences between the enantiomers after a single dose?
    c. Using the single dose data, calculate the peak steady-state concentration ($C_{max, ss}$) you would expect from (−)-MQ on a once-weekly regimen. Assume an intravenous bolus for the problem. Show your calculations. How does your estimate compare with the observed $C_{max,ss}$?
    d. The drug (racemate) was given for 13 weeks. Is this time long enough to assure achievement of steady state for both enantiomers in *all* subjects? Briefly discuss.
    e. Based on the single dose data, calculate an accumulation index for (−)-MQ on administering the racemate once weekly.

TABLE 12-7 | Mean (±SD) Pharmacokinetic Measures and Parameters Obtained for Racemate (Rac-MQ) and (+) and (−) Isomers of Mefloquine (MQ).

	Rac-MQ	(+)-MQ	(-)MQ
After a Single 250-mg Dose of the Racemate			
C_{max} (mg/L)	0.52 ± 0.18	0.12 ± 0.02	0.36 ± 0.09
t_{max} (hr)	27 ± 24	18 ± 16	30 ± 31
AUC (0–∞) (mg-hr/L)	223 ± 118	20 ± 5	190 ± 63
Half-life (hr)	400 ± 275	128 ± 50	409 ± 166
AUC (0–7 d) (mg-hr/L)	56 ± 14	12 ± 2	45 ± 12
At Steady State (13 wk) After Weekly 250-mg Doses of the Racemate			
$C_{max,ss}$ (mg/L)	1.68 ± 0.24	0.26 ± 0.05	1.42 ± 0.19
$C_{min,ss}$ (mg/L)	1.12 ± 0.29	0.11 ± 0.04	1.01 ± 0.26
$C_{av,ss}$ (mg/L)	1.35 ± 0.27	0.18 ± 0.05	1.17 ± 0.22
t_{max} (hr)	12 ± 8	15 ± 11	12 ± 2.6
AUC (0–7 d)	227 ± 45	30 ± 9	197 ± 37
After Last Dose (mg-hr/L)			
Half-life (hr)	421 (±157)	173 (±57)	430 (±255)

Data from Gimenez F, Pennie RA, Koren G, et al. Stereoselective pharmacokinetics of mefloquine in healthy Caucasians after multiple doses. *J Pharm Sci* 1994;83:824–827.

f. Determine the relative fluctuations of the plasma concentrations for (+)-MQ, and (−)-MQ at steady state. How do you explain the difference in the values for the two enantiomers?

g. When given to treat patients with malaria, the dosage regimen is five 250-mg tablets (1250 mg) in a single dose. For prevention of malaria, it is recommended that a traveler take 250 mg once weekly for 2–3 weeks before going to the endemic area, and that the weekly doses be continued while traveling and after returning home. Do these regimens seem reasonable to you? Briefly discuss from a pharmacokinetic point of view.

SECTION IV

Individualization

CHAPTER 13

Variability

OBJECTIVES

The reader will be able to:

- Define the terms: additivity of response, adherence to prescribed dosage, adult dosage regimen, allele, coefficient of variation, dominant trait, extensive metabolizers, genotype, genetic polymorphism, heterozygous, homozygous, interindividual variability, intraindividual variability, monogenic, pharmacogenetics, pharmacogenomics, phenotype, polygenic, polymodal frequency distribution, poor metabolizers, population pharmacodynamics, population pharmacokinetics, recessive trait, renal function, synergism, unimodal frequency distribution.
- List six major sources of variability in drug response.
- Evaluate whether variability in drug response is primarily caused by variability in pharmacokinetics, pharmacodynamics, or substantially by both, given response and pharmacokinetic data.
- State why variability around the mean of a parameter is as important as the mean itself.
- Give three examples each of inherited sources of variability in pharmacokinetics and pharmacodynamics.
- Describe the likely changes in the pharmacokinetics of a drug with age, from newborn to elderly patients.
- List and briefly discuss the pharmacokinetic parameters that are often altered in patients with a chronic renal disease.
- Discuss the graded nature of drug interactions.
- Give three examples in which the pharmacokinetics of one drug is altered by concurrent administration of another drug, food, or a herbal preparation.

Thus far, in the context of drug dosage, all patients have been assumed to be alike. Yet, we know that people differ in their response to drugs. Accordingly, there is often a need to tailor drug administration to the individual patient. A failure to do so can lead to ineffective therapy in some patients and toxicity in others.

This section of the book is devoted to treating the individual patient. A broad overview of the subject is presented in this chapter. In particular, evidence for and causes of variation in drug response are examined. The next, and last, chapter deals with the use and implementation of such information in the initiation and maintenance of drug therapy.

Before proceeding, a distinction needs to be made between an individual and the population. Substantial differences in response to drugs commonly exist among patients. Such ***inter*individual variability** is often reflected by the availability of a variety of marketed dose strengths of a drug. For example, diazepam, used in the management of some anxiety disorders, is marketed as 2-, 5-, and 10-mg tablets for oral administration. Because variability in response within a subject from one occasion to another (***intra*individual variability**) is generally smaller than interindividual variability, there is usually little need to subsequently adjust an individual's dosage regimen, once an optimal one is well established. Clearly, if intraindividual variability were large and unpredictable, finding and maintaining dosage for an individual would be an extremely difficult task, particularly for a drug with a low therapeutic index.

Many patients stabilized on one medicine receive another for the treatment of the same or a concurrent condition or disease. Sometimes, the second drug affects the response to the first. The change in response may be clinically insignificant for most of the patient population, with the recommendation that no adjustment in dosage be made. However, a few individuals may exhibit an exaggerated response to the first drug when coadministered with a second one, which could even prove fatal unless dosage for these individuals is reduced. The lesson is clear: average data are useful as a guide, but, ultimately, information pertaining to the individual patient is all-important.

EXPRESSIONS OF INDIVIDUAL DIFFERENCES

Evidence for interindividual differences in drug response comes from several sources. Variability in the dosage required to produce a given response in an adult population is illustrated in Fig. 13-1, which shows the wide range in the daily dose of (racemic) warfarin needed to produce a similar degree of anticoagulant control. Fig. 13-2 shows frequency distribution histograms of the plateau plasma concentration of the antidepressant drug nortriptyline following an oral regimen of 25-mg three times daily,

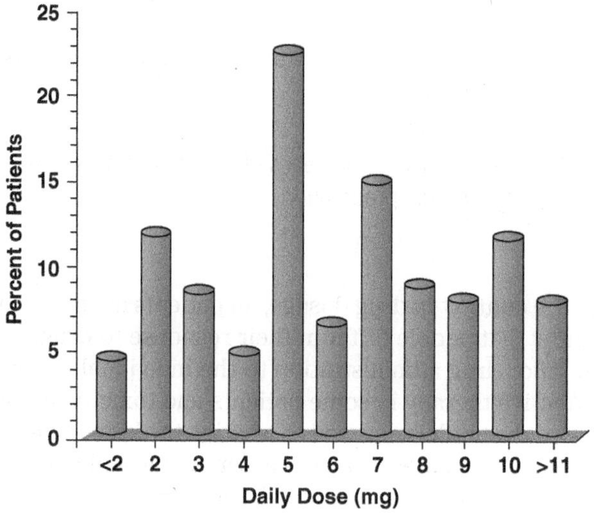

FIGURE 13-1 The daily dose of (racemic) warfarin required to produce a similar degree of anticoagulation in 200 adult patients varies widely. (Redrawn from Koch-Weser J. The serum level approach to individualization of drug dosage. *Eur J Clin Pharmacol* 1975;9:1–8.)

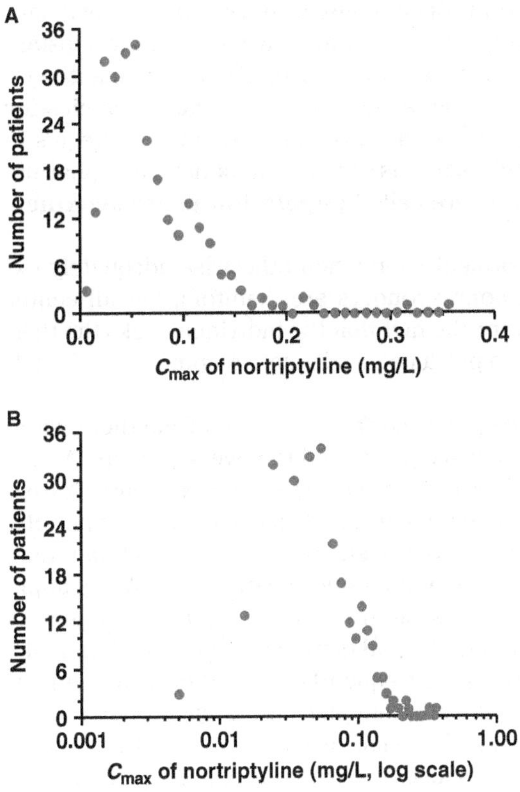

FIGURE 13-2 The maximum plasma concentration of nortriptyline at plateau ($C_{max,ss}$) varies widely in 263 patients receiving a regimen of 25-mg nortriptyline orally three times daily. **A.** Plot of the frequency against the plasma concentration shows a skewed distribution. **B.** The same data plotted against the logarithm of the concentration showing an essentially symmetrical distribution, indicating that the distribution is lognormal. (Redrawn and calculated from Sjoqvist F, Borga O, Orme MLE. Fundamentals of clinical pharmacology. In: Avery GS, ed. *Drug Treatment.* Edinburgh, Scotland: Churchill Livingstone, 1976;1–42.)

thus demonstrating wide interpatient variability in the dose–exposure relationship. Variability in pharmacokinetics is also illustrated by the wide scatter in the plateau plasma concentration of phenytoin seen after various daily doses of this drug (see Fig. 1-7), even when dosage is standardized to body weight. On the other hand, the data in Fig. 13-3, showing the plateau unbound plasma concentration of the more

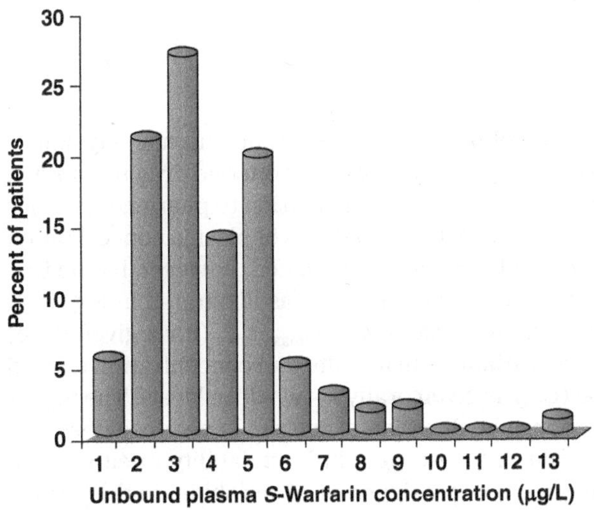

FIGURE 13-3 There is considerable interindividual pharmacodynamic variability in response to the oral anticoagulant warfarin, as demonstrated by the substantial spread in the unbound concentration of the active *S*-isomer associated with a similar degree of anticoagulation in a group of 97 patients on maintenance therapy. (Abstracted from the data of Scordo MG, Pengo V, Spina E, et al. Influence of CYP2C9 and CYP2C19 genetic polymorphisms of warfarin maintenance dose and metabolic clearance. *Clin Pharmacol Ther* 2002;72:702–710.)

active *S*-warfarin enantiomer required to produce a similar degree of anticoagulant control following maintenance therapy with (racemic) warfarin, demonstrate substantial interpatient variability in exposure–response for this drug. Clearly, substantial interindividual variability exists in both pharmacokinetics and pharmacodynamics for warfarin, and measurement of (preferably unbound) drug in plasma is a prerequisite to be able to separate the two. The characterizations of pharmacokinetic and pharmacodynamic variabilities within a population are called **population pharmacokinetics** and **population pharmacodynamics**.

Some patients fail to respond to treatment even when otherwise adequately exposed to the drug. The causes of such nonresponders are manifold, but all center around either misdiagnosis of the disease or the fact that the individual lacks the therapeutic target or expresses one that fails to produce an adequate response (see Genetics later in chapter).

The examples of variability in drug response so far have been of the therapeutic effect, or a surrogate, but the situation applies equally well to adverse effects. As the intensity of an adverse effect in individuals as a function of systemic exposure is rarely studied, adverse events are usually quantified by their incidence in the patient population. Sometimes, however, the intensity of the adverse effect is quantified by examining the incidence of increasingly intense measures of the same general effect. An example is that of phenytoin in which central nervous system depression, a graded effect, is quantified by the incidences of nystagmus, ataxia, and mental changes (see Fig. 10-4). Some relatively minor side effects may occur as frequently as the therapeutic effect, particularly when they are associated with the inherent pharmacologic property of the drug, such as dryness of mouth that occurs with the use of sympathomimetic nasal decongestants. More severe adverse effects may also be frequently experienced. Such is the case for patients undergoing chemotherapy during cancer treatment who tolerate the toxicity because the benefit of the drug outweighs its harm.

Occasionally, a very severe and unusual adverse effect occurs, but its incidence may be so low that only when tens of thousands, if not millions, of patients have been treated with the drug is it detected with any statistical significance. Such adverse effects are most often **idiosyncratic** in nature, that is, they are peculiar to the individual and are genetic in origin. The intensity of these effects, too, has some relationship with systemic exposure in the affected individual, but both the effect itself and the exposure at which it occurs are very different from those observed in the rest of the patient population.

Quantifying Variability

The magnitude and relative contribution of pharmacokinetics and pharmacodynamics to variability in response within a patient population differ from one drug to another. In clinical practice, an attempt to assign the relative contribution to pharmacokinetics and pharmacodynamics is often based on direct observations of plasma concentration and response. Such an assignment could be strongly influenced, however, by the timing of the observations and the magnitude of the response, as illustrated in Fig. 13-4. Here, a drug that displays little interpatient variability in C_{max}, t_{max} (for a given dose) and in maximum effect, E_{max}, but large variability in half-life and concentration needed to produce 50% maximum response (C_{50}), is given orally at two dose levels. The higher dose achieves close to maximal response in all patients, and the lower dose does not. At the higher dose, observations made at t_{max} suggest little variability in either concentration or response, with perhaps a greater assignment of variability to the former,

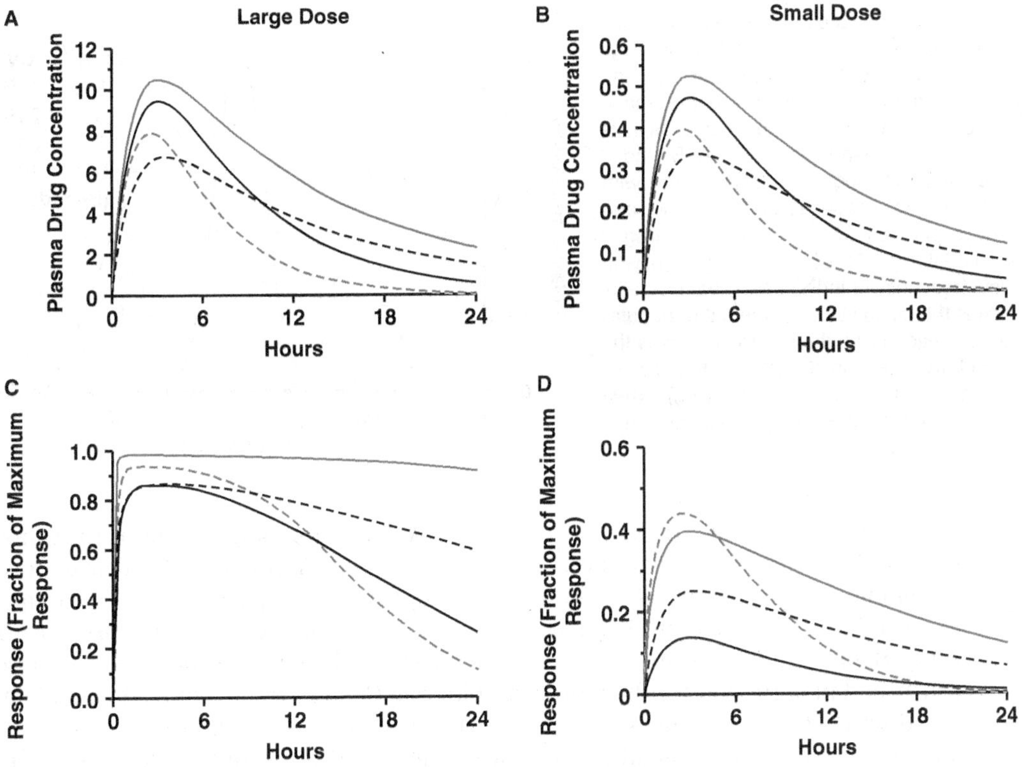

FIGURE 13-4 The interindividual variability in concentration and response varies with dose and time of observation. Shown are plasma concentrations **(A and B)** and responses **(C and D)** following large (*left*) and small (*right*) doses of a drug that displays little interpatient variability in C_{max}, t_{max} and maximum response, E_{max}, but large interpatient variability in both half-life and concentration needed to produce 50% maximum response (C_{50}). Each line corresponds to the value with time in an individual patient. **Observations after large dose:** at t_{max}, there is little variability in C_{max} (**A**) or in response (**C**), as the maximum response is produced in all patients. **Observations after small dose:** at t_{max}, variability in C_{max} (**B**) is still relatively low, but that in response (**D**) is now considerable. Greater variability in concentration and response is seen at later times for both large and small doses.

because variation in plasma concentration produces relatively little change in response. At later times after this higher dose, substantial variability is observed in both concentration and response. In contrast, for the lower dose, at t_{max}, there is still little interpatient variability in C_{max}, but now there is considerable variability in response. This dependence on dose and time in the assignment of variability is minimized by expressing variability not in terms of observations but rather in terms of the parameter values defining pharmacokinetics and pharmacodynamics, that is, in F, k_a, CL, and V for pharmacokinetics, and in E_{max}, C_{50}, and the steepness factor (γ) for pharmacodynamics (Chapter 3). Once variability in each of these parameters, together with any correlation between them, is defined, the expected variability in concentration and response within the patient population at any time associated with a given dosage regimen can be calculated.

Describing Variability

Knowing how a particular pharmacokinetic or pharmacodynamic parameter varies within the patient population is important in therapy. To illustrate this statement, consider the frequency distributions in, for example, clearance of the four hypothetical

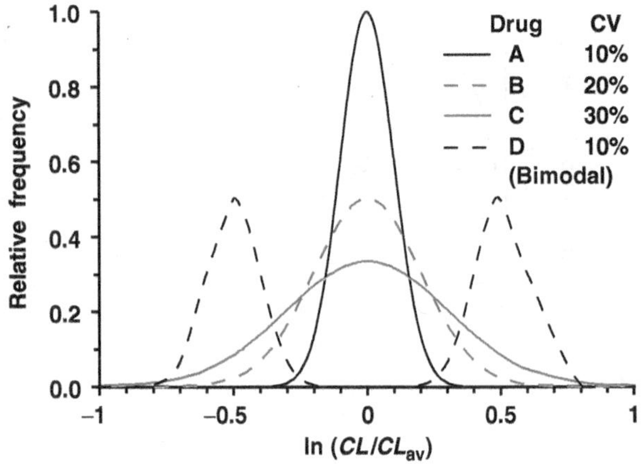

FIGURE 13-5 As the frequency distributions for the clearance of four hypothetical drugs (A, B, C, D) show, it is as important to define variability around the mean and the shape of the frequency distribution curve as it is to define the mean itself. Drugs A, B, and C exhibit unimodal lognormal distributions with coefficients of variation (CV) of 10%, 20%, and 30%, respectively. The distribution for drug D is bimodal (CV = 10% in each subgroup), with a low frequency of individuals in whom clearance is the mean value for the entire population. For each drug, the horizontal axis is the logarithm of the ratio of clearance to the average value within the population (CL_{av}). When clearance equals the average value, the ratio is 1, and its logarithm equals 0.

drugs shown in Fig. 13-5. The mean, or central tendency, for all four drugs is the same, but variability about the mean is very different. For drugs A, B, and C, the distributions are unimodal and lognormal; here, the mean represents a typical value of clearance expected in the population. Because variability about the mean is much greater for drugs B and C than for drug A, one has much less confidence that the mean for these drugs, and in particular for the more variable drug C, applies to an individual patient. For drug D, distribution in clearance is bimodal, signifying that there are two major subgroups within the population: those with high and those with low clearances. Obviously, in this case, the mean is one of the most unlikely values to be found in this patient population.

A comment on the quantitation of variability is needed here. **Coefficient of variation** is widely used to express relative variability when comparing different measures, such as clearance and volume of distribution. Specifically, it is the standard deviation (square root of variance) normalized to the mean. Thus,

$$\text{Coefficient of Variation}(\%) = \frac{\text{Standard Deviation}}{\text{Mean}} \times 100 \quad \textbf{Eq. 13-1}$$

Subsequently, the terms *high variability* and *low variability* refer to distributions that have high and low coefficients of variation, respectively. Typically, a coefficient of variation of a parameter of 10% or less is considered low, 20% moderate, and above 30% high. Although these values do not appear too dissimilar, examination of the three unimodal distributions in Fig. 13-5 with these respective coefficients of variation illustrates, however, just how variable a distribution with a coefficient of variation of 30% (drug C) truly is.

WHY PEOPLE DIFFER

The reasons why people differ in their responsiveness to a given dose, or regimen, of a drug are manifold, and include genetics, disease, gender, race, diet, activity, age, body weight, concomitantly administered drugs, and a variety of behavioral and environmental factors. Age, body weight, disease, and concomitantly administered drugs are important because they are sources of variability that can be readily determined and taken into account. Diet and activity are often harder to evaluate. Although inheritance accounts for a substantial part of the differences in response among individuals for many drugs, and as noted below many advances in genetic aspects have been made in recent years, much of this source of variability is still largely unpredictable, particularly in regard to their pharmacodynamics. Gender-linked differences in hormonal balance, body composition, and activity of certain enzymes manifest themselves in differences in both pharmacokinetics and responsiveness, but overall, the effect of gender is relatively small.

Genetics

Inheritance accounts for a large part of both the striking and the subtle differences among individuals, including much of the variation in response to an administered drug. Our knowledge of this area is expanding very rapidly with the characterization of the human genome. **Pharmacogenetics** is the study of inherited variations in drug response. **Pharmacogenomics** is the application of genomic information to the identification of putative drug targets and to the causes of variability in drug response. Before proceeding to specific examples, some definitions are important to an understanding of the subject.

The basic biological unit of heredity is the gene. **Genotype** is the fundamental assortment of an individual's genes—the blueprint—whereas **phenotype** is the outward characteristic expression of an individual, such as the color of a person's eyes or his or her drug-metabolizing activity. The mode of inheritance is either **monogenic** or **polygenic**, depending on whether it is transmitted by a gene at a single locus or by genes at multiple loci on the chromosomes. Monogenically controlled conditions are often detected as a dramatic and abnormal drug response. They may also be detected in population studies by a **polymodal frequency distribution** of the characteristic or some measure of it, as depicted for the clearance of drug D in Fig. 13-5 with 50% in each subpopulation. Quite often, however, a characteristic of an individual, like that of clearance, is controlled or influenced by many genes, with the overall result being its having an apparent **unimodal frequency distribution** in the general population.

The human genome consists of more than 1.5 million single nucleotide polymorphisms (SNPs) along DNA. The alternate forms, each occupying corresponding positions on paired chromosomes, one inherited from the male and the other from the female, are called **alleles.** Different alleles produce variation in inherited characteristics such as hair color or blood type. An allele is **dominant** if it expresses itself phenotypically, and **recessive** if it does not. An individual possessing a pair of identical alleles, either dominant or recessive, is **homozygous** for the gene. A union of a dominant with a recessive allele produces a **heterozygous** individual for that characteristic. Both homozygous individuals with dominant alleles and heterozygous individuals show the same phenotype, and homozygous individuals with recessive alleles show another. Alleles are often characterized using the * notation. For example, a gene denoted by *1/*1 is homogeneous, and one by *1/*3 is heterogeneous, for allele 1, where allele 1 is often the wild-type, or the most common allele, for the gene found in the population studied. The numbering generally follows the chronologic order that an allele was identified. Sometimes, it is a set of nearby SNPs on the same chromosome that is inherited as a block, a **haplotype**, rather than a single SNP, which determines phenotypic behavior.

Historically, the role of genetics in drug response has been shown by the observation that the differences in phenotypic behavior in identical twins is much smaller than those in either nonidentical twins or between any two randomly selected age-, gender-, and weight-matched subjects. Although this approach in identifying the relative importance of genetics is helpful, today more definitive data concerning mechanisms are obtained by genomic profiling using molecular biology techniques.

Because the approximately 30,000 genes contain multiple SNPs, identification of the most relevant ones affecting disease susceptibility and drug response holds the promise

TABLE 13-1 | Frequency of Genetic Polymorphisms Producing Slow Metabolism in Some Drug-Metabolizing Enzymes and Representative Substrates

Enzyme	Frequency of Poor Metabolizer	Drug Substrates[a]
Phase I Reactions		
CYP2D6	5%–10% Caucasians 3.8% Blacks 0.9% Asians 1% Arabs	Bufurolol, codeine, dextromethorphan, encainide, flecainide, metoprolol, nortriptyline, timolol
CYP2C9	1%–3% Caucasians	Celecoxib, fluvastatin, glyburide, *S*-ibruprofen, tolbutamide, phenytoin, *S*-warfarin.
CYP2C19	3%–5% Caucasians 16% Asians	Diazepam, lansoprazole, omeprazole, pantoprazole.
Butylcholinesterase	Several abnormal genes; most common disorder 1 in 2500	Succinylcholine
Phase II Reactions		
Thiopurine *S*-methyltransferase	0.3% Caucasians 0.04% Asians	Azathioprine, mercaptopurine.
N-acetyltransferase (NAT2)	60% Caucasians, African Americans 10%–20% Asians	Amrinone, hydralazine, isoniazid, phenelzine, aminosalicylic acid.
Uridine diphosphate glucuronosyltranferase		
1A1	11% Caucasians 1%–3% Asians	Irinotecan
2B7	29% Caucasians 7% Asians	Flurbiprofen

Generally results in enhanced or prolonged effect following standard dose of drug.
[a]A major pathway for the elimination of compound.

of predicting these for individual patients. Tables 13-1 and 13-2 list **genetic polymorphisms** that affect the pharmacokinetics and pharmacodynamics of some drugs.

Inherited Variability in Pharmacokinetics

Examples of inherited variability in pharmacokinetics have been mostly restricted to drug metabolism. However, there is increasing evidence of genetic polymorphism in drug transporters, which impact to varying degrees on drug absorption, drug distribution, and renal or biliary excretion. For example, genetic polymorphisms have been identified in organic anion-transporting polypeptide 1B1 (OATP1B1) responsible for the hepatic uptake of a variety of drugs, including statins. These drugs act in the liver to lower cholesterol, but also have the potential to induce skeletal muscle weakness and inflammation. Normally, the orally administered statin is avidly taken up by OATP1B1 into the liver and maintained there, with little escaping into the systemic circulation. However, the 2% of the patient population who are homozygous for the inefficient

TABLE 13-2 | Some Genetic Polymorphisms in Pharmacodynamics

Target	Drug(s)	Drug Effect Linked With Polymorphism
Therapeutic Effects		
ACE[a]	ACE inhibitors (e.g., enalapril)	Lowering of blood pressure, renoprotective effects
VKORC1[b]	Warfarin	Variation in sensitivity to oral coumarin anticoagulants. Pronounced resistance very rarely encountered
β_2-adrenergic receptor	β_2-agonists (e.g., albuterol)	Bronchodilatation, cardiovascular effects
Dopamine receptors (D_1, D_2, D_3)	Antipsychotic agents (e.g., clozapine)	Antipsychotic response
Estrogen receptors	Conjugated estrogens	Increase in bone mineral density
HERG2[c]	Trastuzumab	Treatment of breast cancer
EGFR-TK[d]	Gelfitinib, erlotinib	Treatment of small-cell lung cancer
ABL1[e]	Dasatinib, imatinib	Treatment of chronic myeloid leukemia (CML)
Adverse Effects		
Glucose-6-phosphate dehydrogenase (G6PD)	Variety of drugs (e.g., primaquine, nitrofurantoin)	Favism or drug-induced hemolytic anemia in those with G6PD deficiency. Affects approximately 100 million worldwide; high frequency in African Americans.
Bradykinin B_2 receptor	ACE[a] inhibitors	ACE inhibitor–induced cough
HLA-B*1502[f]	Carbamazepine	Dangerous or even fatal reactions, exclusively in broad area of Asia, including South Asian Indians.
Dihydropyridine Ca^{2+} channel receptors	Volatile anesthetics	Malignant hyperthermia, a rare potentially fatal reaction.

[a]Angiotensin-converting enzyme.
[b]Vitamin K epoxide reductase
[c]Human ether-a-go-go related gene
[d]Epidermal growth factor receptor tyrosine kinase
[e]ABL(Abelson) proto-oncogene 1, non-receptor tyrosine kinase
[f]Human leucocyte antigen, class B, marker for Stevens-Johnson syndrome

allele of this transporter are much more prone to muscle problems, owing to the much higher systemic (and hence muscle) exposure of the statins, resulting from reduced uptake into the liver during their oral absorption in such patients. When polymorphism in a transporter affects the distribution to the site of action, such as the liver or brain, or a site of potential toxicity, modifying the unbound concentration and effect there, without materially affecting the unbound plasma concentration, the effect tends to be defined as an example of an inherited variation in pharmacodynamics, either efficacy or safety, even though the cause is a pharmacokinetic one. Clearly, in the absence of knowing the unbound concentration at the active site, which is rare clinically, correct assignment as to the cause of such variability cannot be made with confidence.

Several genetic polymorphisms of drug metabolism have now been identified, primarily involving oxidation, but also S-methylation, glucuronidation, acetylation, and hydrolysis (Table 13-1). Most were initially detected by adverse reactions occurring in a distinct group within the population termed **poor metabolizers**, following normal doses of the archetypic drugs. Some examples follow.

Oxidation

Debrisoquine, an antihypertensive agent no longer in use, was the first drug shown to exhibit genetic polymorphism in oxidation. There is a deficiency in the metabolism of this drug in 5%–10% of Caucasians, poor metabolizers, with wide differences in frequency in other ethnic groups (Table 13-1). It is a recessive trait, caused by a specific deficient variant of CYP2D6. Of the remainder of the population, often referred to as **extensive metabolizers**, some are ultrafast metabolizers because they possess up to 13 copies of the normal gene within the population, commonly referred to as the wild type. This is clearly expressed phenotypically in the strong inverse correlation between the number of copies and the AUC of nortriptyline, another substrate predominantly cleared via CYP2D6 oxidation (Fig. 13-6). This variation is the main reason for the wide spread in the steady-state plasma nortriptyline concentrations among patients receiving the same regimen of nortriptyline (Fig. 13-2). Recall from Chapter 6, although comprising only approximately 2% of the total hepatic CYP 450 content, CYP2D6 is the major enzyme responsible for the metabolism of approximately 25% of prescribed small molecular weight drugs, particularly basic compounds, including the β-blocker metoprolol and the antidepressants doxepin and paroxetine.

Genetic polymorphism is not restricted to CYP2D6. Although the wide variation in the daily maintenance dose of warfarin has been known for many years, only more

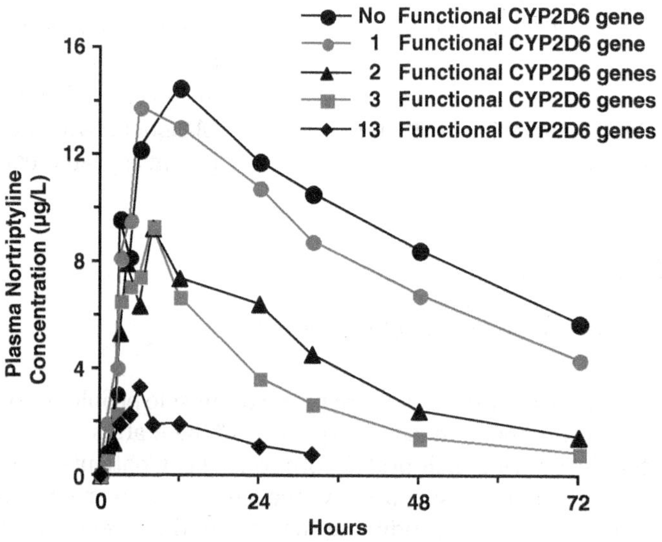

FIGURE 13-6 Strong genetic influence in the pharmacokinetics of nortriptyline is clearly demonstrated by the high correlation between the plasma concentration–time profile and the number of functional *CYP2D6* genes possessed by an individual; the larger the number of functional genes, the higher is the clearance, and the lower is the exposure profile after a single 25-mg dose of nortriptyline. (Redrawn from Dalen P, Dahl ML, Ruiz MLB, et al. 10-Hydroxylation of nortriptyline in white persons with 0, 1, 2, 3, and 13 functional CYP2D6 genes. *Clin Pharmacol Ther* 1998;63:444–452.)

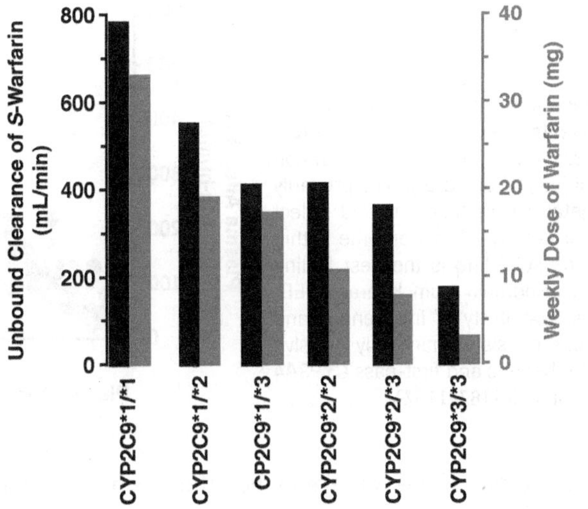

FIGURE 13-7 Genetics plays a significant role in the maintenance dose requirement of warfarin used in the treatment of a variety of cardiovascular diseases. Shown is the unbound clearance of *S*-warfarin (*black*) in groups of patients with different *CYP2C9* genotypes, all titrated and stabilized to a narrow target INR (International normalization ratio, a measure of anticoagulation) range of between 2 and 3, and the mean weekly maintenance dose (obtained by summing the daily dose over 1 week, *in color*). Warfarin is administered in its racemic form, with most of the therapeutic effect associated with the more active *S*-isomer, which is primarily eliminated by CYP2C9-catalyzed metabolism. Patients with two wild-type alleles (denoted by CYP2C9*1/*1) have the highest *S*-warfarin clearance and require the highest maintenance dose, and those with two of the most deficient alleles (CYP2C9*3/*3) have the lowest clearance and need the smallest maintenance dose. However, as noted in Fig. 13-3, there is still considerable interindividual variability in pharmacodynamics of this compound. (Abstracted from the data of Scordo MG, Pengo V, Spina, E, et al. Influence of CYP2C9 and CYP2C19 genetic polymorphisms of warfarin maintenance dose and metabolic clearance. *Clin Pharmacol Ther* 2002;72:702–710.)

recently has it become clear that a significant contribution to this variability is mutation of the *CYP2C9* gene, primarily responsible for the metabolism of the more potent *S*-isomer of this racemically administered drug (Fig. 13-7). Other drugs that are predominantly metabolized by CYP2C9, and for which clearance is reduced between 2 and 10 fold of the wild type in poor metabolizers include celecoxib, *S*-ibuprofen, losartan, phenytoin, tolbutamide, and torsemide.

Many drugs are oxidized with widely differing efficiencies by the different forms of cytochrome P-450 in addition to CYP2D6 and CYP2C9, such as CYP2C19 (Table 13-1). The clearance values within the population associated with the oxidation of certain drugs cosegregate, in that, for example, a poor metabolizer of midazolam is also a poor metabolizer of alfentanil (Fig. 13-8, next page). This indicates that they are substrates for the same enzyme—in this case CYP3A4 (Fig. 13-9, next page). There is also considerable overlap in the structural specificity of some of these enzymes, such that a drug may be a substrate for more than one of them. The majority of oxidatively metabolized drugs are substrates for CYP3A4, the most abundant cytochrome (Fig. 6-9). Commonly, there is marked variability in clearance of such substrates within the population, with a coefficient of variation of 30%–40% owing to variation in enzymatic activity. One might expect to demonstrate a genetic influence in the clearance of substrates of this enzyme, but no such relationship has been clearly demonstrated. Unlike CYP2D6 and CYP2C9, CYP3A4 (and the efflux transporter P-glycoprotein) is inducible by a variety of environmental (nongenetic) factors, weakening any ability

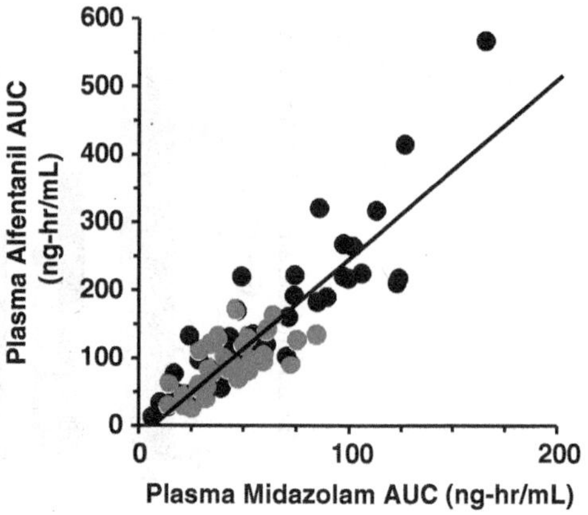

FIGURE 13-8 A high degree of cosegregation exists between midazolam and alfentanil exposures after intravenous (*color circles*) and oral (*black circles*) administration of these drugs to 12 subjects. Both drugs are primarily eliminated by CYP3A4 catalyzed metabolism, and reflect variation in the functional activity of this enzyme within this group of subjects. The solid line is the best fit line to the experimental data. (Redrawn from Kharasch ED, Walker A, Hoffer C, et al. Sensitivity of intravenous and oral alfentanil and papillary miosis as minimally invasive and noninvasive probes for hepatic and first-pass CYP3A4 activity. *J Clin Pharmacol* 2005;45:1187–1197.)

to detect genetic factors. However, even when there is a genetic influence involved in the formation of a metabolite, whether one is likely to detect it based on measurement of drug alone depends on the importance of the affected pathway to the overall elimination of the compound. Examining only half-life or total clearance of the unchanged drug may fail to detect a genetically controlled source of variability of a minor pathway

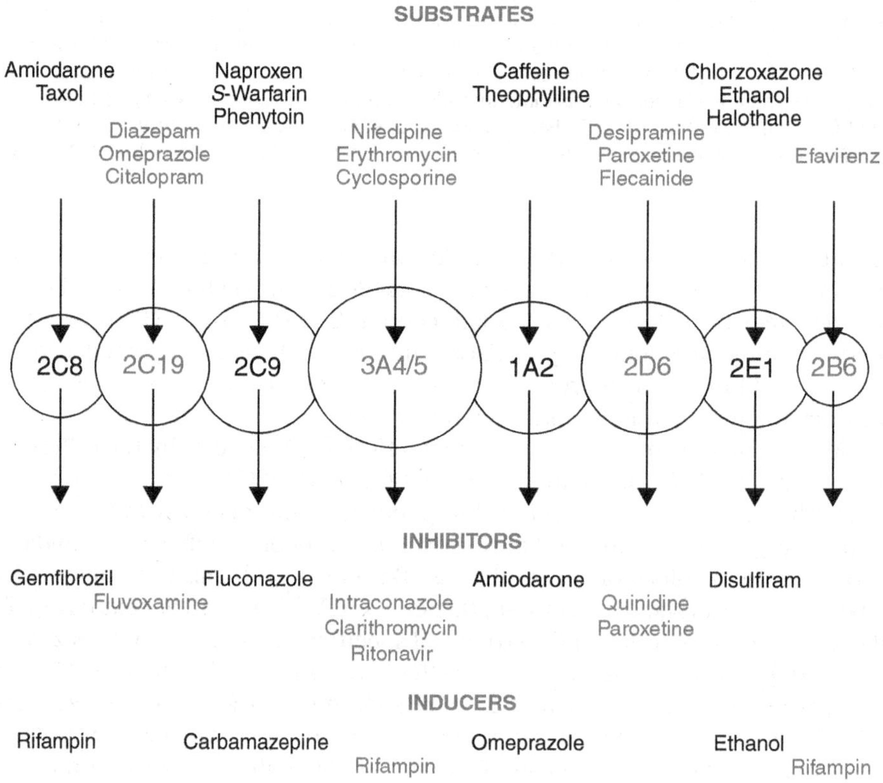

FIGURE 13-9 Graphic representation of the different forms of cytochrome-P450 (*circles*) in humans with different but some overlapping substrate specificities. The arrows indicate single metabolic pathways. Representative substrates are listed above for each enzyme. Also listed are relatively selective and strong inhibitors and inducers of the enzymes.

of metabolism. Yet, if the affected metabolite is very potent or toxic, identifying and quantifying this source of variation may be therapeutically important. This appears to be the case with codeine. Although a generally minor pathway of codeine metabolism, formation of morphine via CYP2D6 oxidation contributes significantly to the analgesic effects following codeine administration. Accordingly, poor metabolizers of codeine via this pathway will derive less analgesic benefit. In contrast, ultrafast metabolizers, having many multiple copies of CYP2D6, form larger than normal amounts of morphine. One particular group vulnerable to such large amounts of formed morphine are suckling neonates, who handle morphine poorly, owing to lack of maturation of the enzymes responsible for the metabolism of this compound, thereby leading to excessively high exposures with potential fatal consequences. Clearly, taking codeine by ultrafast metabolizer breast-feeding mothers is contraindicated. Although rare in Caucasians, this characteristic is relatively common (up to 30%) among some North African communities.

S-Methylation

Thiopurine methyltransferase (TPMT) is the predominant enzyme within hematopoietic cells that inactivates thiopurines by catalyzing their S-methylation. Thiopurine drugs include azathioprine, mercaptopurine, and thioguanine, which are used in the treatment of a number of conditions, such as leukemia and inflammatory bowel disease. TPMT exhibits genetic polymorphism. Approximately 90% of patients inherit high activity; they are homozygous with two high-activity TPMT alleles. Another 10% have intermediate activity; they are heterozygous with one high-activity and one essentially nonfunctional TPMT allele. And 0.3% have minimal to no detectable activity, associated with the inheritance of two nonfunctional TPMT alleles. The last group is at particular risk when given standard doses of the above drugs, resulting in an excessively high intracellular concentration of the corresponding active thioguanine nucleoside, owing to the failure to be removed by S-methylation, and attendant severe hematopoietic toxicity, even sometimes with just one dose. Fortunately, all subjects receiving these drugs can be readily genotyped before treatment, and the dose reduced in the deficient patients, sufficient to achieve adequate therapy without the toxicity, as depicted in Fig. 13-10 (next page).

Conjugation

Irinotecan used in the treatment of metastatic colorectal cancer, is a prodrug hydrolyzed to an active species (SN-38). Some patients manifest severe neutropenia and diarrhea, which can be life threatening, on standard doses of irinotecan while others do not, a difference that appears to be due to genetic polymorphism in uridine diphosphate glucuronosyltranferase (UGT)1A1, the enzyme that catalyzes the conjugation of SN-38 to its inactive glucuronide, its primary route of elimination. The specific mutation (UGT1A1*28) has been identified; it has a lower catalytic activity than the wild type, resulting in lower clearance of SN-38 and higher exposure in patients that are homozygous for this mutation. UGT1A1 is part of a superfamily of glucuronosyl transferases, and while some others also show genetic polymorphism, many do not.

Gluronidation is a common conjugation mechanism of drugs and metabolites. **Acetylation** is much less common, but for those drugs that depend heavily on this pathway, evidence of genetic polymorphism is clear. Included among these is the antitubercular drug isoniazid, which, in fact, was the first identified case of genetic control of drug metabolism. Isoniazid is primarily acetylated in the liver to *N*-acetylisoniazid, a precursor of a hepatotoxic compound; differences in the elimination kinetics of

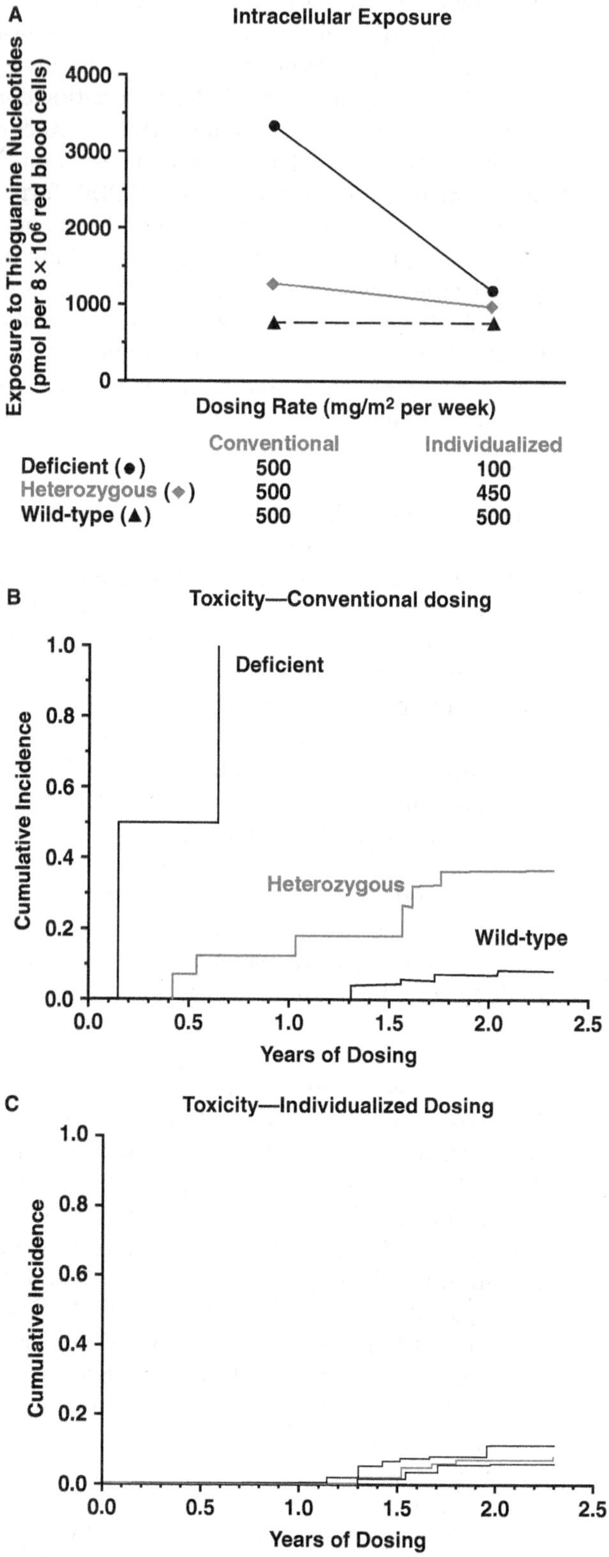

FIGURE 13-10 Genetic polymorphism of TPMT plays a major role in determining the dose of thiopurine drugs (azathiopurine, mercaptopurine, and thioguanine) required for optimal therapy. When all patients receive the same conventional dose of these drugs (**A,** values on left), the systemic exposure of the active thioguanine nucleotides in blood cells is about fivefold higher in the homozygous TPMT-deficient patients than in the wild type, with an associated much higher toxicity experienced by such patients. At the same conventional dose, heterozygous patients have an intermediate systemic exposure and toxicity (**B**). In contrast, when the dosage is individualized based on genotypic status before therapy, systemic exposure is similar across all patients (**A**), and severe acute toxicity is virtually avoided (**C**). (Redrawn from Evans WE. Thiopurine *S*-methyltransferase: a genetic polymorphism that affects a small number of drugs in a big way. *Pharmacogenetics* 2002;12:421–423.)

isoniazid reflect polymorphism of a particular *N*-acetyltransferase, NAT2, a cytosolic enzyme, of which there are many variants, and which show large genetically controlled ethnic differences in the distribution of acetylator status. Both Caucasians and blacks have approximately equal numbers of slow and fast acetylators, but in Asian and Eskimo populations, the percentage of slow acetylators is much smaller.

Interest in acetylation polymorphism is not just academic. Peripheral neuropathy, associated with elevated concentrations of isoniazid, occurs more prevalently in slow acetylators unless an adjustment is made in the dosage of isoniazid or vitamin B_6 is concomitantly administered to offset this effect. Awareness of the prevalence of homozygous and heterozygous rapid acetylators may also be clinically relevant, as they appear to differ in their susceptibility to adverse reactions, such as isoniazid-induced hepatic damage. Acetylation polymorphism also occurs and is important for several other drugs, such as hydralazine and amrinone (Table 13-1). For both drugs the *N*-acetyl derivative is the major metabolite. A systemic lupus erythematosus-like syndrome, a generalized inflammatory response, can limit the use of hydralazine; it develops more rapidly in slow rather than rapid acetylators. The mechanism remains obscure, but does appear to be associated with elevated plasma concentrations of parent compound. In contrast, rapid acetylators require higher doses of hydralazine to control hypertension.

Unusual for drug-metabolizing enzymes, expression of NAT2 activity is under monogenic control. Generally, the frequency of occurrence of an allele is linked with other factors, such as gender. Also, several subgroups within the general population are often of a given ethnicity. These effects make it difficult to calculate the genotype frequency. However, notwithstanding the difficulties in making precise calculations, knowledge of the existence of large ethnic differences in pharmacokinetics, such as seen with isoniazid and some other drugs, is clearly important for the optimal use of drugs. This is particularly true for drugs prescribed worldwide or used in a multiracial society.

Additional Clinical Considerations

Several additional points need to be made. First, the clinical implications of genetic polymorphism in drug metabolism depend on whether activity lies with the affected substrate or with the metabolite, as well as the importance of the pathway to overall elimination. For drugs such as nortriptyline, activity resides predominantly with the drug, and elimination is almost completely restricted to the affected pathway. In such cases, unless the dose is reduced, more pronounced and sustained effects may occur together with potentially more frequent adverse reactions in poor metabolizers. A contrasting and interesting situation is seen with codeine, as mentioned above for the infants of breast-feeding mothers. Many other scenarios can be envisaged, depending on the relative contribution of the affected pathway to total elimination and whether drug, metabolite, or both contribute to activity or toxicity, or both.

Second, part of the large interindividual variability in the degree of drug interactions involving inhibition and induction (increased synthesis) of drug-metabolizing enzymes (see also Interacting Drugs later in this chapter) is under genetic control and is increasingly predictable. For example, quinidine is a potent inhibitor of CYP2D6 and therefore inhibits the formation of all metabolites that are produced from substrates of this enzyme (see Fig. 13-8). Quinidine effectively converts a normally extensive metabolizer of CYP2D6 to a functionally enzyme-deficient one (poor metabolizer).

Inherited Variability in Pharmacodynamics

It is not uncommon for about 30% of a patient population to fail to respond to drug treatment. Reasons for this are many, but one of them is lack of the target receptor. For example, trastuzumab is a humanized monoclonal antibody used in the treatment of primary breast cancer. It has a high affinity for, and effectively inhibits, the proto-oncogene *HER2*, a promoter of cancer. However, HER2 protein overexpression is observed in only 24%–30% of primary breast cancers. Because trastuzumab is not without adverse effects and is expensive, it is inappropriate to administer this drug to patients who will derive no benefit from it. The solution has been to screen all patients with a diagnostic genomic test and give the drug only to patients who overly express the receptor. Other examples are gefitinib (Iressa) and vemurafenib (Zelboraf). Gefitinib, used in the treatment of patients with non–small-cell lung cancer, inhibits epidermal growth factor receptor tyrosine kinase (EGFR-TK), an important mediator of growth factor signaling pathways that regulate key cellular functions. Patients with tumors that have certain somatic mutations of EGFR-TK show a much more marked beneficial response to gefitinib. These susceptible mutations occur more frequently in Japanese than in Caucasians. Used in the treatment of advanced malignant melanoma, vemurafenib inhibits the B-Raf enzyme (involved in cell signaling and growth) and works only in patients who have the BRAF V600 mutation. This approach of stratification of patients into groups based upon some diagnostic, often genomic, screen is being increasingly adopted both during clinical development of a drug, to help identify patients who might best benefit from a new drug and so improve the efficiency of the clinical trial, and in its subsequent therapeutic use. Currently, these and most of the current examples of stratified medicine are in oncology and involve expensive drugs. However, it is envisaged that stratified medicine will become more widespread as our understanding of the molecular basis of disease improves and the price of genomic profiling drops.

Another example of genetically determined variation in pharmacodynamics is illustrated in Fig. 13-11, which shows differences in the FEV_1 (forced expiratory volume in 1 second), which is a measure of respiratory function, in patients following a single oral dose of the β-adrenergic agonist albuterol. Yet another is seen with warfarin. As previously noted, patients vary in the daily dose of warfarin needed to produce adequate anticoagulant control, some of which is due to differences in pharmacodynamics (Fig. 13-3). Warfarin acts by lowering the concentration of reduced vitamin K

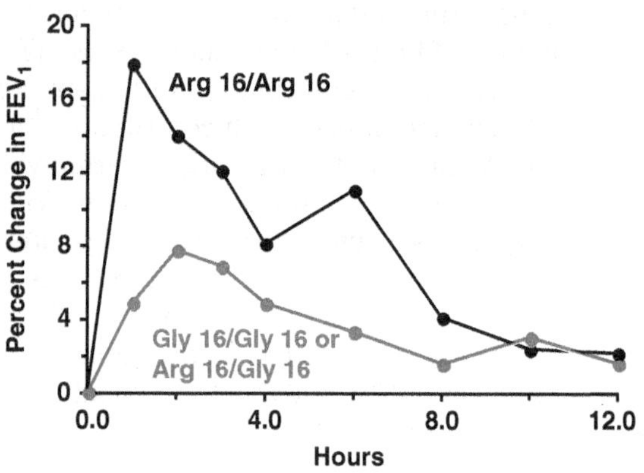

FIGURE 13-11 Functional pharmacodynamic consequences of genetic polymorphisms in the β_2-adrenoreceptor is seen by differences in FEV_1 (forced expired volume in 1 second), a measure of respiratory function, in patients in response to a single 8-mg oral dose of the β-agonist albuterol. Note that the response is greater in those homozygous with arginine (*black*) than with glycine or heterozygous with arginine and glycine (*color*) on position 16 of the gene encoding for the receptor. (Redrawn from Lima JJ, Thomason DB, Mohamed MH, et al. Impact of genetic polymorphisms of the β_2-adrenoreceptor on albuterol bronchodilator pharmacodynamics. *Clin Pharmacol Ther* 1999;65:519–525.)

within the liver by decreasing its regeneration from the inactive vitamin K epoxide pool in the vitamin K cycle, through inhibition of vitamin K epoxide reductase (VKOR). Vitamin K is an essential cofactor for the synthesis of the vitamin K–dependent clotting factors (Factors II, V, IX, and X) as well as the anticoagulant proteins C and S. Certain polymorphisms in the *VKORCI* gene have now been associated with lower dose requirements for warfarin. While, understandably, attention has been focused on patients needing low doses, to minimize the risk of overanticoagulation, some patients are resistant to warfarin and require massive doses (up to 180 mg weekly, compared with the normal range 7–50 mg) to achieve a therapeutic response; failure to do so brings the risk of a thromboembolism. The high resistance is conferred by a particular abnormal variant of the *VKORC1* haplotype, which although rare among most populations, is relatively common (15%) in specific ethnic groups (e.g., of Ethiopian ancestry). Knowledge of the *CYP2C9* and *VKORC1* genotypic status of a patient helps to identify the loading dose of warfarin, especially for those likely to be at the extremes of dose requirement. Because of the ease of measurement of prothrombin complex and its usefulness in guiding therapy, adjustment of the maintenance dose continues to be based on measures of the individual's degree of anticoagulation.

Genetic control is not restricted to therapeutically beneficial effects, but is increasingly being identified as a major source of variability in adverse effects. One clear example is seen with abacavir (Ziagen), a guanosine reverse-transcriptase inhibitor used as part of anti-HIV treatment. In Caucasians, 5%–8% experience severe, and potentially fatal, immunologically determined adverse reactions, including fever, rash, and severe gastrointestinal and respiratory distress when treated with abacavir. These patients carry the HLA (human leukocyte antigen)-B*5701 allelic variant, which is highly predictive of these severe reactions. HLA-B*5701 has been proposed as a screening biomarker to limit the use of abacavir to HLA-B*5701-negative patients, in whom it is relatively safe.

Some other examples of genetically determined variation in pharmacodynamics are given in Table 13-2. Although the number of examples is still currently small, the importance of such sources of variability in response, when coupled with an appropriate diagnostic test, is likely to play a more dominant role in future drug therapy.

Age and Weight

Age is an additional source of variability in drug response, and, as a result, the usual adult dosage regimen may need to be modified, particularly in the young and the very old, if optimal therapy is to be achieved. Furthermore, it is the very young and the aged who often are in most critical need of drugs.

The life of a human is commonly divided into various stages. In this book, the various stages are defined as follows: *neonate*, up to 1 month post utero; *infant*, between the ages of 1 month and 2 years; *child*, between 2 and 12 years; *adolescent*, between 13 and 17 years; *adult*, between 18 and 75 years; and *elder*, a person older than 75 years of age. It is recognized, however, that this stratification of human life is arbitrary. Life is a continuous process with the distinction between one period and the next often ill defined.

Expediency and practicality dictate against the wide use of longitudinal studies in individuals to examine for the influence of age, which would involve studying an individual for many years, if not a lifetime. Rather, single observations are made in many individuals of differing ages. The information obtained therefore pertains to the population and does not necessarily reflect how a specific individual may change with age.

A Point of Reference

Throughout this and the next chapter, reference is made to the "(usual) **adult dosage regimen.**" This phrase needs to be defined. The word *adult* refers here to the typical adult patient with the disease or condition requiring the drug. The "(usual) adult dosage regimen" is defined as that regimen which, when given to this typical patient, achieves therapeutic success. Clearly, the characteristics of the adult patient population differ with the disease being treated. Age is certainly one of these characteristics. In the case of antibiotics, because anyone in the adult population may suffer an infection, the typical age may be close to the mean age of the adult population, 39 years old, whereas patients requiring a drug to treat incontinence are often 80 years or older, and patients with asthma tend to be between 15 and 30. Overall, however, most patients requiring drugs tend to be about 60–70 years or more. For didactic purposes, we will subsequently use 60 years as the age of a typical patient.

Pharmacodynamics

Data on the influence of age on pharmacodynamics are limited. For antiepileptic drugs and digoxin, effective plasma drug concentrations appear to be the same in both children and adults, although children appear to tolerate a higher concentration of these drugs before any toxic manifestations become apparent. However, differences in pharmacodynamics with age are likely to exist for certain drugs. For example, the observed increased sensitivity of elderly patients to the central nervous system effects of benzodiazepines and general anesthetics, such as desflurane (see Fig. 1-8) and propofol (Fig. 13-12), and their decreased sensitivity to the cardiovascular effects of β-adrenergic agonists and antagonists, cannot be explained on the basis of differences in pharmacokinetics of this group of drugs.

Pharmacokinetics

Drug absorption does not appear to change dramatically with age. Most of the change in systemic exposure with age is due to a change in disposition kinetics. Consider, for example, data on diazepam, a drug eliminated primarily by hepatic metabolism. As seen in Fig. 13-13, diazepam half-life is longer in the neonate and in adults older than 55 years of age than in children or young adults. Infants eliminate the drug the most rapidly. To rationalize these observations, it is helpful to first express the dependence

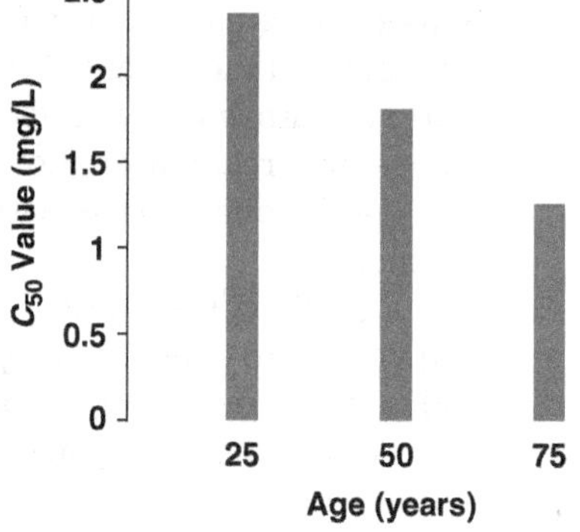

FIGURE 13-12 Steady-state propofol concentration at which 50% (C_{50}) lose consciousness during infusion of the drug decreases with advancing age, a clear indication that the sensitivity to the drug increases with age. (Data from Schneider TW, Minto CF, Shafer SL, et al. The influence of age on propofol pharmacokinetics. *Anesthesiology* 1999;90(6):1501–1516.)

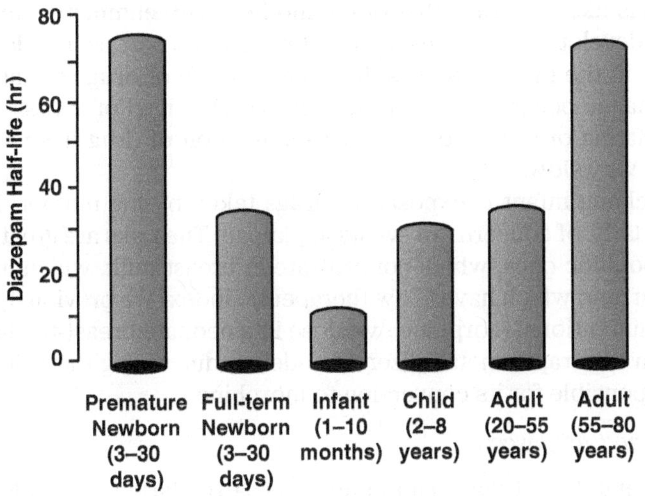

FIGURE 13-13 Half-life of diazepam is shortest in the infant and longest in the premature newborn and the elderly. (Adapted from the data of Morselli PL. *Drug Disposition During Development.* New York, NY: Spectrum Publications, 1977;311-360, 456; and from the data of Klotz U, Avant GR, Hoyumpa A, et al. The effect of age and liver disease on the disposition and elimination of diazepam in adult man. *J Clin Invest* 1975;55:347-359.)

of half-life on clearance and volume of distribution, and then divide each parameter by body weight, *W*; namely,

$$t_{1/2} = 0.693\frac{V}{CL} = 0.693\frac{\left(V/W\right)}{\left(CL/W\right)} \quad \text{Eq. 13-2}$$

The reason for normalizing to body weight is, first, to acknowledge the vast range in body weight, from neonates, who weigh 2 kg or less, to adults, who weigh 70 kg or more. The second reason is to recognize that both volume of distribution, which depends on the size of the tissues, and clearance, which depends on the amount of enzyme or transporter (when it rate limits clearance) and hence the size of the liver (or size of the kidney for renally excreted drug), vary with body weight.

The Newborn

With diazepam, the long half-life in the newborn, especially the premature, reflects an immature drug-metabolizing activity, expressed as a low clearance per kilogram body weight. Metabolic activity may take many months postpartum to mature; the time to do so varies with the enzyme system. That the premature neonate has the longest half-life of diazepam is not surprising in that the metabolic activity is then only in the early stages of its development. This observation stresses an important point: chronologic and functional age must be distinguished, especially in neonates. Unfortunately, changes occur so rapidly in these early stages of life that it is impossible to predict clearance, and hence the required dosage regimen for individual neonates, with confidence. Caution must clearly be exercised in administering drugs to this patient population, particularly drugs with a low therapeutic index.

A comment is needed about the incidental exposure of fetus and suckling infant to drugs taken by the mother. For drugs that are able to pass the placenta, the exposure in the fetus is likely to track that of the mother. With eliminating mechanisms generally poorly developed, the fetus, acting for the most part as an additional "tissue" of distribution in the mother, shows the same half-life of drug as that in the mother. A dramatic change occurs, however, on delivery. Deprived of access to the fully developed eliminating organs of the mother, elimination of drug from the newborn child now can be very slow.

The suckling infant is exposed to drugs taken by the mother. Because suckling occurs regularly, of concern are events at plateau. The risks are greatest for drugs, particularly lipophilic ones, which concentrate in breast milk, which are poorly cleared by the infant, and which have a low therapeutic index. We previously considered such a case of unintentional morphine overdose in a neonate breast-feeding from a mother who was an ultrarapid metabolizer of codeine, due to high activity of CYP2D6, the enzyme responsible for its conversion to morphine.

The Infant, Child, and Adolescent

The shorter half-life of diazepam in infants (particularly those older than 6 months) and young children in general than that in the 20- to 55-year-old adult group at first may seem surprising. It is explained by a higher clearance per kilogram of body weight, since separate studies show that the volume of distribution per kilogram of this drug is approximately the same (1.2 L/kg) in both groups. This trend in both clearance and volume of distribution is commonly seen with other drugs. Had clearance and volume of distribution both been directly proportional to body weight, then no change in half-life would have been anticipated on growing to adulthood (see Equation 13-1). The explanation for the higher clearance per kilogram of body weight in the young is mainly due to a higher liver weight per kg body weight, decreasing from about 4% in infants to 2% of body weight in adults. The metabolic enzyme activity per gram of liver is close to that in adults by the time an infant reaches 1 year. Experimentally, this change in clearance (a measure of function) with age from 2 through adolescence tends to be more closely correlated with body surface area than body weight. This applies also to some other physiological functions, such as glomerular filtration rate and cardiac output, and explains why these are often expressed per unit body surface area when making comparisons among individuals with widely differing body weights. Finally, because the ratio of surface area to body weight is higher in a small than in a large person, so, too, is clearance per kilogram of body weight. This analysis also serves to show that, during development to adulthood, body size largely accounts for age effects. And since, for any particular age, body size varies considerably within the infant and adolescent population, in practice, body size is used to guide dosage.

This relationship with body size has two important consequences. First, because dosing rate and clearance control the average plasma concentration at steady state (Equation 12-6), it follows that for drugs for which the therapeutic average steady-state concentration does not vary with age, as a reasonable approximation, the dosing rate needed in children is given by:

$$\text{Dosing rate in child} = \left[\frac{\text{Surface area of child}}{\text{Surface area of adult}}\right] \times \text{Dosing rate in adult} \qquad \textbf{Eq. 13-3}$$

The body surface area in a 70-kg adult is 1.73 m^2. This value in a child can be estimated from his or her body weight (in kg) and height (in cm) by the relationship:

$$\text{Surface area of child (m}^2\text{)} = \left(W^{0.425} \times H^{0.728}\right) \times 0.007184 \qquad \textbf{Eq. 13-4}$$

For a child of average weight for height, the surface area ratio, child to adult, can be approximated from:

$$\frac{\text{Surface area of child}}{\text{Surface area of adult}} = \left(\frac{\text{Weight of child (kg)}}{\text{Weight of adult (kg)}}\right)^{0.75} \quad \textbf{Eq. 13-5}$$

Second, because the half-life is shorter in children, particularly the very young, than in adults, for a low therapeutic index drug, it may be necessary to shorten the dosing interval of the regimen in line with half-life to keep the plasma concentration within the therapeutic window.

The Adult and the Elderly

Prolongation of diazepam half-life in later years of adulthood requires some discussion. The primary reason for this observation is diminished capacity for hepatic metabolism of diazepam, which occurs primarily by CYP2C19, with advancing age. A similar decrease in the elderly has been found with most other drugs, particularly those eliminated principally by oxidation. As a rough general guide, it is useful to characterize hepatic clearance as decreasing, based on both body and liver weight, by approximately 1%/year beyond 20 years.

Generalizing beyond hepatic elimination, drugs predominantly eliminated by renal excretion tend to display a similar pattern of change in pharmacokinetics with age, as seen with diazepam. This is because the renal clearances of drugs tend to parallel the changes in hepatic clearance observed for diazepam. Poor in the newborn, especially the premature newborn, renal clearance increases during the early months of life as renal function develops, then increases in line with body surface area during infancy and adolescence, and thereafter declines again by approximately 1% /year with advancing years beyond 20 years. By age 90, renal clearance is down, on average, to only 30% of that of a young 20-year-old adult.

The elderly constitute an increasingly greater proportion of the total population in much of the world. They also consume more prescription and over-the-counter drugs per capita than do people at any other age. As a broad generalization, dosage should be reduced in elderly patients, reflecting the general decline in body functions with age. A reduction is particularly needed in a weak, infirm, and frail elderly patient. How much it should be reduced depends on the age of the reference population with the indication for which the drug was specifically developed, the age of the patient, and his/her clinical status. In addition, such a patient often suffers from several diseases, receives multiple drugs, and has many bodily functions that have decreased sharply with advancing years. Certainly, the marked and progressive decrease in renal function implies that dosage regimens of drugs that are predominantly excreted unchanged should be reduced in the elderly population. For example, a 70-kg, 90-year-old patient requires, on average, only 63% of the usual dosage of a 60-year-old. The dose required may be even less in a small elderly patient and even less yet in a small, weak, infirm, and frail elderly patient. A depressed clearance without dose adjustment, as has been the common practice, probably contributes, along with an increased number of drugs taken, to the increased frequency and severity of adverse drug effects often noted in elderly patients.

Disease

Concurrent disease is an added source of variability in drug response. Response has been shown to change in cardiovascular disease, in respiratory disease, and in certain endocrine diseases, such as thyroid disease. The most common and consistent conditions for which a change is seen are those in which hepatic or renal functions are impaired, resulting in a diminished ability to eliminate drugs. Changes in pharmacodynamics may also occur, such as the increased sensitivity in emphysema patients to respiratory depression produced by morphine. However, generally our current knowledge in this area is limited.

There are a variety of conditions in which hepatic and renal functions are diminished. Disorders of the liver include cirrhosis, obstructive jaundice, and acute viral hepatitis. Renal disorders include acute glomerular nephritis, nephrotic syndrome, and chronic renal disease. Each disease or condition affects various levels of tissue organization and function to a different extent. By far the most important and common of these conditions are chronic alcoholic cirrhosis and chronic renal disease. Hepatic clearance (metabolism and biliary excretion) of drugs tends to decrease in cirrhosis, whereas renal clearance (including renal metabolism) is decreased in chronic renal disease. Whether these decreases in hepatic and renal clearance manifest in significant variability in total clearance depends on the relative importance of these pathways to total elimination of the drug. Consider, for example, the data in Fig. 13-14 for the antiviral compound ganciclovir. Shown is its pharmacokinetics after a single dose in subjects with different values of creatinine clearance. Creatinine, produced endogenously and readily measured in serum or plasma, is the end product of muscle catabolism; it is renally excreted entirely unchanged and offers a clinically convenient measure of **renal function.** The lower the creatinine clearance, the ratio of urinary excretion rate and serum creatinine, the lower the renal function. Notice that the total clearance of ganciclovir, inversely reflected by an increase in AUC and a commensurate prolongation in half-life, shows large interpatient variability, decreasing in line with renal function. This observation is explained by the fact that ganciclovir is almost totally eliminated by renal excretion (i.e., *fe* is close to 1), so its clearance depends almost entirely on renal function. The same applies to the intravenously administered anticoagulant, desirudin (Iprivask), as shown in Table 13-3. Of interest here is the decrease in metabolic clearance. As this drug is a relatively small protein (7000 g/mol), it is filtered in the kidneys and partially metabolized in the renal tubule. In common with

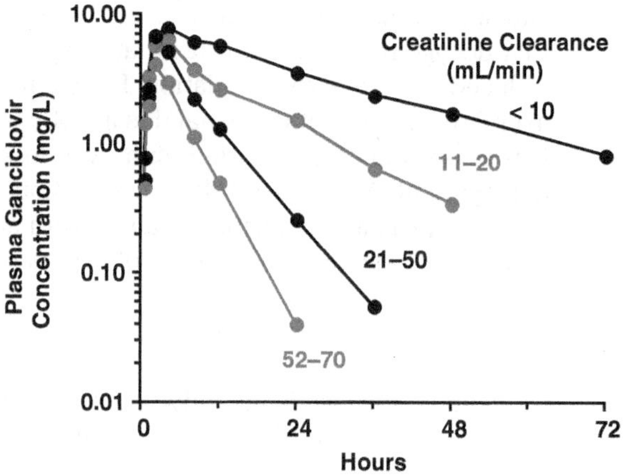

FIGURE 13-14 Mean plasma concentration with time of ganciclovir in groups of subjects classified into various ranges of renal function, as assessed by creatinine clearance. A marked decrease in clearance of ganciclovir is seen (manifested by an increase in AUC and half-life) as renal function decreases. This large variability within the subject population and the dependence of clearance on renal function arise primarily because ganciclovir is totally dependent on renal excretion for its elimination. Each subject received a 900-mg oral dose of valganciclovir, an ester prodrug that is completely hydrolyzed to ganciclovir on passage across the intestinal wall. (Redrawn from Czock D, Scholle C, Rasche FM, et al. Pharmacokinetics of valganciclovir and ganciclovir in renal impairment. *Clin Pharmacol Ther* 2002;72:142–150.)

TABLE 13-3 | Influence of Renal Impairment on Clearance of Desirudin, a Recombinant Hirudin

Participants in Study	Number	Creatinine Clearance (mL/min, range)	Total Clearance (mL/min)[a]	Renal Clearance (mL/min)[a]	Metabolic Clearance[b] (mL/min)[a]
Healthy volunteers	8	93–126	165	98	67
Patients with renal insufficiency	4	64–83	129	72	57
	5	36–57	51	29	22
	6	12–27	19	11	8

[a]Mean listed.
[b]Difference between total clearance and renal clearance.
Fischer K-G. Hirudin in renal insufficiency. *Semin Thromb Hemost* 2002;28:467–482.

many relatively small, glomerularly filtered, protein drugs, the kidney is the primary organ of both excretion and metabolism. In patients with renal disease, filtration and therefore both excretion and renal metabolism of such drugs are reduced. Clearly, serious consideration to reducing the usual dosage of ganciclovir and desirudin would need to be made in patients with severe renal impairment if excessive accumulation of drug, and potentially greater adverse effects, are to be avoided. In contrast, for drugs such as diazepam, in which very little is excreted unchanged and renal metabolism does not occur (*fe* is close to 0), no change in clearance and hence dosage adjustment is anticipated in patients with poor renal function. Although not strong, there are emerging data suggesting that even for some drugs primarily eliminated by the liver, clearance is reduced in chronic renal impairment, perhaps due to the accumulation of inhibitors of hepatic uptake or metabolism, reminding us that an end-stage disease in one organ can be manifested in the function of others.

Another important source of variability in response in renal disease is the formation of active metabolites. For some drugs, one or more of their metabolites can account for most of the therapeutic response, as is clearly the case for prodrugs; for others, metabolites account for the adverse effects. Metabolites tend to accumulate excessively in patients with poor renal function when they are primarily eliminated by this route. The consequence of renal disease therefore depends on the contribution of the renal route to total elimination for both the drug and any active metabolite and on their involvement in producing therapeutic and adverse responses. For example, patients with impaired renal function tend to experience more severe and prolonged respiratory depression when treated with normal doses of morphine, which has been found to be due to the excessive accumulation of the pharmacologically active metabolite morphine-6-glucuronide, which depends on renal excretion for its elimination. The concentration of morphine, which is mostly metabolized, is only modestly changed in such patients. Thus, this active metabolite must be taken into account when considering dose adjustment of morphine in this patient subpopulation, and, indeed, the general principles above apply to all drugs with active metabolites.

Interacting Drugs

Patients commonly receive two or more drugs concurrently; inpatients on average receive five drugs during a hospitalization, and many, particularly elderly, patients may be concurrently taking eight or more drugs. The reasons for multiple-drug therapy are many. One reason, as discussed in Chapter 10, is that drug combinations have been found to be beneficial in the treatment of some conditions, including a variety of cardiovascular diseases, infections, and cancer. Another reason is that patients frequently suffer from several concurrent diseases or conditions, and each may require the use of one or more drugs, in which case the number of drugs concurrently taken can become huge. Furthermore, drugs are prescribed by different clinicians, and each clinician may be unaware of the other's therapeutic maneuvers, although this problem is being addressed in settings in which the patient's medication record is made available to all of the patient's clinicians. However, unbeknown to any of the clinicians, the patient may be also taking a variety of over-the-counter medicines, or herbal products containing interacting constituents.

The potential for interactions among drugs within the body are almost limitless and can be a major source of variability in drug response. Yet for many of these interactions, the resultant change in exposure is too small to be clinically important. However, in a sufficient number of cases, the change in exposure is sufficiently large to cause a clinically significant interaction, and in these cases a cautionary note is warranted for those situations in which the two drugs need to be coprescribed.

Occasionally, the magnitude of an interaction is so great as to contraindicate the simultaneous use of the drugs. Some examples are listed in Table 13-4; in most cases, the interaction results in an exaggerated response of the affected drug, but not always so. Reduced activity can arise because the perpetrating drug is an antagonist, reduces bioavailability, or increases clearance. Occasionally, the interaction has been so severe, and the likelihood of the combination being inadvertently given so great, that it has caused either the affected or the offending drug to be removed from the market, at least in some countries. Some examples are the antihistamine terfenadine, the antihypertensive mebifredril, and cisapride, which was used to treat heartburn.

In pharmacodynamic interactions, when the mechanism of action of each compound is known, the interaction is generally predictable and, if undesirable, is avoidable. As with pharmacodynamic interactions, pharmacokinetic ones can also be beneficial, and combinations of fixed doses are used, although in such cases there is commonly only one active principle. The second compound interacts to overcome an existing limitation in one or more aspects of the pharmacokinetics of the affected drug to increase its exposure–time profile at the target site for a given dose. Also, by inhibiting a normally substantial and highly variable pathway of elimination, such as CYP3A4-mediated metabolism, interindividual variability of an affected drug can be significantly reduced in the presence of the inhibitor. Examples of pharmacokinetically driven beneficial combination products are listed in Table 13-5 (p. 280).

Before considering specific examples of drug interactions, a final general comment needs to be made regarding the sequence of drug administration. A drug interaction is likely to be detected in clinical practice only when the interacting drug is initiated or withdrawn during therapy with the other. For example, given the usual large degree of variability in patients' responses to drugs, a drug interaction is unlikely to be detected if the affected drug is administered to a patient already stabilized on the drug causing the interaction. Certainly, the dosage regimen of the affected drug would be different in *that* patient than would otherwise be the case, but the resulting regimen may still be within the normal range. In this case, only if the offending drug is withdrawn first when the patient is stabilized on the drug combination would the interaction be seen. The interaction would also have been detected if the interacting drug had been administered to the patient already stabilized on the original drug.

TABLE 13-4 | Classification and Examples of Drug Interactions to Be Avoided

	Response[a]	Example	Comment
		Pharmacodynamic Interactions	
	↑[a]	Diphenhydramine ↔[b] alcohol	Mutual sedative effects
	↓	Naloxone →[c] fentanyl	Naloxone antagonizes the analgesic effect of the opioid fentanyl and can precipitate withdrawal symptoms.
		Pharmacokinetic Interactions	
Parameter			
Oral bioavailability	↑	Saquinavir → midazolam	Saquinavir inhibits intestinal CYP3A4-mediated metabolism of midazolam, increasing its systemic exposure and hypnotic response.
	↓	Antacids → chloroquine	An interval of at least 4 hours is needed to avoid reduced absorption of chloroquine.
Volume of distribution	↓	Quinidine → digoxin	Quinidine reduces the tissue distribution of digoxin, causing need to reduce loading dose.
Metabolic clearance	↑	Rifampin → warfarin	Rifampin strongly induces hepatic microsomal enzymes, increasing warfarin clearance and dose requirements of this anticoagulant.
	↓	Erythromycin → sildenafil	Erythromycin strongly inhibits CYP3A4, major enzyme responsible for sildenafil metabolism, causing it to have excessive exposure.
Renal clearance	↓	Diuretics → lithium	By causing increased sodium ion loss, diuretics can reduce the renal clearance of lithium, and increase lithium retention, with potential toxicity.

[a]↑, denotes increase, ↓, decrease in pharmacodynamic response or pharmacokinetic parameter value.
[b]↔, denotes a mutual interaction, each affecting the other.
[c]→, denotes a unidirectional interaction; the arrow points to affected drug.

A pharmacodynamic interaction can arise for a variety of reasons. These include the interacting drug complementing the action of the other, such as the use of a thiazide diuretic and a β-blocker, each acting by different mechanisms to lower blood pressure. Alternatively, the interacting drug may act as an antagonist or agonist at the same receptor site as the other drug. If the drug is an agonist, it may act additively or synergistically. The effect is **additive** if the combined effect is that expected based on the concentration–response curves for each drug given independently. **Synergism** occurs when the effect produced with the two drugs is even greater than that expected had the effect been additive.

TABLE 13-5 | Pharmacokinetically Driven Combination Products

Drug Combination	Indication	Rationale for Combination
Lopinavir/ ritonavir	HIV/AIDS	Ritonavir increases the systemic exposure and decreases interpatient variability of lopinavir by increasing its oral bioavailability and decreasing its clearance, by inhibiting its CYP3A4-catalyzed metabolism. It also allows for a reduced daily dose of lopinavir and a decrease in the frequency of dosing—every 12 vs. 8 hr.
L-Dopa/ carbidopa	Parkinson's disease	Carbidopa increases the systemic exposure, and decreases interpatient variability, of L-dopa by inhibiting the decarboxylase enzyme responsible for L-dopa metabolism in intestinal, hepatic, and renal tissues. It allows for a reduced dosage of L-dopa and a more prolonged systemic exposure.
Imipenem/ cilastatin	Urinary tract infection	By inhibiting renal dehydropeptidase, which is responsible for metabolism of imipenen in the kidney, cilastatin increases the urinary tract concentrations of this antibiotic.
Amoxicillin/ clavulanate	Systemic infection	Some microorganisms are resistant to amoxicillin; they produce β-lactamases that destroy this antibiotic locally. Clavulanate overcomes this resistance by inhibiting β-lactamases, thereby increasing the local antibiotic exposure.

A pharmacokinetic interaction can occur by the second drug altering the absorption, distribution, or elimination of the affected drug, such as those listed in Table 13-4; sometimes, more than one process is altered. The most profound interactions are those affecting oral bioavailability and clearance, particularly by affecting drug metabolism. Drugs can act as inhibitors or inducers of the various enzymes responsible for drug metabolism. Many of them, particularly inhibitors, act specifically on one enzyme, as indicated by the examples in Fig. 13-9. How substantial an interaction can be is illustrated in Fig. 13-15 involving midazolam and the antifungal agent itraconazole, both given orally.

Midazolam is a short-acting hypnotic, owing to its rapid absorption and elimination. Its rapid elimination is attributable to its being an excellent substrate for CYP3A4-mediated metabolism, resulting in a moderately high hepatic extraction ratio (0.4–0.5). Unlike most of the other CYP450 enzymes, CYP3A4 resides in the intestinal epithelium as well as in the liver; consequently, midazolam has a low oral bioavailability because of substantial first-pass loss on passage through both these organs (see Table 8-4). Notice the almost sevenfold increase in the AUC of midazolam in the presence of itraconazole, a specific and strong inhibitor of CYP3A4. Calculations show that a large part of the increase in midazolam AUC is due to an increase in its oral bioavailability, caused by the presence of high concentrations of itraconazole in the intestinal lumen and portal blood entering the liver during its oral absorption. This inhibition manifests in the almost threefold increase in midazolam C_{max}, with only a minor change in t_{max}. Once absorbed systemically, circulating intraconazole also inhibits hepatic metabolism of midazolam, but the inhibition now, as manifested by a change in clearance (and half-life), is more modest, owing in part to the lower systemic concentrations of itraconazole resulting from its extensive distribution into

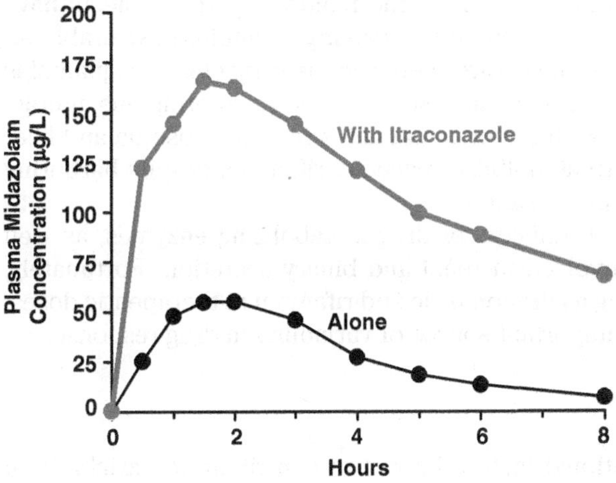

FIGURE 13-15 Mean plasma midazolam concentration with time after a single 15-mg oral dose alone (*black*) and after a 7.5-mg dose given on day 4 of 200-mg daily itraconazole treatment (*color*). The plasma concentrations following the 7.5-mg dose have been doubled to allow comparison between the two treatments. Notice the almost threefold increase in C_{max} and sevenfold increase in AUC caused by itraconazole inhibiting the first-pass metabolic loss and systemic clearance of midazolam. (Redrawn from Backman JT, Kivistö KT, Olkkola KT, et al. The area under the plasma concentration-time curve for midazolam is 400-fold larger during treatment with itraconazole than with rifampicin. *Eur J Clin Pharmacol* 1998;54:53–58.)

tissues (volume of distribution is very high, 1000 L). An additional factor is that being of intermediate hepatic extraction ratio, clearance of midazolam is less sensitive to the reduction in its hepatocellular activity than had it been a low extraction ratio drug. The clinical consequence of this interaction is a more profound and prolonged sedative effect of oral midazolam in the presence of itraconazole. For this reason, the combination is contraindicated.

Enzyme induction can produce as dramatic an effect as can inhibition, but the consequence is a decrease, not an increase, in systemic exposure of the affected drug. This is illustrated in Fig. 13-16, which shows the profound impact of coadministration of the antibiotic rifampin, a strong enzyme inducer, on the plasma concentration of praziquantel (Biltricide), an anthelmintic drug. This figure illustrates two points: (1) a profound reduction in the systemic exposure of praziquantel and (2) the substantial

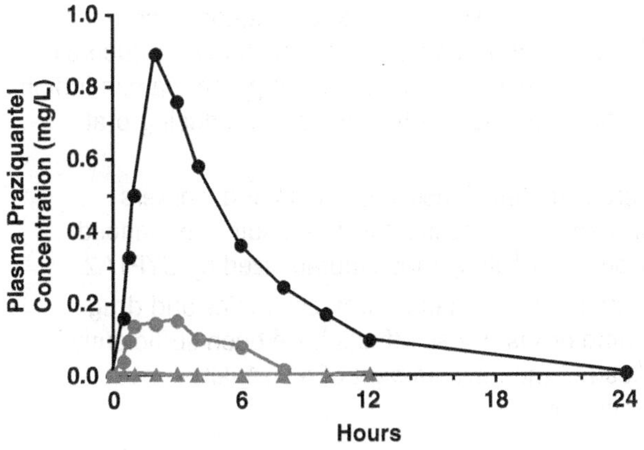

FIGURE 13-16 Mean plasma concentration versus time plot of the anthelmintic agent praziquantel in 10 subjects following the administration of 40-mg/kg praziquantel alone (*black circle, black line*) and after 5 days of treatment with 600-mg oral rifampin once daily (*color circle, color line*). In all subjects, induction by rifampin caused a large reduction in the plasma concentration of praziquantel. In 7 of the 10 subjects, the effect was so pronounced that the concentrations were below the limits of detection of the assay (*color triangle*). The mean of the other 3 subjects is shown by the middle curve. (Redrawn from Ridtitid W, Wongnawa M, Mahatthanatrakul W, et al. Rifampin markedly decreases plasma concentrations of praziquantel in healthy volunteers. *Clin Pharmacol Ther* 2002;72:505–513.)

interindividual variability in the effect. Although the majority of the subjects have no measurable praziquantel concentrations after receiving rifampin, measurable effects , but very low, plasma concentrations are seen in some subjects. Praziquantal is given for both intestinal and systemic parasitic diseases. Clearly, ignoring this interaction can mean that those patients with systemic parasites (e.g., shistosoma and liver flukes) may well be ineffectively treated if also receiving rifampin, despite harboring parasites normally susceptible to praziquantel.

There are many inhibitors and inducers of drug-metabolizing enzymes, as well as those affecting transporters involved in renal and biliary secretion. Fortunately, relatively few of them are as strong as itraconazole and rifampin at therapeutic doses. Still, drug interactions remain an important source of variability in drug response.

Adherence to Regimen

Table 13-6 lists examples of additional factors known to contribute to variability in drug response. Undoubtedly, the most important of these is the ubiquitous lack of **adherence** to the prescribed regimen. This lack includes the taking of drug at the wrong

TABLE 13-6 | Additional Factors Known to Contribute to Variability in Drug Response

Factor	Comments
Lack of adherence and persistence in taking a dosage regimen	A major problem in clinical practice; solution lies largely in patient motivation.
Route of administration	Patient response can vary when changing the route of administration. Particularly noticed when speed of absorption and bioavailability are route dependent.
Food and diet	Rate and occasionally extent of absorption can be affected by eating. Effects depend on composition of food, in particular, the presence of a high-fat meal, which markedly slows gastric emptying. Severe protein restriction may reduce the rate of drug metabolism, and increase urine pH, which will affect the renal clearance of urine pH-sensitive drugs. Constituents in grapefruit and cranberry juices are inhibitors of intestinal CYP3A4.
Herbs	Certain herbs contain constituents that can enhance or antagonize the effect of drugs or act as inhibitors or inducers of drug-metabolizing enzymes. Constituents in green tea can inhibit the intestinal uptake transport of some drugs, reducing oral bioavailability.
Pollutants	Drug effects are sometimes less in smokers and workers occupationally exposed to pesticides, the result of enhanced drug metabolism, particularly those metabolized by CYP1A2.
Time of day and season	Circadian variations are seen in pharmacokinetics and drug response of some drugs. These effects have been sufficiently important to lead to the development of a specialty—chronopharmacology.

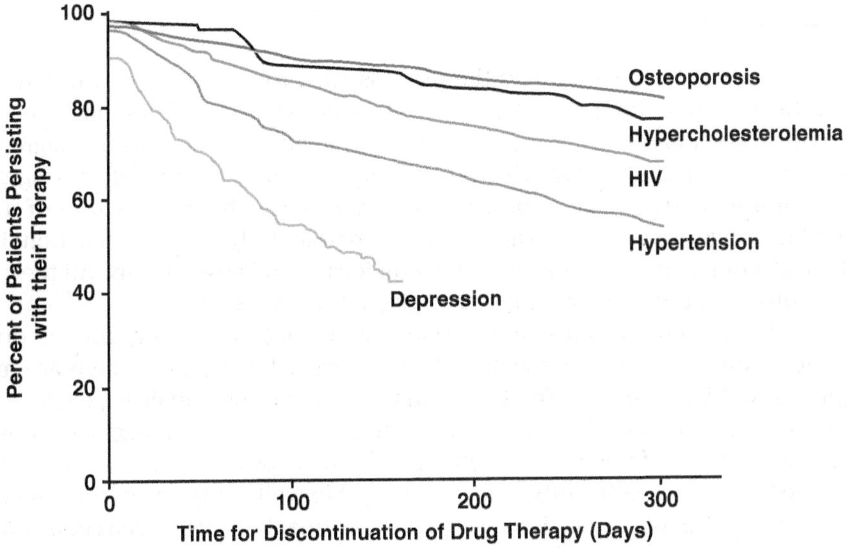

FIGURE 13-17 The decline in the percentage of patients persisting with drug treatment varies with the disease condition, being particularly rapid and extensive in patients being treated for mental disorders and hypertension. Also noticeable is the higher, and significant, percentage of patients with mental disorders who failed even to initiate drug treatment. Data were gathered using electronic monitoring devices that detect each time the patient opens the container to take the drug. (Redrawn from Blaschke TF, Osterberg L, Vrejens B, et al. Adherence to medications: Insights arising from studies on the unreliable link between prescribed and actual drug dosing histories. *Annu Rev Pharmacol Toxicol* 2012;52:275–301.)

time, the omission or supplementation of the prescribed dose, and premature stopping of therapy. Nonadherence is especially noticeable when reliance is placed on patients themselves to adhere to their drug treatments, particularly when dealing with oral dosage forms, and it has a strong behavioral component. Whereas some patients are compulsive in taking their medicines, most do so much less reliably. Nonadherence is much less of a problem in institutional settings and when patients have to attend clinics to be administered drugs parenterally, such as intravenous or subcutaneous administration of many protein drugs. As shown in Fig. 13-17, the disease or condition itself can also have a strong influence on the **persistence** of drug therapy, that is, the time between the first-taken dose and the last-taken dose, however well or poorly the patient adheres to the regimen in between. Notice that persistence is a problem in all patient groups, but is particularly the case in those treated for hypertension, and is even more so in patients suffering with mental disorders, in whom it can be seen that approximately 10% fail to even start the drug treatment, while a further 50% have stopped taking the prescribed drug after 6 months of treatment. There are many reasons for nonadherence to drug therapy besides behavioral traits. If patients suffer adverse effects, particularly if they perceive that they are deriving no benefit, or if they perceive that the cause of the problem has been resolved, they tend to stop medication before the end of the prescribed treatment. Whatever the reason, if adherence to the full course of treatment is important, the solution in large part lies in the area of patient counseling to enhance motivation to take the daily regimen as prescribed and to persist in taking the full course of treatment.

Additional Factors

Pharmaceutical formulation and the process used to manufacture a product can be important because both can affect the rate and extent of release, and hence entry, into the body (Chapter 8). A well-designed formulation diminishes the degree of variability in the release characteristics of a drug in vivo. Good manufacturing practice, with careful control of the process variables, ensures the manufacture of a reliable product. Drugs are given enterally, topically, parenterally, and by inhalation. Route of administration can affect the concentration locally and systemically. All these factors can profoundly affect the response to a given dose or regimen.

Food—particularly fat—slows gastric emptying and absorption of drug. The extent of absorption is not usually affected greatly by food, but there are many exceptions to this statement. Food is a complex mixture of chemicals, each potentially capable of interacting with drugs. For example, alendronate, a bisphosphonate used to reduce the risk of bone fracture in the elderly, needs to be taken on a fasting stomach because food significantly reduces its oral bioavailability. In contrast, nelfinavir, a lipophilic, sparingly soluble drug used in the treatment of AIDS, needs to be taken with food because food substantially improves its oral bioavailability, as explained for such compounds in Chapter 8. Recall also that grapefruit juice contains compounds that inhibit, particularly intestinal, CYP3A4 and so increase the hepatic and systemic exposure of compounds, such as simvastatin (an agent used to reduce cholesterol) and felodipine (a calcium channel–blocking agent used in the treatment of hypertension), which normally exhibit a low oral bioavailability due to extensive CYP3A4-catalyzed metabolism during absorption across the intestinal wall (Fig. 8-6). Diet may also affect drug metabolism. Enzyme synthesis is ultimately dependent on protein intake. When protein intake is severely reduced for prolonged periods, particularly because of an imbalanced diet, drug metabolism may be impaired. Conversely, a high-protein intake may cause enzyme induction.

To many, herbal preparations and other plant extracts are believed to be both efficacious in ameliorating or curing diseases and devoid of adverse effects because they are "natural products." However, it is well to remember that these preparations contain many constituents about which little to nothing is known and that many potent and potentially toxic compounds, including morphine, atropine, and digoxin, are derived from plants, namely opium poppy, deadly nightshade, and foxglove, respectively. Many plant constituents also have the potential to interact with prescribed drugs. Fig. 13-18 illustrates the magnitude of such an interaction with one example, St. John's wort (*Hypericum perforatum*), a popular herbal preparation used to treat depression. The substantial decrease in systemic exposure of midazolam arises because this herb contains compounds that are powerful inducers of CYP3A4. The result is a tendency for a decrease in the effectiveness of CYP3A4 substrate drugs that can have severe consequences. For example, taking St. John's wort has been reported to precipitate organ rejection in patients stabilized on cyclosporine, an immunosuppressive agent used to minimize the risk of organ rejection. Cyclosporine has a narrow therapeutic window and is eliminated almost entirely via CYP3A4-mediated metabolism; its metabolites are either less active than cyclosporine itself or inactive. St. John's wort also induces P-glycoprotein, particularly in the intestinal wall, and in doing so, decreases the oral bioavailability of compounds such as fexofenadine, a relatively polar nonmetabolized drug, used to treat allergic ailments such as hay fever and rhinitis. Its absorption is limited due to efflux by this transporter (Fig. 13-18). Another example, shown in Fig. 13-19, is the dramatic reduction in the plasma concentration of the β-adrenergic

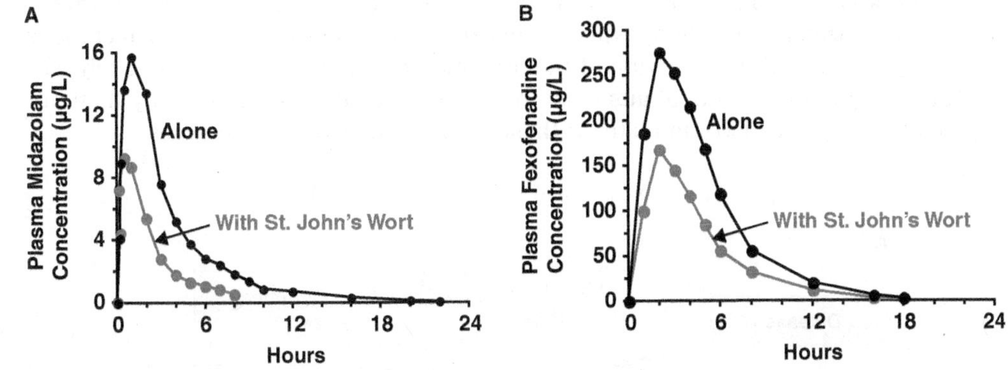

FIGURE 13-18 Mean plasma concentrations with time of midazolam (**A**) and fexofenadine (**B**) following a single oral dose of 4-mg midazolam and 180-mg fexofenadine, respectively, alone (*black*) and after 11-day treatment with 300-mg St. John's wort three times daily (*color*). Notice the reduction in the AUC of both midazolam (2.7-fold) and fexofenadine (1.9-fold) caused by St. John's wort inducing CYP3A4 and P-glycoprotein, respectively. (Redrawn from Dresser GK, Schwarz UI, Wilkinson GR, et al. Coordinate induction of both P4503A and MDR1 by St John's wort in healthy subjects. *Clin Pharmacol Ther* 2003;73:41–50.)

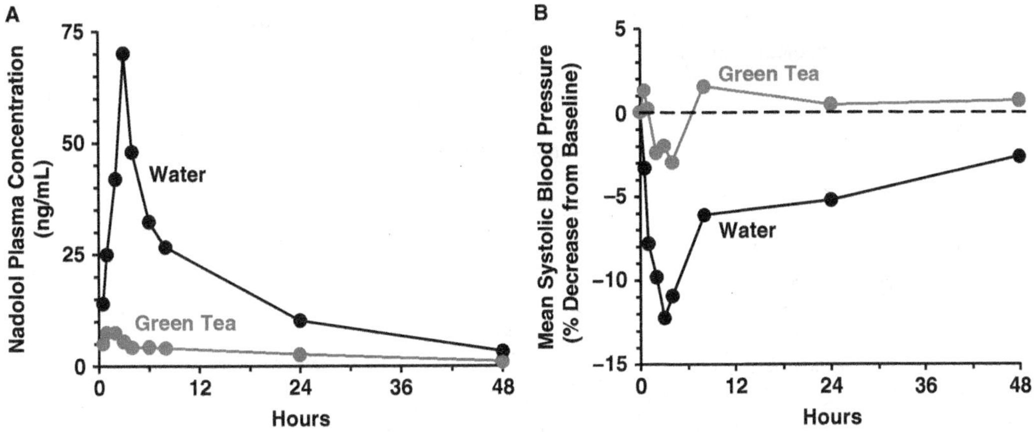

FIGURE 13-19 **A.** Both C_{max} and AUC of the β-adrenergic blocking agent nadolol are reduced by 85% when 30 mg are taken orally after repeated consumption of green tea (700 mL/day) for 14 days, compared with when taken with the same volume of water. The mechanism involves inhibition by constituents in green tea of the intestinal uptake transporter OATP1A2 needed to ensure the normally good oral bioavailability of nadolol. **B.** Associated loss in the nadolol-induced lowering of the mean systolic blood pressure. (Redrawn from Misaka S, Yatabe J, Müller F, et al. Green tea ingestion greatly reduces plasma concentrations of nadolol in healthy subjects. *Clin Pharmacol Ther* 2014:95:432–438.)

blocking agent nadolol, with a commensurate loss in its therapeutic effect of lowering systolic blood pressure, when taken with green tea. The mechanism appears to be inhibition by constituents in green tea of the intestinal uptake transporter OATP1A2, essential for the normally high oral bioavailability of nadalol, a relatively small hydrophilic compound with low passive permeability. Interestingly, these inhibitors are relatively stable in hot water. The message from these two examples is clear. Herbal preparations can significantly affect the pharmacokinetics, and possibly the pharmacodynamics, of drugs with adverse consequences.

Cigarette smoking tends to reduce clinical and toxic effects of some drugs, including diazepam and theophylline. The drugs affected are extensively metabolized by hepatic oxidation; induction of the drug-metabolizing enzymes is the likely cause. Many environmental pollutants exist in higher concentrations in the city than in the country; they can also stimulate synthesis of hepatic metabolic enzymes.

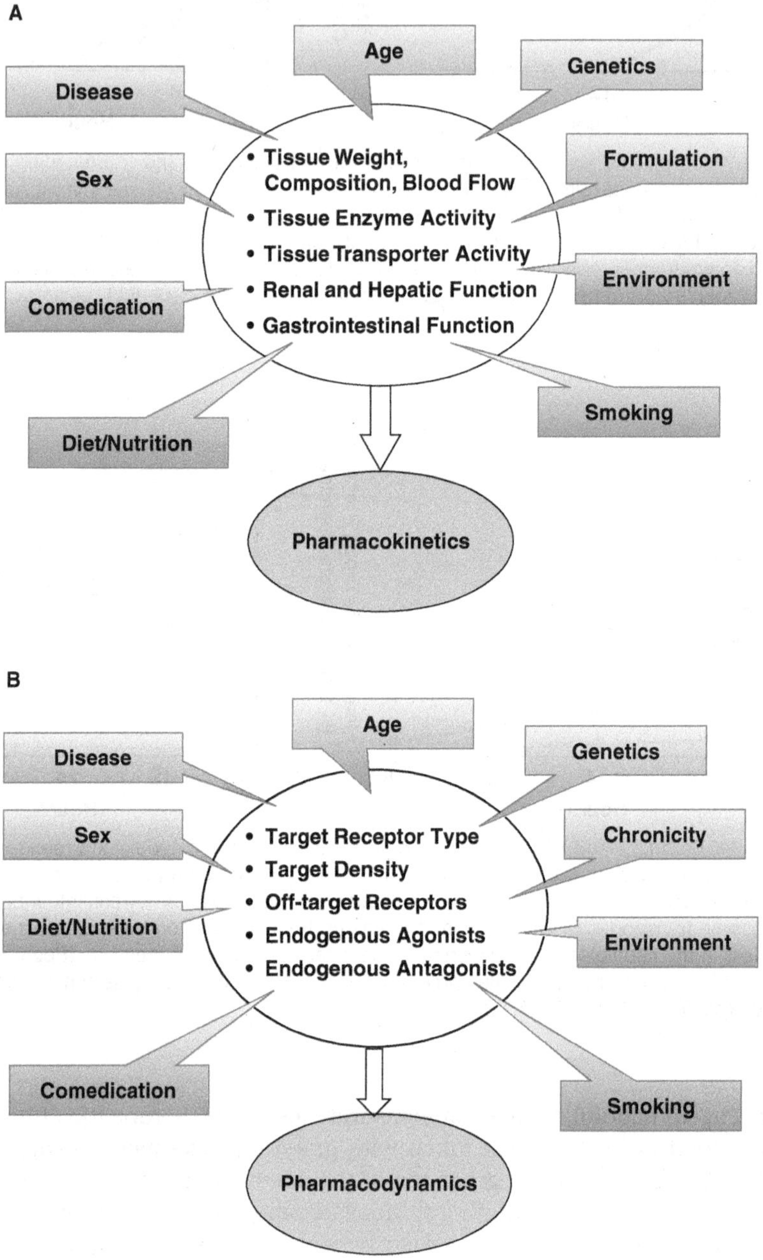

FIGURE 13-20 Variability in observed pharmacokinetics (**A**), and pharmacodynamics (**B**) of a drug within and among patients is influenced to varying degrees by many factors that not only impact the underlying controlling processes but also are often themselves highly correlated (such as predisposition of chronic diseases in the elderly).

Variability is a major issue in drug therapy. This chapter has provided evidence for, and identified causes of, variability in drug response. Each cause has been considered separately for didactic purposes. However, it is important to stress that in reality, not only does each affect the underlying processes controlling the pharmacokinetics (Fig. 13-20A), and also the pharmacodynamics (Fig. 13-20B) of a drug to varying degrees, as indicated in the figure, but many are themselves significantly correlated, such as advancing age and changes in cardiovascular, renal, and hepatic functions, resulting in a complex interplay that determines both inter- and intrapatient variability. How this information is used in practice is considered in the last chapter, Initiating and Managing Therapy.

SUMMARY

- Variability in drug response is caused by variability in both pharmacokinetics and pharmacodynamics.
- Population pharmacokinetics and population pharmacodynamics are terms used to characterize how parameters in these areas vary within the population.
- Distinction should be made between intraindividual variability and interindividual variability; generally, intraindividual variability is the smaller of the two.
- Coefficient of variation is a useful statistical measure for comparing variability among the same and different types of parameters.
- Genetics, age, body weight, disease, concomitant drugs, and lack of adherence to the prescribed dosage regimen are major sources and correlates of variability in drug response.
- Pharmacogenetics is the study of inherited variations in drug response. Pharmacogenomics is the application of genomic information to the identification of putative drug targets and to the causes of variability in drug response.
- Genetic polymorphisms exist in drug metabolism and transport, in target receptor sensitivity, and in sensitivity of nontarget receptors.
- A drug idiosyncrasy is a rare, often dramatic adverse reaction usually under monogenetic control.
- Hepatic and renal functions vary with age, being poorly developed in the newborn, and declining with advancing age in the elderly.
- The "adult" of the "usual adult dosage regimen" is the typical patient in the adult population with the disease or condition for which a drug is indicated.
- Organ eliminating function is low in newborns and early infants, and increases with maturation toward normal adult values per gram of organ over the first year of life.
- During childhood and adolescence, much of the variability in pharmacokinetics with age can be accommodated for by body size.
- Beyond 30 years of age, clearance of drugs tends to decrease by approximately 1%/year.
- Drug interactions are graded responses the intensity of which varies with the concentration of the interacting drugs and hence with their dosage regimens and time.
- Drug interactions involving pharmacokinetics and pharmacodynamics are causes of failure of drug therapy. Those involving drug metabolism and transporters are frequently produced by increasing drug exposure, and thereby increasing adverse effects, and occasionally by reducing exposure leading to ineffective therapy.
- Food and herbal preparations can interact with drugs.

KEY TERM REVIEW

Additivity of response
Adherence to prescribed dosage
Adult dosage regimen
Age
Allele
Body weight
Coefficient of variation
Disease
Dominant
Drug combinations
Drug interactions
Extensive metabolizer
Genetic polymorphism
Genetics
Genotype
Haplotype
Heterozygous
Homozygous
Idiosyncrasy
Intraindividual variability
Interindividual variability
Mean
Monogenic
Persistence
Pharmacogenetics
Pharmacogenomics
Phenotype
Polygenic
Polymodal frequency distribution
Poor metabolizers
Population pharmacodynamics
Population pharmacokinetics
Recessive
Renal function
Synergism
Unimodal frequency distribution

KEY RELATIONSHIPS

$$\text{Dosing rate in child} = \left[\frac{\text{Surface area of child}}{\text{Surface area of adult}}\right] \times \text{Dosing rate in adult}$$

$$\text{Surface area of child } (\text{m}^2) = \left(W^{0.425} \times H^{0.728}\right) \times 0.007184$$

$$\frac{\text{Surface area of child}}{\text{Surface area of adult}} = \left(\frac{\text{Weight of child (kg)}}{\text{Weight of adult (kg)}}\right)^{0.75}$$

STUDY PROBLEMS

1. Which one or more of the following is (are) likely to be a cause(s) of decreased response to midazolam during its chronic administration?
   I. Coadministration of itraconazole
   II. Coadministration of clarithromycin
   III. Coadministration of rifampin

   A. I only
   B. II only
   C. III only
   D. I and II
   E. I and III
   F. II and III
   G. All
   H. None

2. Whether eliminated by metabolism or excretion, a drug's clearance tends to change with age. Which of the following approximations is (are) commonly used to describe this tendency?

I. Clearance increases in proportion to body surface area during childhood.
II. Clearance decreases by about 1%/year in adults, that is, after age 20.
III. Clearance decreases by about 1%/year from birth to old age.

A. I only	**E.** I and III
B. II only	**F.** II and III
C. III only	**G.** All
D. I and II	**H.** None

3. Which of the following statements is (are) correct?
   I. Pharmacogenomics is the application of genomic information to the identification of putative drug targets and to the causes of variability in drug response.
   II. The coefficient of variation is the standard deviation (square root of variance) of a measured value normalized to its mean.
   III. Occasionally, a very severe and unusual adverse effect occurs, but its incidence is so low that only when tens of thousands, if not millions, of patients have been treated with the drug is it detected with any statistical significance. Such adverse effects are most often idiosyncratic in nature, that is, they rarely occur, and the cause of them is generally unknown.

A. I only	**E.** I and III
B. II only	**F.** II and III
C. III only	**G.** All
D. I and II	**H.** None

4. Which *one* of the following statements is *incorrect*?
   a. A drug interaction is likely to be detected in clinical practice only when the interacting drug is initiated or withdrawn during therapy with the other drug, and is unlikely to be detected if the affected drug is administered to a patient already stabilized on the drug causing the interaction.
   b. A pharmacodynamic interaction can arise if the interacting drug complements the action of the other drug or if the interacting drug acts as an antagonist or agonist at the same receptor site as the other drug.
   c. The most profound pharmacokinetic drug interactions are those affecting oral bioavailability and clearance, particularly by affecting drug metabolism.
   d. Enzyme induction can produce as dramatic an effect as can inhibition, but the consequence is an increase, not a decrease, in systemic exposure of the affected drug.
   e. A response is said to be additive if the combined effect of two drugs is that expected based on the concentration–response curves for each drug given independently. Synergism occurs when the effect produced with the two drugs is even greater than that expected had the effect been additive.
5. List six major sources of variability in drug response.
6. Why is variability in response so important in drug therapy, and why does distinction need to be made between intraindividual and interindividual variability?
7. Age, weight, and renal disease are known to affect renal function. Briefly discuss, from a pharmacokinetic point of view, when changes in renal function are most likely to be clinically important for a specific drug. For example, consider an individual patient whose renal function is reduced to 20% of that in a typical patient. Would you expect it to be prudent to reduce drug administration to the patient if:
   a. All the activity (beneficial and harmful) resides with the drug, and $fe = 0.96$.
   b. All the activity (beneficial and harmful) resides with the drug, and $fe = 0.02$.

TABLE 13-7 | Pharmacokinetic Data Following Intravenous Infusion to Steady State

Subject	1	2	3	4	5
Steady-state plasma concentration (mg/L)	2.5	1.6	3.0	1.5	2.3
Postinfusion half-life (hr)	1.4	1.9	1.7	3.0	2.8
Fraction unbound	0.1	0.15	0.09	0.16	0.12

c. All the activity resides with a metabolite, which is the sole route of drug elimination, and the metabolite is exclusively eliminated by the renal route.

d. All the activity resides with a metabolite, which is the sole route of drug elimination, and the metabolite is entirely eliminated by further metabolism to inactive metabolites.

8. Discuss how pharmacodynamic sources of variability can be distinguished from pharmacokinetic sources, and give three examples of inherited variability in pharmacokinetics and three in pharmacodynamics.

9. The data in Table 13-7 were obtained in a study to provide a preliminary assessment of the pharmacokinetic variability of a drug that is predominantly excreted unchanged, $fe = 0.99$. The drug was infused intravenously in five subjects at a constant rate of 20 mg/hr for 48 hours. The fraction unbound was found to be independent of drug concentration, but did vary among the subjects.

   a. From the values above, calculate the values of Cu_{ss}, CL, and V missing in the table below for each of the patients in the study.

Subject/Parameter	1	2	3	4	5
Cu_{ss} (mg/L)	0.25	0.24			0.28
CL (L/hr)		12.5	6.7	13.3	
V (L)		34.3		57.7	35.1

   b. The coefficients of variation (standard deviation/mean) for the measured and derived values in the two previous tables are summarized in Table 13-8.

      (1) Which of the measures or parameters is the most and which is the least variable?

      (2) What do these data imply with respect to the source of the pharmacokinetic variability in the most variable measure or parameter (answer to 1.)?

   c. Discuss briefly the therapeutic implications of these data with regard to the rate of attainment and maintenance of a "therapeutic" concentration in the various subjects during a constant-rate intravenous infusion.

10. Montelukast sodium is a leukotriene receptor antagonist, used to treat asthma and seasonal allergic rhinitis. The package insert recommends once-daily oral administration of the drug as shown in Table 13-9.

TABLE 13-8 | Variability in Plasma Concentration and Pharmacokinetic Parameters and Measures

Measure or Parameter	C_{ss}	$t_{1/2}$	fu	Cu_{ss}	CL	V
Coefficient of variation	0.29	0.39	0.25	0.07	0.30	0.54

TABLE 13-9 | Demographic Data and Dosage Regimens of Montelukast

Patient	Typical Weight (kg) and (Mean Age in years)	Recommended Daily Dose	Predicted Daily Dose (mg)
Young adult ≥18 years	66 (22)	10-mg tablet	10
Child			
6–14 years of age	33 (10)	5-mg chewable tablet	
2–5 years of age	16 (3.5)	4-mg chewable tablet or 4-mg oral granules	
12–33 months of age	12 (1.5)	4-mg oral granules	

a. Compare the package insert recommendations for the dosage in children with those that you would predict based on the adult dose (assume a typical patient is a 22-year-old, 66-kg young adult) and their body surface areas. Make your comparison by completing the last column of Table 13-9. To do so, use the relationship below, given in the chapter, which is based on an approximation for how body surface area varies with body size in children from 2 to 18 years of age. Use the mean ages and weights given for the groups shown.

$$\text{Child's Dosage} = \left(\frac{\text{Weight of child (kg)}}{70\,\text{kg}}\right)^{0.75} \times \text{Adult Dose}$$

b. In the case of many diseases, the typical age of an adult patient is close to 60. Do you think a typical patient on montelukast is 60 years old? Briefly comment.

c. What assumptions have been made in calculating the child's dosing rate?

d. Is there a need to consider more frequent administration than once daily in a young patient, 2–5 years old?

11. Verapamil, a calcium ion antagonist with antiarrhythmic, antianginal, and coronary and peripheral vasodilator properties, has been studied in patients with hepatic cirrhosis. The study was conducted using a double isotope technique in which both intravenous and oral doses were concurrently administered. The intravenous dose of 10 mg was given via a 5-minute infusion of the unlabelled drug. The oral doses of 40 mg (given to the cirrhotic patients) and 80 mg (given to the normal subjects) consisted of verapamil with three deuterium atoms on the methoxy group attached to the benzene ring. Verapamil and deuterated-verapamil were analyzed concurrently in plasma using mass fragmentography. Fig. 13-21 (next page) shows the concentration–time profiles in one of the control healthy subjects and in one of the patients with hepatic cirrhosis following the intravenous and oral doses. The mean data of the seven cirrhotic subjects and the six healthy subjects are listed in Table 13-10 (next page). The average of the plasma-to-blood concentration ratio was 0.85. About 3.5% of an intravenous dose was excreted unchanged in the urine.

a. How do you explain the rapid *initial* decline in the plasma concentration after the intravenous doses, but not after the oral doses, in both the cirrhotic patients and the normal subjects?

b. From the intravenous data in healthy subjects, do you expect the drug to have a high or low hepatic extraction ratio. Hepatic blood flow is 1.35 L/min. Briefly discuss.

TABLE 13-10 | Verapamil Pharmacokinetics in Healthy Subjects and Cirrhotic Patients

	V (L/kg)	*fu*	Terminal Half-life (hr)	Dose/AUC (L/min)	
Healthy Subjects					
Intravenous dose	6.15	0.08	3.7	1.33	–
Oral dose	–	–	3.5	6.4	0.22
Cirrhotic patients					
Intravenous dose	9.17	0.08	14.2	0.62	–
Oral dose	–	–	13.9	1.3	0.55

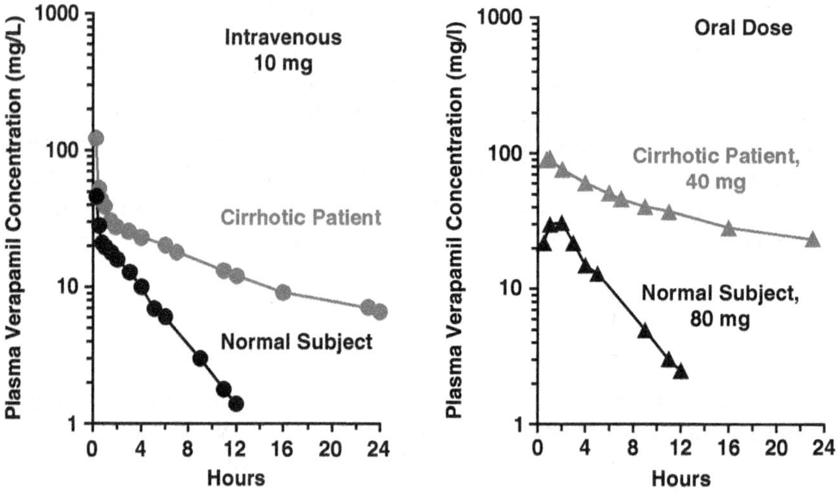

FIGURE 13-21 Plasma verapamil concentration-time profiles after intravenous (*panel on left*) and oral (*panel on right*) administrations in normal subjects (*black lines*) and cirrhotic patients (*colored lines*). The intravenous dose was 10 mg in both groups, while 80 mg and 40-mg doses were given to normal subjects and cirrhotic patients, respectively. (From Somogyi A, Albrecht M, Kliems G et al. Pharmacokinetics, bioavailability and ECG response of verapamil in patients with liver cirrhosis. Br J Clin Pharmacol 1981;12:51-60).

c. Why is the ratio of Dose/AUC values for the oral and intravenous doses so much lower in the cirrhotic patients (2.1 L/min) than in the healthy subjects (4.8 L/min)?

d. The fraction unbound in plasma was not affected by hepatic cirrhosis. How would you explain the increase in *V* (assuming that the change in *V* is statistically significant)?

CHAPTER 14

Initiating and Managing Therapy

OBJECTIVES

The reader will be able to:

- Suggest an approach for initiating a dosage regimen for an individual patient, given patient population pharmacokinetic and pharmacodynamic data and the individual's measurable characteristics.
- Describe why a pharmacokinetic or pharmacodynamic parameter in an individual patient is predictable when the value in a typical population is known and its variability is small, and the converse.
- Discuss why loading doses are sometimes given for drugs with half-lives in minutes and not given for other drugs with half-lives in days.
- State why several sequential doses, instead of just one, are sometimes used as a loading dose.
- Explain why plasma concentration monitoring is useful for some low therapeutic index drugs, but not for others in this same category.
- Briefly discuss how tolerance to therapeutic and adverse effects can influence the chronic dosing of drugs.
- Discuss why adherence to the prescribed regimen is so important in drug therapy.
- Discuss why, for some drugs, the dosage needs to be tapered downward gradually when discontinuing therapy.

Drug therapy is one of several options in the treatment of patients. Other options include surgery, physiotherapy, and counseling or a combination of these options. In selecting drug therapy, the decision is made that this is the most appropriate option to achieve a therapeutic objective. Once this objective is defined, a drug and its dosage regimen are chosen for a patient with the condition for which the drug is indicated. This choice is based on the assumption that the diagnosis is correct. Increasingly, although still uncommonly, genomic or phenotypic information about the patient is used to help to refine the diagnosis, such as the determination of overexpression of human epidermal growth factor receptor 2 protein, HER2, to determine whether a patient's breast cancer is likely to be successfully treated with trastuzumab. Recall, from Chapter 13, this applies to only 30% of breast cancer patients. In the remainder, trastuzumab is ineffective. Subsequently, drug therapy is often initiated and managed by one of two strategies, as shown schematically in Fig. 14-1 (next page). Management is usually, to one degree or another, accomplished by monitoring the incidence and intensity of therapeutic and adverse effects. In the first strategy, a "usual"

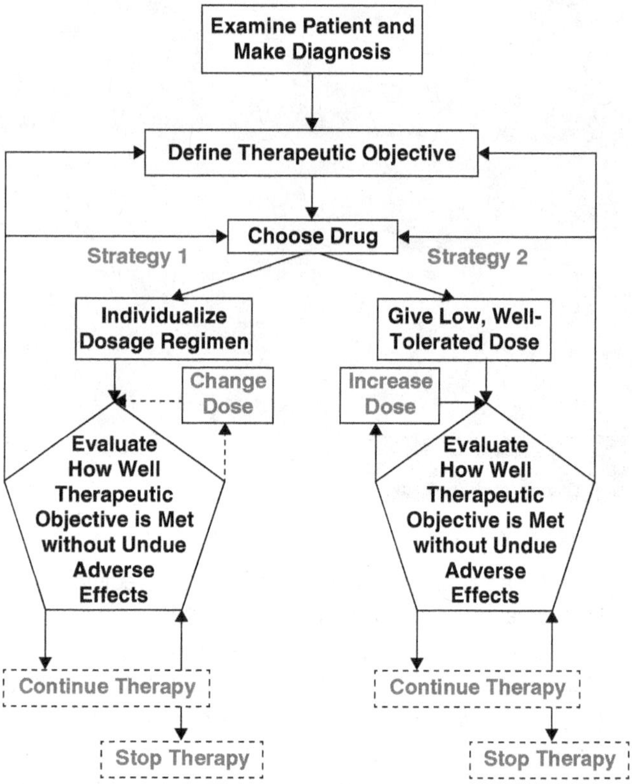

FIGURE 14-1 Scheme showing two strategies for initiating and managing drug therapy. The dashed line in Strategy 1 indicates that changes in dosing rate may be carried out, but the main expectation is that the regimen has already been tailored to the needs of the individual patient. This is in contrast to Strategy 2, in which the dosing rate is escalated to find the patient's dosage requirement.

dosage regimen anticipated for the patient is administered and maintenance therapy adjusted only if the desired response is inadequate or the adverse response excessive. In the second strategy, an individual's dosage requirements are established by starting the patient on a low dose and then titrating the dose upward, if needed, based on assessment of therapeutic and/or adverse end points. Both strategies probably reach a similar optimal dosage regimen; only the method of getting there differs.

The first strategy is primarily based on population pharmacokinetics and pharmacodynamics, that is, on what is known about the general tendencies and variabilities in the dose–exposure (pharmacokinetics) and exposure–response (pharmacodynamics) relationships. This strategy also allows a degree of individualization based on specific information about the individual patient, especially in assigning the appropriate initial regimen for a given patient. Most of the subsequent discussion revolves around this strategy. The second strategy, involving dose escalation to measured effects, clearly is also a means of individualizing dosage and managing therapy.

This chapter examines pharmacokinetic and pharmacodynamic issues in the initiation and management of drug therapy in both the patient population in general and in the individual patient. It brings together from previous chapters many points presented in other contexts.

ANTICIPATING SOURCES OF VARIABILITY

Choosing the right dose, or dosing rate, for patients with a given disease or condition is best accomplished when the sources of variability in the response to a drug are well understood and when there are good correlates between response and easily measured patient characteristics. First, consider the issue of the causes of variability.

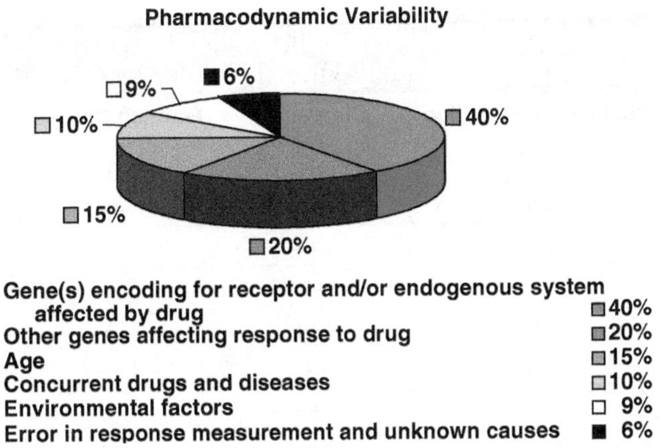

FIGURE 14-2 Schematic representation of the pharmacodynamic variability in drug response within the patient population. The variability occurs for a variety of reasons. In this analysis, six categories causing the variability are identified along with the percentage of the total variability associated with each category.

Obviously, the desired therapeutic objective would be most efficiently achieved if the individual's dosage requirements could be established *before administering the drug*. Without the required information in the patient, one must often rely on knowledge from a typical patient population. In Chapter 13, we examined variability in drug kinetics and response. The question before us now is how to handle this information from the patient population studies to treat an individual patient.

Pharmacodynamic Variability

In the pie chart of Fig. 14-2, the sources of pharmacodynamic variability of a hypothetical drug are indicated. For this drug, it is apparent that most (60%, first two categories) of the variability in response at a given exposure is genetically related. Clearly, pharmacogenomic correlates of exposure and response could be very useful to guide therapy. Such information may be used to identify individuals who are unlikely to respond, and so would not be given the drug or who are likely to respond differently (have a different dosage requirement, exhibit a peculiar adverse event, or show an increase in the incidence of usual adverse events) to a typical systemic exposure to the drug. As an example, recall from Chapter 13, the β-agonist albuterol in which response has been found to correlate with genotypic status. Knowing a patient's genotype may well help in selecting an appropriate dosage regimen for this patient.

The data in the pie chart also suggest that individualization of the exposure–response relationship may be helped if information about the individual, such as age, concurrent diseases, and environmental factors are taken into account, but only about one-third of the pharmacodynamic variability (15% + 10% + 9%) can be captured with this information, at best. If both the genotypic and the factors mentioned above are taken into account, one should be able to obtain a good estimate of the individual's response to a given exposure. To date, individualizing dosage based on patient-specific information affecting the pharmacodynamics of a drug has not been as successful as that affecting a drug's pharmacokinetics, our next topic.

Pharmacokinetic Variability

Drug administration–exposure relationships have an impact on the overall response to drugs. Again, one may be able to predict the exposure in an individual patient at a given dose based on patient-specific information. The general approach is to move from average or typical population pharmacokinetic parameter estimates to those most likely to be present in the individual patient.

TABLE 14-1 | Degree of Variability in the Oral Absorption and Disposition of Representative Drugs Within the Patient Population

Drug	Bioavailability	Volume of Distribution	Clearance	Fraction Unbound
Alendronate	++++	++	++	+
Amiodarone	++	+++	++	++
Atorvastatin	+++	++	+++	+
Cyclosporine	++	+	++	+
Digoxin	+++	++	+++	+
Ibuprofen	+	+++	++	++
Lithium	+	+	+++	+
Nortriptyline	+++	+++	+++	++
Phenytoin	+	++	++++	++
Propranolol	+++	+++	+++	+++
Sitagliptin	+	+	+++	++
Theophylline	+	+	+++	+
Trastuzumab	N/A	+	+	N/A
Warfarin	+	+	++	+

+, little; ++, moderate; +++, substantial; ++++, extensive; N/A, not applicable.

The first step is to identify the most variable parameters within the patient population. Variability in pharmacokinetic parameters within the patient population differs widely among drugs, as shown in Table 14-1 for a number of representative drugs. Some drugs, such as digoxin and propranolol, have substantial variability in absorption, but for different reasons. With digoxin, the variability in absorption is caused primarily by differences in pharmaceutical formulation and efflux transport (involving P-glycoprotein) of the drug in the intestines; with propranolol, it is caused by differences in the extent of first-pass hepatic metabolism. For other drugs, such as sitagliptin, used in the treatment of mature onset diabetes, the only substantial source of variability is clearance. It is well absorbed and totally renally eliminated unchanged. With others, the antiviral protease inhibitors and the statins included, significant variability exists in both absorption and disposition parameters.

The next step is to accommodate as much of the pharmacokinetic variability as possible with measurable characteristics. If the characteristic is discrete and independent, this can be achieved by partitioning the population into subpopulations. For example, as illustrated for clearance of the hypothetical drug in Fig. 14-3, the discrete characteristics are hepatic disease and smoking. Chronic hepatic disease typically reduces drug metabolism, sometimes dramatically, as previously stated in Chapter 13. Cigarette smoking induces the metabolism of some drugs, for example, theophylline, caffeine, tacrine, haloperidol, pentazocine, propranolol, flecainide, clozapine, and other drugs that are substrates of CYP1A1 and CYP1A2. For our example, the population might be divided into four categories: those who smoke and have no hepatic disease; those who smoke and have hepatic disease; those who have hepatic disease but do not smoke; and those who neither have hepatic disease nor smoke. The frequency distribution for the entire population is determined from the relative size (each area is proportional to the number of individuals) and shape (measure of variability) of the distribution curve of each subpopulation. If, on the other hand, the measurable

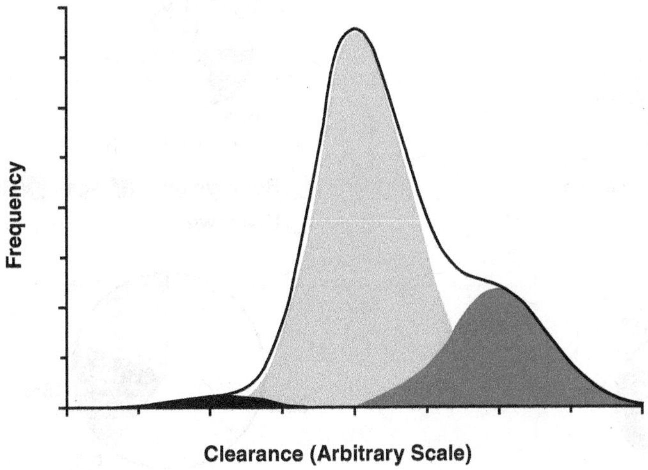

FIGURE 14-3 The frequency distribution of clearance of a drug within a patient population (*heavy line*) is a function of the shape of the frequency distribution within the various subpopulations that make up the total patient population and the relative sizes of each of these subpopulations. In this simulation, the variables are cigarette smoking and hepatic disease, and the subpopulations are those who neither have hepatic disease nor smoke (75%, the majority) (*shaded gray*); those who smoke but have no hepatic disease (22.5%) (*colored area*); those who have hepatic disease but do not smoke (2%) (*black*); and those who both smoke and have hepatic disease (0.5%). The size of the last population is too small to be readily seen in this figure. The average values for clearance in the four subpopulations were set at 1, 1.5, 0.5, and 0.75 units, respectively, assuming that smoking increases clearance by enzyme induction and that clearance is reduced in hepatic disease.

characteristic is continuous, such as age, body weight, or renal function, it may be possible to find a functional relationship with one or more pharmacokinetic parameters, such as that seen between the renal clearance of ganciclovir, an antiviral agent, and creatinine clearance, a graded measure of renal function (Fig. 14-4). Clearly, consideration needs to be given to reducing the dosing rate of this drug, and others, including sitagliptin, whose clearance depends heavily on renal function, in patients with impaired renal function to avoid excessive adverse effects.

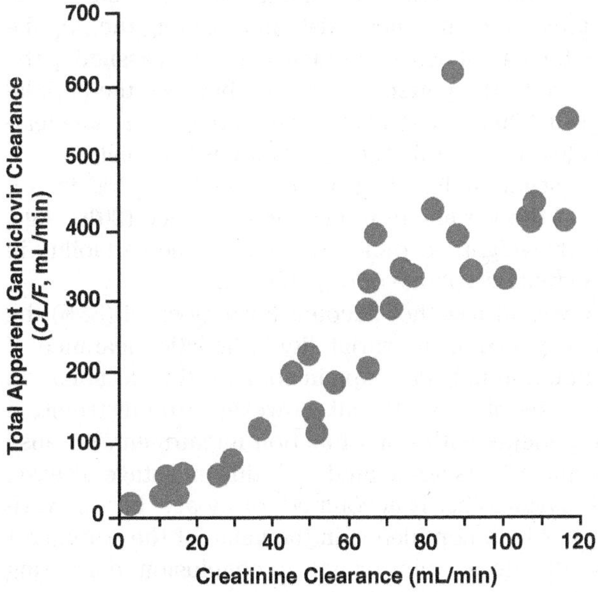

FIGURE 14-4 The apparent total body clearance (Dose/AUC or *CL/F*) of ganciclovir after oral administration of its prodrug, valganciclovir, increases linearly with creatinine clearance, a measure of renal function. Note that there is very little clearance when the renal function approaches zero (no creatinine clearance), indicating that this drug depends almost completely on renal excretion for its elimination. To maintain a comparable systemic exposure to the drug in patients with renal function impairment, the dosage of the drug needs to be decreased in proportion to the creatinine clearance. (From Czock D, Scholle C, Rasche FM, et al. Pharmacokinetics of valganciclovir and ganciclovir in renal impairment. *Clin Pharmacol Ther* 2002;72:142–150.)

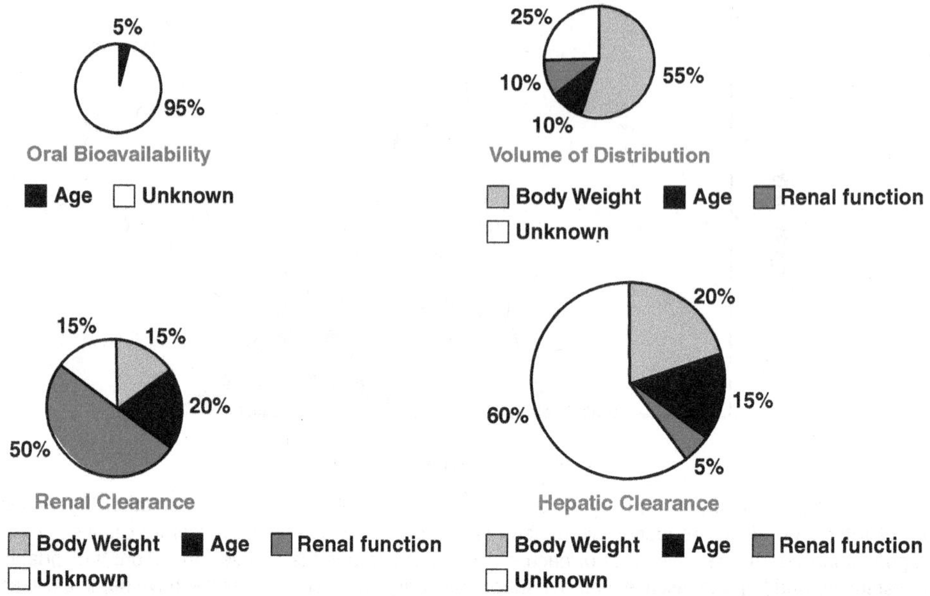

FIGURE 14-5 Schematic representation of variability in various pharmacokinetic parameters within a population. The size of each tablet is related to the degree of variability in the parameter. The portion of each tablet labeled with body weight (*gray*), age (*black*), and renal function (*colored*) reflects the fraction of total variability captured by each of these patient-specific measures. The portion of the variability not accounted for by these measures is indicated in white.

To envisage how the entire strategy would work, consider the information in Fig. 14-5 for a drug partly metabolized in the liver and partly excreted unchanged in the urine for which average population pharmacokinetic parameters are: oral bioavailability, 0.73; volume of distribution, 83 L; renal clearance, 2.7 L/hr; and metabolic clearance, 14.1 L/hr. Depicted are four tablets, representing oral bioavailability, volume of distribution, renal clearance, and metabolic clearance. The size of each tablet is a measure of variability (coefficient of variation) of that parameter within the patient population. For this drug, oral bioavailability is the least and hepatic clearance is the most variable. Stated differently, greatest confidence exists in assigning the population value of oral bioavailability to the patient; least confidence exists in assigning the population value of hepatic clearance to the patient. Moreover, because the population value for hepatic clearance (14.1 L/hr) is much greater than that for renal clearance (2.7 L/hr), variability in total clearance within the population is also high.

Not unexpectedly, body weight accounts for most of the variability (55%) in volume of distribution and for some of the variability in hepatic clearance (20%). Age, separated from its influence on body weight, accounts for some of the variability in hepatic clearance and, to a lesser extent, in volume of distribution.

Renal function, age, and body weight together account for almost all (85%) the variability in renal clearance, but only 40% of the variability in hepatic clearance. It is surprising, perhaps, that renal function helps to explain some of the variability in metabolic clearance and volume of distribution. Recall, however, drug distribution and metabolism can be altered in patients with renal function impairment, because such patients manifest many systemic effects associated with this end-stage disease. Only 5% of the variability in oral bioavailability is accounted for by age, but the variability is small, and therefore one has high confidence in the value of the parameter in the patient, whether one takes age into account or not. In conclusion, correcting

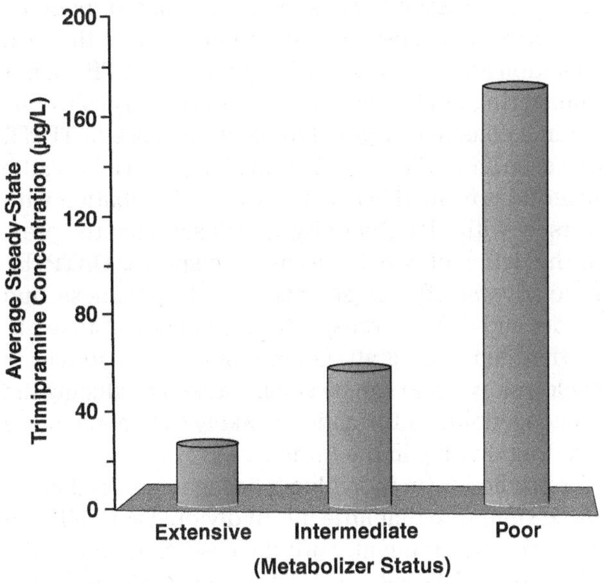

FIGURE 14-6 The daily maintenance dose of the antidepressant trimipramine depends on an individual's genotype. Without adjusting for genotype of CYP2D6, the average steady-state concentration of trimipramine and its active metabolite, desmethyltrimipramine, vary greatly between the genotypes, identified here as extensive, intermediate, and poor metabolizers. The concentrations are calculated from single-dose data for a regimen of 75 mg twice daily. The metabolite concentration (not shown) also goes up in the groups with intermediate and poor metabolism, a result of the demethylation reaction forming the metabolite (catalyzed by CYP2C19) not being affected by the genotype of CYP2D6, the enzyme responsible for hydroxylation of both trimipramine and desmethyltrimipramine. (Values calculated from data in Kirchheiner J, Müller G, Meinke I, Wernecke K-D, et al. Effects of polymorphisms in CYP2D6, CYP2C9 and CYP2C19 on trimipramine pharmacokinetics. *J Clin Psychopharmacol* 2003;459–466.)

the population pharmacokinetic parameters for the patient's weight, age, and renal function should give reasonable individual estimates of F, V, and CL_R, for this drug, but little confidence in the estimate of CL_H and hence total clearance.

Finally, the inability of age, weight, and renal function to account for most of the variability in metabolic clearance should be noted. Genetics, concurrent disease(s), and the simultaneous administration of other drugs undoubtedly play a role, but the variability in hepatic clearance produced by them may not yet be accounted for by known patient-specific information about the drug in question.

Markers of genetic control of drug metabolism have been developed for some drugs; this helps to explain much of their inherited interindividual differences in metabolic clearance (Chapter 13). An example (Fig. 14-6) is that of the antidepressant trimipramine. Like nortriptyline, this drug is primarily eliminated by CYP2D6-catalyzed metabolism. The patient population can be divided into four groups: poor metabolizers (5%–10% of population), intermediate metabolizers (10%–15%), extensive metabolizers (65%–80%), and ultra-rapid metabolizers (5%–10%). The group to which an individual belongs can be determined by genotyping (pharmacogenomic test), which is becoming increasingly available and applied in circumstances where such stratification is beneficial and cost-effective. For example, the assignment of the initial dose of eliglustat (Cerdelga), used for the treatment of patients with Gaucher disease and heavily dependent in its clearance on CYP2D6 activity, is based on genotyping (Chapter 13). The initial recommended dosage regimen for extensive and intermediate metabolizers is 100-mg tartrate salt (84-mg base equivalence) twice daily, whereas that for poor metabolizers is 100 mg once daily. The alternative to genotyping is phenotyping. Both methods may become more common in the future. An example of characterizing an individual's CYP2D6 phenotypic status involves a urine test of drug/metabolite ratio determined after a single dose of a suitable probe drug (substrate) of this enzyme, such as sparteine, debrisoquine, or dextromethorphan—the higher the ratio, the lower the amount of metabolite formed and the poorer the metabolic status of the individual.

Another example is that of patients placed on thiopurine drugs (Chapter 13), for which measurement of thiopurine *S*-methyltransferase (TPMT) activity can identify patients who are likely to show severe adverse effects to drugs in this class unless the normal dose is reduced accordingly. An issue here is the prevalence of patients with the genotypic status that is of concern, against the risk of failing to do the test. Recall, only 0.3% of the patient population are homozygous for the deficient TPMT, but the risk of severe toxicity on administering normal doses of thiopurine drugs to this patient group is so high that it warrants considering genotyping. In the case of TPMT, an alternative is phenotyping, in this case an in vitro test that involves determining the concentration of 6-thioguanine nucleotides formed in erythrocytes on incubation with azathioprine, which correlates inversely with TPMT activity. Recall also that the prevalence of patients homozygous for the deficient hepatic uptake transporter OATP1B1 allele is also very low (0.2%), but the adverse effects (skeletal muscle weakness, and damage) in patients on statins that depend on this transporter for hepatic uptake are not considered sufficiently severe that genotyping all patients prior to treatment is warranted. The adverse effects develop slowly and can be ameliorated by reducing the dose. Still, the application of pharmacogenomic information is likely to become more commonly applied to diagnosis and drug therapy in the future.

The approach just presented for predicting an individual's dosage regimen before administering a drug is based on the assumption that little interindividual variability in pharmacodynamics exists. This is, of course, frequently not the case. Sometimes the majority of the variability in drug response following a given dosage regimen is due to variability in pharmacodynamics. Although knowing the mean pharmacokinetic parameters of the drug may help to predict the time course in exposure, quantifying pharmacokinetic variability then adds little to our ability to predict individual dosage. Nonetheless, the basic strategy still holds for both pharmacokinetic and pharmacodynamic variability: to determine the relative contribution of measurable characteristics such as age and body weight to drug response within the patient population and then to use the individual's characteristics to predict his or her therapeutic dosage regimen. Frequently, however, age, weight, and other measurable characteristics fail to account for much of the variability in either pharmacokinetics or pharmacodynamics. Then, there is little choice but to start the individual patient on a typical dosage regimen (*Strategy 1* in Fig. 14-1), which may be far from the individual's requirement, and to monitor and adjust the regimen based on the patient's response to the drug. When the drug has a low therapeutic index, it may be prudent to start therapy with a low, generally safe dose and titrate to the patient's need for the drug (*Strategy 2* in Fig. 14-1). The choice between the two strategies also depends on the urgency of initiating therapy. Let us now apply these concepts to initiating and managing drug therapy.

INITIATING THERAPY

The first dose given depends on the strategy used to treat a patient, the patient's total therapy, and on the specific drug. There are situations in which the first dose needs to be smaller than the maintenance dose. For other drugs, a loading dose larger than the maintenance dose may be appropriate.

Choosing the Starting Dose

Let us examine situations requiring a starting dose different from the maintenance dose and the determinants of its size. The argument was presented in Chapter 12 that a priming, or loading, dose may be needed to rapidly achieve a therapeutic response. There are times when this strategy is appropriate and times when it is not.

When Is a Loading Dose Needed?

One consideration is the urgency of drug treatment. Recall from Table 12-3 that a loading dose is recommended for esmolol, a drug used to treat life-threatening supraventricular tachycardias. With a half-life of only 9 minutes, one would expect steady state to be reached in about 30 minutes; however, this is too long to wait in this emergency situation. By giving a loading dose at the time the infusion is started, effective systemic concentrations can be achieved within a few minutes. The infusion thereafter maintains therapy. This strategy is common to many drugs given by intravenous infusion (see Table 11-1) for which there is an urgent need to achieve the therapeutic response rapidly.

There may also be a need for a loading dose when the drug accumulates extensively, that is, when the dosing interval is short compared with the half-life and the same dose is repeatedly given. When a loading dose is required, it may be given all at once. Consider the choice of a loading dose for the antimalarial agent, mefloquine hydrochloride. To treat patients with mild to moderate malaria caused by *Plasmodium vivax* or mefloquine-susceptible strains of *Plasmodium falciparum*, a loading dose of 1250 mg (five 250-mg tablets) is recommended. No maintenance dose is required because the drug has a 3-week half-life, a period of time sufficient to cure the patient. This loading dose might be compared to the maintenance dose of mefloquine as a prophylaxis for the prevention of malaria, which is 250 mg once weekly, starting 1 week before going to areas where malaria is endemic, and continuing for 4 weeks after returning from the area. The *accumulation* index of this drug on this weekly regimen is 5 (Equation 12-10). Thus, the amount of mefloquine in the body at steady state is about 1250 mg, the level found to be effective for treating an acute episode of malaria.

Adverse reactions often give rise to no loading dose being used or to the need to administer the loading dose over a period of time, but a short time relative to the drug's half-life. Another antimalarial drug serves as a good example of this situation. For treating an acute attack of chloroquine-sensitive malaria, chloroquine phosphate is given in a loading dose of 1000 mg initially, followed by 500 mg in 6–8 hours, then 500 mg on each of 2 successive days for a total of 2500 mg. Again, this treatment completes therapy because the half-life of the drug is about 6 weeks. The reason for the divided loading dose is to reduce adverse effects (headache, drowsiness, visual disturbance, nausea, and vomiting, which in the worst scenario may lead to cardiovascular collapse, shock, and convulsions). These effects can occur within minutes of ingestion of a single 2500-mg loading dose.

The need for a loading dose is also a question of the kinetics of the pharmacodynamic response. Certainly, a loading dose is unnecessary for antidepressants, antihyperlipidemic agents, and agents used to treat and prevent osteoporosis. For these drugs, the therapeutic response takes from weeks to months to fully develop. Although a loading dose may somewhat shorten the time to achieve a therapeutic response, the major cause of the delay is in the response of the body to the drug. An example of a drug in this category is alendronate, an agent used to treat and prevent osteoporosis in postmenopausal women. As shown in Fig. 14-7, the increase in bone mineral density, a likely surrogate end point of the therapeutic use of the drug, namely, a reduction of bone fracturing, takes months, if not years, to fully develop.

What Should the Loading Dose Be?

A loading dose is a consideration for drugs with half-lives of 24 hours or more when they are administered in a convenient once-a-day or twice-a-day regimen. In these

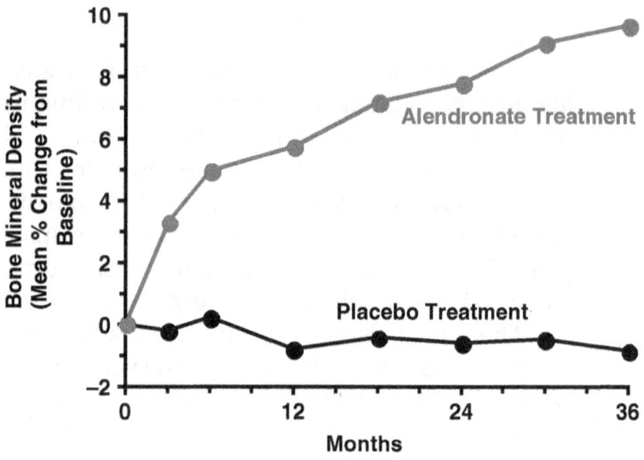

FIGURE 14-7 Time course of the change from baseline in bone mineral density after 10 mg of alendronate sodium daily in postmenopausal women with osteoporosis. Mean data for both treated (*color*) and placebo (*black*) groups are shown. Note the long time required for development of the effect, a surrogate of the desired reduction in frequency of bone fractures. (*Physicians' Desk Reference*. Montvale, NJ: Thomson PDR, 2005 Edition:2051.)

situations, the size of the loading dose may be anticipated from a pharmacokinetic perspective. The loading dose can be approximated from the amount accumulated in the body at plateau on chronic dosing and knowledge of the drug's bioavailability. It might also be estimated, if applicable, from the window of concentrations associated with optimal therapy. As an example, consider the individual patient needing the drug for which population data were presented in Fig. 14-5. As the ratio F/V strongly influences the peak plasma concentration after a single dose, and shows little interpatient variability, reasonable confidence can be expected in estimating the patient's loading dose based on body weight, if required. This particularly applies to the administration of drugs to both very small and very large adults and to infants and children for whom the volume of distribution is expected to deviate substantially from that of a typical patient, but to vary proportionally with body weight. This approach, however, would not be very helpful if most of the variability in the response to the drug lay in its pharmacodynamics.

Dose Titration

For drugs that do not require an immediate response, a logical and safe procedure to initiate therapy is to titrate the dosage in the individual. Dosage is adjusted upwards until the desired therapeutic response is obtained without undue adverse effects. This procedure is recommended for a number of drugs. Flecainide acetate is an example of a drug dosed in this manner. For patients with paroxysmal supraventricular tachycardia, the recommendation is to start with 50 mg every 12 hours. Doses are then increased in 50-mg increments every 4 days until an optimal response in the individual patient is obtained. The 4-day interval between changing the dosing rate is based on the observation that at least 2–4 days is required to achieve a steady state of drug effect. This is not surprising from a pharmacokinetic point of view because the half-life of the drug ranges from 12 to 27 hours in patients.

Another example is valproic acid, an agent used in treating complex partial seizures. When given alone, therapy is initiated with 10–15 mg/kg/day in divided doses. The dosage is increased by 5–10 mg/kg/week until optimal control of seizures is achieved. Optimal clinical response is usually achieved with daily maintenance doses below 60 mg/kg/day. With terazosin, an agent used to symptomatically treat patients with an enlarged prostate and sometimes to treat hypertension, the recommendation is similar. The initial dose is 1 mg taken at bedtime. The dose is increased in a stepwise fashion, based on blood pressure response, to 2, 5, or 10 mg once daily until the desired improvement in urine flow rate is achieved by relaxing the smooth muscles in the bladder neck. Daily maintenance doses of 10 mg are typically required. Accumulation of this drug is not very extensive on once-daily administration of a fixed regimen because the half-life is about 12 hours. Careful and slow upward titration of dosage reduces the incidence of severe postural hypotension and syncope and explains, in part, why weeks to months of treatment are often required to achieve the optimal response.

MANAGING THERAPY

For some drugs, there is a standard dosage regimen that works in almost all patients, other than those at the extremes of the population, namely, infants, children, and perhaps the elderly, especially those who are frail. Adherence is the main issue for these drugs. For other drugs, therapy is frequently monitored, and dosage is optimized by continual assessment of clinical responses, surrogate end points, biomarkers, or adverse effects, or combinations of them. Still, for some others, measurement of plasma drug concentration is incorporated into the strategy for drug utilization. One of the key considerations that determine how therapy is managed is the therapeutic index of the drug.

Low Therapeutic Index

Recall from Chapter 10 that a low therapeutic index drug is one for which the dosing rate required for a good therapeutic response in an individual patient is very close to that producing excessive adverse effects. To maintain a reasonably constant therapeutic response in the individual, the drug *must* show relatively little intrasubject variability in both its pharmacokinetics and pharmacodynamics. The dosing rate of such drugs needs to be individualized and the responses monitored more frequently than with high therapeutic index drugs. The degree of individualization and monitoring required depends on intersubject variability. As shown in Table 14-2, there may be

TABLE 14-2 | Interpatient Variability and Monitoring of a Low Therapeutic Index Drug

Source of Interpatient Variability		
Pharmacokinetics	**Pharmacodynamics**	**Monitoring**
High	High	Full and continuous monitoring is required. If no good biomarkers or surrogate end points are available, the drug may not be useful.
Low	Low	Generally, there is less need for monitoring of the individual, and the doses needed across the population are more similar.
Low	High	Assessment of therapeutic and/or adverse responses is essential. Little benefit is obtained by monitoring the plasma concentration of the drug.
High	Low	Although monitoring of responses is important, concentration monitoring may also be useful to aid in tailoring dosage to the individual patient.

less need for monitoring if intersubject variability is low in both the drug's pharmacokinetics and pharmacodynamics. If the interpatient pharmacodynamic variability is high and pharmacokinetic variability low, then monitoring response is essential to establish the proper dose. If, on the other hand, the interpatient variability between dose and response lies primarily in pharmacokinetics, which cannot be readily predicted from the patient's characteristics, then a strong case can be made for using plasma concentration monitoring to aid in managing therapy with the drug. For such drugs, a therapeutic window of concentrations determined for the patient population then applies to the individual patient, and plasma concentrations obtained at one or more appropriate times can be used as a supplementary piece of information to guide the adjustment of dosage for the individual patient, as discussed later in this chapter, under Concentration Monitoring.

Use of Biomarkers and Clinical and Surrogate Endpoints

Although preferable, it is not always possible to use a direct measure of the desired effect as a therapeutic end point. Sometimes, adverse effects are used as a dosing guide. Antineoplastic agents such as 5-fluorouracil, and immunosuppressive agents such as cyclosporine are examples. Dosage is increased to levels at which adverse effects are seen, but are kept from being excessive. The expectation is that the likelihood of achieving the therapeutic effect is optimized with this procedure, as it permits the highest dose possible for the patient. In this sense, these are clearly low therapeutic index drugs.

Another example is that of the antiepileptic drug, phenytoin. The therapeutic effect here is the nonoccurrence of seizures. Seizures may be infrequent, and as a result, delays and difficulties exist in assessing therapeutic success. Adverse effects that can be readily measured, such as nystagmus and ataxia, have therefore been used to assist in determining the upper limit of an epileptic patient's dosage requirement (see Chapter 10). Plasma concentration monitoring is a supplementary approach to optimize phenytoin dosage, but it is useful because much of the variability in the response to this drug resides in its pharmacokinetics. Concentration monitoring thus increases the likelihood of achieving therapeutic success without the patient having to endure excessive adverse effects.

Another situation in which the therapeutic objective cannot readily be assessed is the prevention of thromboembolic complications with oral anticoagulants. In this case, an alternative, simple, and rapid laboratory test—the international normalized ratio test, which measures the tendency of blood to clot—is used as a predictor of how well the therapeutic objective is achieved. Similarly, for antihypertensive agents, blood pressure is often considered a reasonable surrogate of clinical outcome, that is, prevention of cardiovascular and renal disease associated with chronic hypertension. For antihypercholesterolemic, hypoglycemic, and uricosuric agents, clinical laboratory tests of lipids and lipoproteins, blood glucose, and serum uric acid, respectively, are used as surrogate end points.

Monitoring of therapeutic response and toxicity is best accomplished when integrated with kinetic concepts. Half-life determines the time course of drug accumulation and hence of the development of responses. It is also a determinant of the time for a toxic response to resolve on reducing or discontinuing therapy. In both these situations, the statement particularly applies when pharmacokinetics rate-limits the time course of response. Time is also a factor in the development of response to many drugs, even when the plasma concentration is constant. For example, the response to warfarin (Chapter 9) is delayed by several days because of the time required for the clotting factors to decline to values that produce an adequate and stable degree of anticoagulation. Tailoring dosage to an individual's needs clearly requires integration of both kinetic and dynamic principles.

Tolerance

Another consideration in managing therapy is the buildup of tolerance to a drug. As discussed in Chapter 11, nitroglycerin, an antianginal agent with a 2- to 4-minute half-life, is an example of a drug to which tolerance to the therapeutic response develops with continuous therapy. The use of transdermal patches to deliver the drug at a constant rate around the clock turned out to be unsuccessful because of the development of tolerance. The problem was, in large part, overcome by administering the patch only during the daytime. The time without the patch during the night appeared to be sufficient to prevent the buildup of tolerance to the therapeutic effect.

Tolerance can also develop to the adverse effects of a drug, as is the case with terazosin as mentioned above. The drug, used to treat benign prostatic hyperplasia, produces hypotension. The adverse hypotensive effect can be kept under control by slowly increasing the dosing rate so that the therapeutic effect can be obtained without undue postural hypotension and syncope. How quickly the dosage can be titrated up to the dose needed chronically is primarily a function of the rapidity of the development of tolerance to the hypotensive effect.

Concentration Monitoring

Another approach more explicitly incorporating kinetic principles is the monitoring of plasma drug concentrations. At a minimum, the plasma concentration serves as an additional piece of information to guide and assess drug therapy. It can also help to distinguish between pharmacokinetic and pharmacodynamic causes of either a lack of response or an excessive response. The application of plasma concentration measurements to therapy involves **target concentration strategy**. The basic idea is to apply a strategy to achieve and maintain a target concentration or a target range of concentrations for an individual patient.

When Is It Useful?

Monitoring of plasma concentrations may be useful when a drug has a low therapeutic index, and pharmacokinetics accounts for much of the interpatient variability in its response (Table 14-2). Concentration monitoring is especially helpful when there are only poor end points/biomarkers to assess response, as is the case for cyclosporine, sirolimus, and other agents used to prevent rejection following organ transplantation.

The Target Concentration

The target concentration initially chosen is the value or range of values with the greatest probability of therapeutic success (Table 10-1), keeping in mind that higher concentrations may be appropriate when the patient's condition is severe, and the converse when the condition is mild. If altered plasma protein binding is anticipated, such as in uremia, after surgery, or when displacing drugs that achieve high concentrations, are also administered, then the target total concentration should be adjusted to attain the same therapeutically important unbound concentration.

In contrast to many endogenous substances, which remain relatively constant, drug concentrations can vary greatly with time. The time of sampling and an appropriate kinetic model are therefore essential to interpret measured concentration(s) correctly. Several kinds of information are needed to evaluate a measured plasma concentration efficiently. A history of drug administration, which includes doses and times of dosing, is mandatory, as are the times of blood sampling.

Frequency of monitoring is a function of the presumed change in the factors that influence drug response. For example, the plasma concentration of sirolimus, an immunosuppressive agent, needs to be monitored only after approximately 7–14 days after changing dosage because of its 3-day half-life. More frequent monitoring may be indicated for this and other drugs when a patient's health is rapidly deteriorating or when therapy with coadministered drugs is altered. For example, weekly monitoring of plasma phenytoin concentrations may be helpful in treating an epileptic patient, when treatment with other drugs, which are inhibitors or inducers of phenytoin metabolism, are changed or withdrawn.

Adherence Issues

The most frequent patterns of nonadherence to prescribed dosage (Table 14-3) are failure to take drug at the times indicated, omitting an occasional dose, failure to take several consecutive doses, and occasional overdosing, particularly with once-daily dosing. Another form of nonadherence is discontinuance of drug therapy for short periods (a few days to a week), the so-called "drug holiday," or completely, before the prescribed duration of treatment, a lack of persistence (as discussed in Chapter 13). A third form of nonadherence is to not start therapy at all, which, although generally uncommon, tends to occur with greater prevalence in some conditions, such as mental depression, than others.

Some drugs are forgiving, that is, occasional nonadherence of the types in the second category of Table 14-3 (deviation to a daily regimen) may have little effect on therapy with the drug. This can occur when the dosing interval is small relative to the half-life, as is the case when using bisphosphonates, with half-lives of months or longer, to treat osteoporosis and amiodarone, with a half-life of about 2 months, used to treat ventricular arrhythmias and atrial fibrillation. It also applies to drugs for which the response persists, relative to drug in the body, as is the case with the statins, a pharmacodynamic rate limitation. On the opposite extreme are drugs that are absolutely unforgiving, as is the case for a drug such as esmolol for which the drug concentration must be rapidly attained and maintained. In this case, the drug is given intravenously, and the clinician rather than the patient must carefully monitor drug administration.

TABLE 14-3 | Patterns of Nonadherence to Prescribed Dosage
Failure to Initiate Therapy
Nonadherence to Dosage Regimen (Daily Deviations)
Change in time of day for taking dose
Omitting 1–3 doses/day
Taking extra doses to make up for missed doses
Lack of Persistence in Dosing
Discontinuing doses for periods of time (vacations, business trips, etc.)
Completely stop taking drug

Consider now the impact of not taking an oral medication as directed from a pharmacokinetic point of view.

Missed Dose(s)

The lack of adherence to the prescribed manner of taking a drug is one of the sources—sometimes the major one—of variability in drug response in clinical practice. It is commonly believed that regimens of multiple (3–4) daily doses tend to produce more frequent missed doses than those in which drug is taken once or twice daily. As shown in Fig. 14-8, such decreases in frequency (with corresponding increase in each dose to keep the same daily dose) may not improve therapy. Note that even when three doses

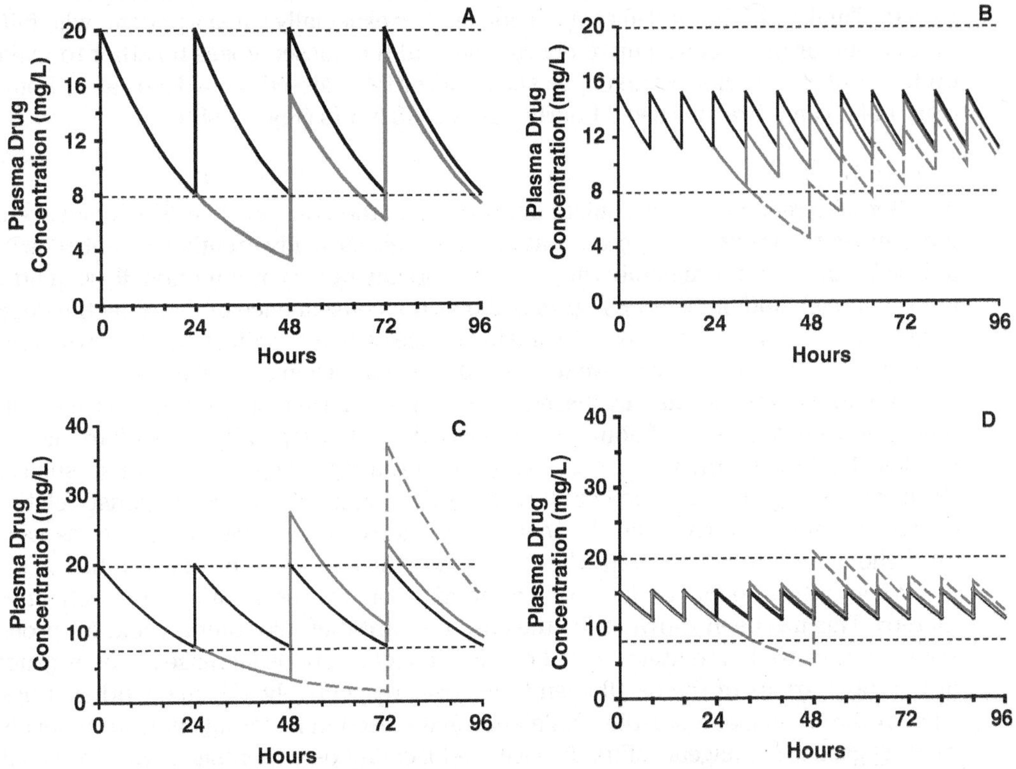

FIGURE 14-8 From a kinetic perspective, the impact of a missed dose is greater, the larger the dose and the less frequent the administration. Consider steady-state multidose conditions for a drug with a therapeutic window of 8–20 mg/L, a volume of distribution of 50 L, and a half-life of 18.2 hours. **A.** When a 600-mg dose is given once daily to maintain therapeutic concentrations (*black line*), a missed dose (*solid colored line*) results in a trough concentration of 3.2 mg/L, a value well below the lower limit of the therapeutic window. **B.** When a 200-mg dose is given every 8 hours (*solid black line*), the lowest concentration after a single missed dose is 8.2 mg/L, a value within the therapeutic window. Even if three consecutive doses are missed (*dashed colored line*), the minimum concentration (5.0 mg/L) is still above that observed 24 hours after a single 600-mg dose is missed. **C.** When a patient attempts to make up for missed doses, the chances of adverse effects are increased, particularly on the once-a-day regimen. When a patient takes twice the daily dose at 48 hours, the peak concentration is increased (*solid colored line*), but not greatly. However, if the patient tries to make up for two missed doses (*dashed colored line*), that is, takes three times the normal dose, adverse effects become more likely. **D.** When the patient takes two 200 mg doses at 32 hours after missing one dose on the 8-hourly regimen (*solid red line*), the plasma concentration returns close to what would have been the case had no dose been missed. Even when four doses are taken at 48 hours after missing three consecutive doses, the peak plasma concentration is only 20.2 mg/L, a value just above the therapeutic window (*dashed colored line*). Note the difference in scales of concentration between the top and bottom panels.

are missed on the three-times-a-day regimen (Fig. 14-8B), the plasma concentration does not go as low as when one dose is missed on the once-a-day regimen (Fig. 14-8A). Clearly, an increase in the incidence of missed doses presumably occurring with an 8-hourly regimen must be balanced against the benefit of less nonadherence on giving the same daily dose once only.

Make-Up Dose(s)

Another issue involving adherence is taking larger doses to make up for missed doses. If one or more doses are missed, should the next dose be increased? Shown in Fig. 14-8C and D are situations in which missed doses are simply added to the dose taken at the next prescribed time. Again, note the greater risk associated with the once-daily regimen (Fig. 14-8C) compared with the three-times-a-day regimen (Fig. 14-8D) with the "make-up" doses. This conclusion applies especially when a patient, who fails to take one or more consecutive doses, takes all the missed doses together to make up for drug not previously taken, as shown after two missed daily doses at 72 hours (Fig. 14-8C) and three missed 8-hourly doses at 48 hours (Fig. 14-8D).

Doubling-Up of Doses

Another adherence issue of clinical importance is the consequence of taking two or more times the recommended dose at one time, either inadvertently (patient repeats a dose because of not remembering the dose already taken) or intentionally (if a little helps; more should be better). Fig. 14-9 shows the consequence of doubling the dose. Clearly, a greater maximal exposure and incidence of adverse effects is likely when the drug is given infrequently, relative to the half-life, than when given frequently.

The above simulations are based on a drug's pharmacokinetic properties. The therapeutic consequence of nonadherence to a drug also depends on the pharmacodynamics of a drug. All the issues previously discussed regarding drug response, such as the pertinent region of the exposure–response curve, a delay in the response relative to the systemic exposure, and the therapeutic index of the drug, apply here as well. They should also be considered when evaluating the consequence of nonadherence.

When critical, patient education and motivation are essential to obtain effective therapy. This has been shown to be the case for antitubercular therapy and for protease inhibitors used in treating AIDS. Low drug concentrations increase the emergence of resistant strains of the bacillus and the virus, respectively. For many other drugs, such as the statins, omeprazole, and alendronate, used in lowering cholesterol levels, treating gastroesophageal reflux disease, and treating osteoporosis, respectively, adherence to the prescribed manner of taking the medication is perhaps not so critical.

Changes in Therapy

In the foregoing discussion, the assumption was generally made that therapy with a drug was initiated and managed in the absence of other drugs and other disease conditions. In practice, a drug is commonly initiated when one or more other drugs are being administered for the same or other conditions. These other drugs and diseases or conditions must be integrated into the evaluation of the individualization process. The pharmacokinetic and pharmacodynamic principles are the same, but an adaptation to the specific therapeutic setting must be made.

Other common scenarios are those in which one or more of the other drugs that a patient is concurrently taking is adjusted in its dosage or withdrawn, or a new medication is added. In all of these and similar situations, drug interactions should be

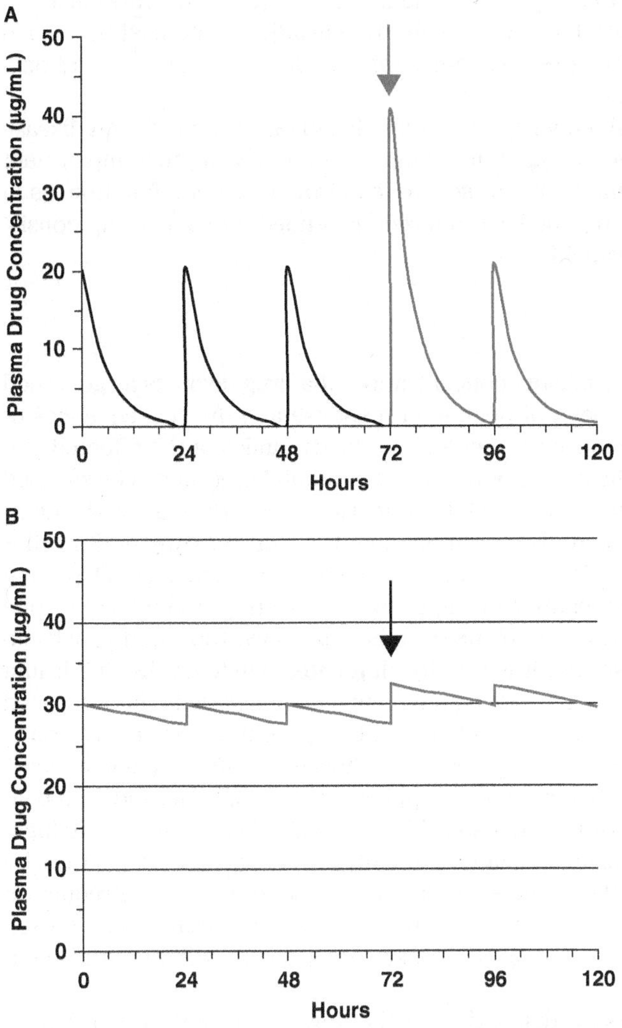

FIGURE 14-9 Another form of nonadherence to the prescribed regimen is when a patient takes more than one dose at essentially the same time. In this example, a patient takes two tablets instead of one at 72 hours (*vertical arrows*), a consequence of forgetting that he had taken his daily dose 15 minutes before. It is also an example of what would happen if the patient does not feel well and believes that an additional dose may help. **A.** When a drug is given infrequently compared with its half-life, the effect of taking multiple doses at once can be dangerous, particularly if the incidence and/or severity of adverse events increases sharply with higher C_{max} values. Note that the peak concentration of this drug, which has a 4-hour half-life, is nearly twice the usual peak concentration. **B.** When the drug is taken frequently compared with its half-life (drug with a half-life of 12 days is now at steady state), the consequences of taking twice the dose (*at arrow*) may be minimal as the extra dose represents only a small fraction of the amount in the body, owing to extensive accumulation on the regimen, so that the peak exposure is not changed much.

considered, not only in terms of the magnitude of the potential effect of the interaction, but also in terms of the time frame for drug accumulation and elimination and the rapidity of gain and loss of drug response. In addition, for drugs prescribed for treatment of chronic disease, the degree of severity of the disease or condition may change with time, requiring an adjustment in the dosage of a drug, as is often the case for drugs used, for example, in treating patients with Parkinson's disease.

DOSE STRENGTHS AND STRATIFICATION OF PATIENTS

Adjustment of either the initial dose or the maintenance dose to meet the requirements of an individual patient cannot be exact. As stated previously (Chapter 13), solid dosage forms of drugs are commonly available in discrete dose strengths, which usually differ from each other by twofold. The number of dose strengths is dictated by the therapeutic index of the drug and the interpatient variability in the dose–response relationship. Simvastatin, for example, is available in 5-, 10-, 20-, 40-, and 80-mg tablets. Occasionally, the dose strengths are closer together as is the case for warfarin, a drug with a low therapeutic index and large interpatient variability, which comes in 1-, 2-, 2.5-, 3-, 4-, 5-, 6-, 7.5-, and 10-mg tablets. Obviously, dosage adjustment must be carried out consistent with the dose strengths available. Some tablets are scored so that one-half of its contents can be taken.

Similarly, there is a clinical tendency to stratify physiologic functions and disease severity that are, in reality, continuous. For example, patients with renal impairment are classified as having mild, moderate, or severe impairment of renal function, as in Fig. 13-14. Here, too, a dosage regimen is often recommended for each group consistent with the dose strengths available.

DISCONTINUING THERAPY

On stopping administration, the plasma concentration of a drug declines as governed by its pharmacokinetics. The speed of decline in response and the consequences of stopping therapy vary. They are often dependent on the dynamics of the affected system as well as the kinetics of the drug. For many drugs, administration can be stopped abruptly without appreciable immediate safety concerns. This is the case with antibiotics, antihistamines, and nonsteroidal anti-inflammatory agents. However, for other drugs, sudden discontinuation of therapy can have serious consequences. This often occurs because the chronic exposure to drug causes a resetting in the level of one or more important body constituents. If the drug is withdrawn too rapidly, particularly if it has a short half-life so that it is rapidly eliminated, an acute disequilibrium occurs within the body with potential adverse effects. One example is the increased β-receptor sensitivity noticed with the sudden withdrawal of β-blockers with sometimes fatal consequences. Another example is the withdrawal of morphine in addicts. A third example is the adverse effects, such as rapid weight loss, fatigue, and joint pain seen on sudden withdrawal of oral corticosteroids, especially following chronic high-dose therapy. In such cases, it is important to gradually reduce the daily dose, thereby allowing the body to adjust to the change in systemic exposure. The rate of reduction and duration of tapering dosage can vary from days to weeks or months, depending on the kinetics of the drug and the dynamics of the key components within the affected system within the body.

With these final comments on discontinuing therapy, it is fitting to end this introductory book on quantitative principles relevant to drug therapy. It is hoped that, armed with these principles, the reader will be in a better position to ensure the optimal administration of drugs for the benefit of the patients taking them.

SUMMARY

- Two basic strategies are used for initiating and maintaining drug therapy. One involves individualizing dosage based on population pharmacokinetics and pharmacodynamics and the patient's characteristics. The other involves titration of dosage to the individual's specific needs, usually by starting with a well-tolerated small dose.
- Doses for a specific patient can be anticipated when sources of variability, good correlates of response, and easily measured patient characteristics are known.
- Whether a loading dose is needed or not depends on the urgency of starting therapy and on the pharmacokinetic and pharmacodynamic properties of a drug.
- Titrating dose to response to achieve optimal therapy requires consideration of the time required for drug in the body and response to drug to adjust to initiating or changing dosage.

- Plasma concentration monitoring can be a useful supplementary procedure to guide therapy for a low therapeutic index drug for which much of the variability in response is associated with variability in its pharmacokinetics.
- Monitoring of drug response should, in general, incorporate knowledge of both pharmacokinetics and pharmacodynamics, especially when concurrently administered drugs are withdrawn or new drugs are added.
- Tolerance, when it occurs, must be taken into account when managing the dosage of a drug showing this behavior.
- The lack of adherence to the prescribed regimen of drug is a major cause of therapeutic failure. The likelihood of failure depends on both the pharmacokinetics and the pharmacodynamics of the drug as well as the dosage regimen. When adherence is critical, every effort must be made to ensure that a patient adheres to the prescribed regimen for the prescribed duration of therapy and that the clinician knows how the patient has been taking the drug. Unfortunately, patients often provide unreliable information about their adherence.
- For some drugs, to avoid undue consequences, dosage must be decreased slowly when discontinuance of the drug is desired. The rate of reduction depends on the kinetics of the drug and the dynamics of the affected system within the body.

KEY TERM REVIEW

Change in therapy
Concentration monitoring
Discontinuing therapy
Dose titration
Initiating therapy
Managing therapy
Pharmacodynamic variability
Pharmacokinetic variability
Population pharmacodynamics
Population pharmacokinetics
Target concentration strategy
Therapeutic index

STUDY PROBLEMS

1. After the third 8-hourly 100-mg dose of gentamicin intravenously, a hospitalized 80-kg patient's plasma gentamicin concentration levels of the drug were reported as follows: Peak (7.2 mg/L, drawn one-half hour after a half-hour infusion); trough (1.8 mg/L, drawn just before the next dose). Which of the following statements is (are) correct, knowing that gentamicin follows first-order kinetics?
   I. The elimination half-life in the patient is about 3.5 hours.
   II. There is insufficient information to be able to crudely estimate a volume of distribution in this patient.
   III. The measured trough concentration is probably a good estimate (>90%) of the trough at steady state.
   A. I only **E.** I and III
   B. II only **F.** II and III
   C. III only **G.** All
   D. I and II **H.** None
2. Which of the following statements is (are) *incorrect*?
   I. The target concentration, or range of concentrations, in drug therapy is the value, or range of values, with the greatest probability of therapeutic success. Higher concentrations may be appropriate when the patient's condition is severe, and the converse when the condition is mild.

II. Monitoring of plasma concentrations may be useful when a drug has a low therapeutic index, and pharmacodynamics accounts for much of the interpatient variability in its response.

III. The lack of adherence to the prescribed manner of taking a drug is one of the sources—sometimes the major one—of variability in drug response in clinical practice. Patterns of nonadherence to prescribed dosage include the failure to take drug at the times indicated, omitting an occasional dose, failure to take several consecutive doses, occasional overdosing, and discontinuance of the drug.

A. I only	**E.** I and III
B. II only	**F.** II and III
C. III only	**G.** All
D. I and II	**H.** None

3. A first dose (loading dose) larger than the maintenance dose is sometimes required in therapy. Which of the following is (are) explanations for giving a loading dose?

I. The drug is typically given in a regimen with a high accumulation index.

II. The response to the drug is pharmacodynamically, not pharmacokinetically, rate limited.

III. Tolerance to the adverse effects of the drug rapidly develops.

A. I only	**E.** I and III
B. II only	**F.** II and III
C. III only	**G.** All
D. I and II	**H.** None

4. Which *one* of the following statements is *correct*?

a. A doubling of doses (such as repeating a dose because one has forgotten that a dose was taken 15 minutes before) is more likely to show greater peak toxicity when the drug is taken frequently than when taken infrequently, relative to the drug's half-life.

b. The dose of terazosin, an agent used to symptomatically treat patients with an enlarged prostate and sometimes to treat hypertension, is increased in a stepwise fashion because it takes a long time for the effect of the drug to develop.

c. For drugs given for conditions that do not require an immediate response, a logical and safe procedure to initiate therapy is to slowly titrate the dosage in the individual upward until the desired therapeutic response is obtained without undue adverse effects. Flecainide acetate is an example of a drug dosed in this manner.

d. Plasma concentration monitoring is a supplementary approach to optimize phenytoin dosage, but it is useful only because much of the variability in the response to this drug resides in its pharmacodynamics.

5. Meloxicam (MW = 351.4) is a nonsteroidal anti-inflammatory agent. It is typically given in a regimen of 7.5 mg once daily, but the dose may be increased to 15 mg daily. It is 99.4% bound to plasma albumin (0.6 mM) at a plasma concentration of 1 mg/L; it has a volume of distribution of 10 L, a half-life of 20 hours, and an oral bioavailability of 0.9.

a. Draw on the graph at the top of the next page the expected amount of meloxicam in the body with time in a subject receiving an oral regimen of one 7.5-mg tablet once daily. Assume that the drug is very rapidly, but incompletely, absorbed (IV bolus model). Be sure to show the salient features (steady state and approach to steady state) of drug accumulation. Use straight lines to connect daily values.

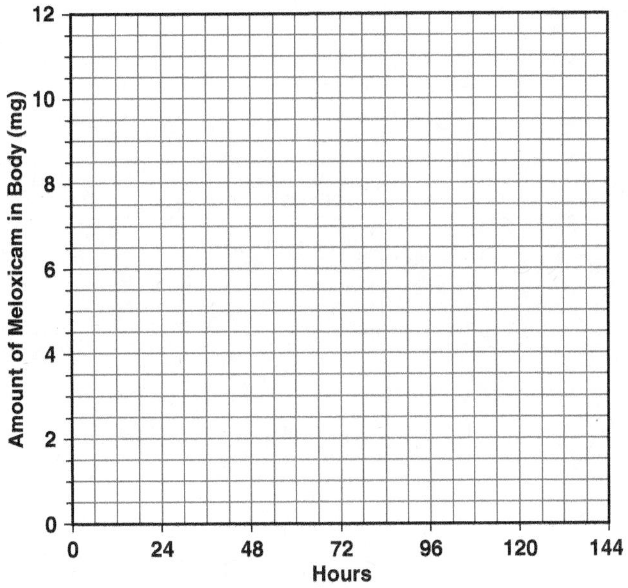

b. Also draw on the graph above (use a dashed line) the amount in the body with time (0–144 hours) had the third and fourth doses both been missed (not taken). Use straight lines to connect daily values.

c. Estimate the average steady-state plasma concentration of meloxicam on a 7.5 mg daily regimen.

d. Only 0.2% of an intravenous dose of meloxicam is excreted unchanged in the urine. Would you expect the drug to be: A. Filtered and neither reabsorbed nor secreted, or B. Extensively reabsorbed in the renal tubule? Explain your answer.

e. From the information provided above, would you expect the binding of meloxicam to plasma proteins to be nonlinear (increase in *fu* with plasma concentration) within the therapeutic range expected following 7.5–15 mg a day? Show how you come to your conclusion. Hint: What is the molar concentration of the drug and its binding protein, albumin?

6. a. Briefly describe the two basic strategies used to determine the optimal regimen of a drug for the treatment of an individual patient, and give examples of each.

   b. Briefly discuss why tailoring a dosage regimen of a drug to an individual patient should be considered before initiating therapy.

7. a. State why several sequential doses, instead of just one, are sometimes used as the loading dose.

   b. Discuss why loading doses are sometimes given for drugs with half-lives in minutes and not given for drugs with half-lives in days.

   c. Briefly comment on why loading doses are sometimes not used for drugs with long (>24-hour) half-lives.

8. Explain why plasma drug concentration monitoring is useful for some low therapeutic index drugs, but not for others.

9. Give one example each of how tolerance to therapeutic and adverse effects can influence how drugs are administered.

10. Describe a situation in which a slow decrease in dosing is needed when discontinuation of drug therapy is desired.

APPENDIX A

Definitions of Symbols

Symbol	Definition, Typical Units
A	Amount of drug in body, mg or µmol.
A_a	Amount of drug at absorption site remaining to be absorbed, mg or µmol.
$A_{av,ss}$	Average amount of drug in body during a dosing interval at steady state, mg or µmol.
A_{inf}	Amount of drug in body during a constant-rate infusion, mg or µmol.
$A_{max,N}$; $A_{min,N}$	Maximum and minimum amounts of drug in body after the Nth dose of fixed size and given at a fixed dosing interval, mg or µmol.
A_{ss}	Amount of drug in body at steady state during constant-rate administration, mg or µmol.
$A_{max,ss}$; $A_{min,ss}$	Maximum and minimum amounts of drug in body during a dosing interval at steady state on administering a fixed dose at a fixed dosing interval, mg or µmol.
AUC	Area under the plasma drug concentration–time curve. Total area from time 0 to ° is implied unless the local context indicates a specific time interval, e.g., a dosing interval, mg-hr/L or µM-hr.
C	Concentration of drug in plasma or reservoir mg/L or µM.
C_{50}	Concentration giving one-half the maximum effect, mg/L or µM.
$C(80\%)$	Plasma concentration on entering from region 3 to region 2 of the response-concentration relationship, mg/L or µM.
$C(0)$	Initial plasma concentration obtained by extrapolation to time 0 after an IV bolus dose, mg/L or µM.
$C_{av,ss}$	Average drug concentration in plasma during a dosing interval at steady state on administering a fixed dose at equal dosing intervals, mg/L or µM.
C_b	Concentration of drug in blood, mg/L or µM.
CL	Total clearance of drug from plasma, L/hr or mL/min.
CL_b	Total clearance of drug from blood, L/hr or mL/min.
CL_{cr}	Renal clearance of creatinine, mL/min or L/hr or mL/min.
CL_H	Hepatic clearance of drug from plasma, L/hr or mL/min.
CL_R	Renal clearance of drug from plasma, L/hr or mL/min.
CL_u	Clearance of unbound drug, L/hr or mL/min.

Symbol	Definition, Typical Units
C_{max}	Highest drug concentration observed in plasma after administration of an extravascular dose, mg/L or μM.
C_{out}	Concentration leaving the extractor in the reservoir model, mg/L or μM.
C_{min}	Concentration of drug in plasma required to give the minimum desired effect, mg/L or μM.
C_{ss}	Concentration of drug in plasma at steady state during constant-rate administration, mg/L or μM.
Cu	Unbound drug concentration in plasma, mg/L or μM.
E	Extraction ratio, no units.
E_H	Hepatic extraction ratio, no units.
E_{max}	Maximum effect, units of response measurement.
F	Bioavailability of drug, no units.
fe	Fraction of drug systemically available that is excreted unchanged in urine, no units.
F_{ev}	Bioavailability of drug after extravascular administration, no units.
F_F	Fraction of an oral dose that dissolves and enters the gut wall no units.
F_G	Fraction of drug entering the gut that passes on through to the portal circulation, no units.
F_H	Fraction of drug entering the liver that escapes elimination on single passage through the organ, no units.
F_R	Fraction of filtered and secreted drug reabsorbed in the renal tubule, no units.
fu	Ratio of unbound and total drug concentrations in plasma, no units.
fu_T	Ratio of unbound and total drug concentrations in tissues (outside plasma), no units.
γ	Steepness factor in concentration–response relationship, no units.
GFR	Glomerular filtration rate, mL/min or L/hr.
k	Elimination rate constant, min^{-1} or hr^{-1}
k_a	Absorption rate constant, min^{-1} or hr^{-1}
K_p	Equilibrium distribution ratio of drug between tissue and blood or plasma, no units
MW	Molecular weight, g/mol
n	A unitless number.
N	Number of doses, no units.
P	Permeability coefficient, cm/sec.
Q	Blood flow, L/min or L/hr.
Q_H	Hepatic blood flow (portal vein plus hepatic artery), L/min or L/hr.
R_{ac}	Accumulation ratio (index), no units.
R_{inf}	Rate of constant intravenous infusion, mg/hr.
SA	Surface area, m^2.
τ	Dosing interval, hr.

Symbol	Definition, Typical Units
t	Time, hr.
t_D	Duration of response, hr.
t_{max}	Time at which the highest drug concentration occurs after administration of an extravascular dose, min or hr.
$t_{1/2}$	Elimination half-life, hr.
$t_{1/2,a}$	Half-life of systemic absorption, hr.
V	Volume of distribution (apparent) based on drug concentration in plasma, L.
V_P	Plasma volume, L.
V_T	Physiologic volume outside plasma into which drug distributes, L.

APPENDIX B

Medical Words and Terms

Word/Term	Definition
Acute supraventricular tachycardia	A rapid heart rhythm originating at or above the atrioventricular node. Supraventricular tachycardias can be contrasted with the potentially more dangerous ventricular tachycardias that originate *within* the ventricles.
Angina	Angina is chest pain or discomfort that occurs when an area of the heart muscle does not get enough oxygen-rich blood.
Asthma	A respiratory condition marked by spasms in the bronchi of the lungs, causing difficulty in breathing. It usually results from an allergic reaction or other forms of hypersensitivity.
Atherosclerosis	A disease of the arteries characterized by the deposition of plaques of fatty material on their inner walls.
Atrial fibrillation	Also known as AF, Afib, or auricular fibrillation, atrial fibrillation is an irregular and often very fast heart rate in which electrical signals are generated chaotically throughout the upper chambers (atria) of the heart and may cause symptoms like heart palpitations, fatigue, and shortness of breath. While the condition is not considered life-threatening, people with AF are 5–7 times more likely to form blood clots and suffer a stroke.
Benign	In medical usage, benign is the opposite of malignant. It describes an abnormal growth that is stable, treatable, and generally not life-threatening.
Benign prostatic hyperplasia	Enlargement of the prostate gland caused by a benign overgrowth of chiefly glandular tissue that occurs especially in some men over 50 years old and that tends to obstruct urination by constricting the urethra.
Chronic bronchitis	Inflammation and swelling of the lining of the airways, leading to narrowing and obstruction, generally resulting in daily cough and breathlessness. The inflammation stimulates production of mucus, which can cause further blockage of the airways. Obstruction of the airways, especially with mucus, increases the likelihood of bacterial lung infection. Chronic bronchitis, defined as a chronic cough or mucus production for at least 3 months in 2 successive years when other causes have been excluded, is common in persons who have smoked for extended periods.

(*continued*)

Word/Term	Definition
Chronic obstructive pulmonary disease (COPD)	This refers to a group of lung diseases that block airflow and make breathing difficult. Emphysema and chronic bronchitis are the two most common conditions that make up COPD.
Congestive cardiac (heart) failure	Heart failure is a condition in which the heart has lost the ability to pump enough blood to the body's tissues. With too little blood being delivered, the organs and other tissues do not receive enough oxygen and nutrients to function properly.
Coronary heart disease	Coronary heart disease is a common term used to describe the buildup of plaque in the heart's arteries that could lead to heart attack.
Deep vein thrombosis	Thrombosis (a clot) in a vein lying deep below the skin, especially in the legs. It is a particular hazard of long-haul flying.
Duchenne dystrophy	A severe progressive form of muscular dystrophy of males that appears in early childhood, affects the muscles of the legs before those of the arms and the proximal muscles of the limbs before the distal ones, is inherited as an X-linked recessive trait, is characterized by complete absence of the protein dystrophin, and usually has a fatal outcome by age 20.
Emphysema	Emphysema is a chronic respiratory disease marked by an abnormal increase in the size of the air spaces of the lungs, resulting in labored breathing and an increased susceptibility to infection. It is also called pulmonary emphysema, which is the most common cause of death from respiratory disease in the United States, and the fourth most common cause of death overall. Smoking is a common cause of emphysema.
Endometriosis	Endometriosis is a condition in which bits of the tissue similar to the lining of the uterus (endometrium) grow in other parts of the body. Like the uterine lining, this tissue builds up and sheds in response to monthly hormonal cycles. However, there is no natural outlet for the blood discarded from these implants. Instead, it falls onto surrounding organs, causing swelling and inflammation. This repeated irritation leads to the development of scar tissue and adhesions in the area of the endometrial implants.
End-stage renal disease (ESRD)	This is the last stage (stage five) of chronic kidney disease, when the kidneys stop working well enough to sustain life without dialysis or a transplant. This kind of kidney failure is permanent and cannot be fixed, except by a kidney transplant. Most cases of ESRD are caused by diabetes or high blood pressure.
Epilepsy	A disorder of the nervous system, characterized either by mild, episodic loss of attention or sleepiness (petit mal) or by severe convulsions with loss of consciousness (grand mal).
Erythropoiesis	The process of erythrocyte (blood red cells) production in the bone marrow involving the maturation of a nucleated precursor into a hemoglobin-filled, nucleus-free erythrocyte that is regulated by erythropoietin, a hormone produced by the kidney.

Word/Term	Definition
Febrile neutropenia (FN)	This is defined as an oral temperature >38.5°C or two consecutive readings of >38.0°C for 2 hours and an absolute neutrophil count $<0.5 \times 10^9$/L, or expected to fall below this value. Despite major advances in prevention and treatment, FN remains one of the most concerning complications of cancer chemotherapy.
Gastroesophageal reflux disease (GERD)	This is a chronic digestive disease in which stomach acid or, occasionally, stomach content, moves back up into the esophagus, irritating its lining.
Gaucher's disease	Gaucher's (go-SHAYs) disease is a rare inherited disorder that affects specific cells and organs in the body. It belongs to a group of disorders called lysosomal storage disorders (LSDs). In Gaucher's disease, an enzyme called glucocerebrosidase is either absent or faulty. This enzyme's job is to break down a fatty substance called glucocerebroside that is normally used or eliminated by the body. When this enzyme does not work properly, glucocerebroside builds up in the cells, where it accumulates extensively in the organs, tissues, and bone marrow—particularly in the spleen, liver, bones, and central nervous system (CNS: in types 2 and 3 Gaucher's disease). This accumulation makes these organs unable to function properly, causing the symptoms of Gaucher's disease.
Glucose-6-phosphate dehydrogenase deficiency	Glucose-6-phosphate dehydrogenase deficiency is an inherited condition caused by a defect or defects in the gene that codes for the enzyme glucose-6-phosphate dehydrogenase (G6PD). It can cause hemolytic anemia, varying in severity from lifelong anemia to rare bouts of anemia to total unawareness of the condition.
Hairy cell leukemia	Hairy cell leukemia is a disease in which a type of white blood cell, called the lymphocyte, present in the blood and bone marrow, becomes malignant and proliferates. It is called hairy cell leukemia because the cells have tiny hair-like projections when viewed under the microscope.
Hematocrit	The ratio of the volume of red blood cells to the total volume of blood as determined by separation of red blood cells from the plasma usually by centrifugation.
Hemolytic anemia	Hemolytic anemia is a disorder in which the red blood cells are broken down at a faster rate than the bone marrow can produce new ones. Hemoglobin, the component of red blood cells that carries oxygen, is released when these cells are destroyed. In acute hemolytic anemia, the breakdown is very fast, leading to an increase in the degradation products of hemoglobin.
Hemorrhagic shock	Hemorrhagic shock is a condition of reduced tissue perfusion resulting in inadequate delivery of oxygen and nutrients that are necessary for cellular and organ function. The condition results from a rapid loss of circulating blood volume from clinical etiologies, such as penetrating and blunt trauma, gastrointestinal bleeding, and obstetrical bleeding.

(continued)

Word/Term	Definition
Hepatic cirrhosis	Hepatic cirrhosis is a chronic degenerative disease characterized by scarring (fibrosis) of the liver caused by many diseases and conditions, such as hepatitis and chronic alcohol abuse. Normal liver tissue is replaced by scar tissue and regenerative nodules (lumps that occur due to attempted repair of damaged tissue). As cirrhosis progresses, more and more scar tissue forms, making it difficult for the liver to function and eventually becoming life-threatening.
Hypersensitivity	A state of altered reactivity, including allergies and autoimmunity, in which the body reacts with an exaggerated immune response to what it perceives as a foreign substance. These reactions may be uncomfortable, damaging, or occasionally fatal.
Malignant	The term literally means growing worse and resisting treatment. It is used as a synonym for cancerous and connotes a harmful condition that generally is life-threatening.
Myocardial infarction	Myocardial infarction, commonly known as a heart attack, occurs when blood stops flowing properly to a part of the heart, and the heart muscle is injured as a result of it not receiving enough oxygen, usually because one of the coronary arteries that supplies blood to the heart develops a blockage. The event is called "acute" if it is sudden and serious.
Neoplasm	An abnormal new growth of tissue that grows by cellular proliferation more rapidly than normal, continues to grow after the stimuli that initiated the new growth cease, shows partial or complete lack of structural organization and functional coordination with the normal tissue, and usually forms a distinct mass of tissue that may be either benign or malignant.
Neutropenia	The presence of abnormally few neutrophils in the blood, leading to increased susceptibility to infection. It is an undesirable side effect of some cancer treatments.
Nonmyeloid malignancies	Any type of cancer, except myeloid leukemia (also called myelocytic leukemia).
Oncolytic	Pertaining to, characterized by, or causing the destruction of tumor cells.
Osteoarthritis	A disease of the entire joint involving the cartilage, joint lining, ligaments, and underlying bone. The breakdown of these tissues eventually leads to pain and joint stiffness. The joints most commonly affected are the knees, hips, and those in the hands and spine.
Parkinson's disease (PD)	This is a progressive degenerative disorder of the central nervous system marked, early in the course of the disease, by shaking, rigidity, slowness of movement and difficulty with walking. Later, thinking and behavioral problems develop, with dementia and depression commonly occurring in the advanced stages of the disease. The motor symptoms result from the death, of unknown etiology, of dopamine-generating cells in the midbrain.
Paroxysmal supraventricular tachycardia	Paroxysmal supraventricular tachycardia (PSVT) refers to episodes of rapid heart rate that originate in a part of the heart above the ventricles. "Paroxysmal" means from time to time.

Word/Term	Definition
Postural hypertension	Postural hypertension, or orthostatic hypertension, is a medical condition consisting of a sudden increase in blood pressure when a person stands up. It is diagnosed by a rise in systolic blood pressure of 20 mm Hg or more when standing.
Postural hypotension	Postural hypotension, or orthostatic hypotension, is a form of low blood pressure that happens when you quickly stand up from a sitting, supine, or prone position. Orthostatic hypotension can make you feel dizzy, or lightheaded, and maybe even faint.
Prostate cancer	Prostate cancer is a malignancy of the prostate, a male sex gland about the size of a walnut and lying between the bladder and the penis and just in front of the rectum.
Pseudomembranous colitis	Pseudomembranous colitis is an inflammatory condition of the colon that occurs in some people who have taken antibiotics. It is sometimes called antibiotic-associated colitis or C. difficile colitis, as it is almost always associated with an overgrowth of the bacterium *Clostridium difficile.*
Rheumatoid arthritis	Rheumatoid arthritis, an autoimmune disorder in which your immune system mistakenly attacks your own body's tissues. It typically affects the small joints in your hands and feet. Unlike the wear-and-tear damage of osteoarthritis, rheumatoid arthritis affects the lining of your joints, causing a painful swelling that can eventually result in bone erosion and joint deformity and can sometimes affect other organs of the body—such as the skin, eyes, lungs, and blood vessels.
Rhinitis	Rhinitis is an inflammation of the mucous membrane of the nose, caused by a virus infection (e.g., the common cold), a bacterial infection, or an allergen. The general symptoms of rhinitis are a stuffy nose, a runny nose, and a postnasal drip. The most common kind of rhinitis is allergic rhinitis (hay fever).
Status epilepticus	This is a common, life-threatening neurologic disorder that is essentially an acute, prolonged epileptic crisis. Definitions vary, but currently, it is defined as one continuous, unremitting seizure lasting longer than 5 minutes, or recurrent seizures without regaining consciousness between seizures for greater than 5 minutes.
Stroke	A stroke is the sudden death of brain cells in a localized area when blood flow is interrupted. Without blood to supply oxygen and nutrients and to remove waste products, brain cells quickly begin to die. Depending on the region of the brain affected, a stroke may cause paralysis, speech impairment, loss of memory and reasoning ability, coma, or death.
Supraventricular tachycardia	Supraventricular tachycardia means that from time to time, your heart beats very fast (100 and may reach 300 bpm) for a reason other than exercise, high fever, or stress. For most people who have the condition, the heart still works normally to pump blood through the body, and the condition starts and ends quickly. It becomes a problem when it happens often, or lasts a long time.

(*continued*)

Word/Term	Definition
Syncope	Partial or complete loss of consciousness with interruption of awareness of oneself and one's surroundings. When the loss of consciousness is temporary and there is spontaneous recovery, it is referred to as syncope or, in nonmedical quarters, fainting. Syncope is due to a temporary reduction in blood flow and therefore a shortage of oxygen to the brain. It can be caused by a heart condition or by conditions that do not directly involve the heart.
Tachycardia	A rapid heart rate, usually defined as greater than 100 bpm under resting conditions, but can refer to normal heart rate under exercise conditions.
Thromboembolism	Thromboembolism refers to the formation of a clot (thrombus) in a blood vessel that breaks loose and is carried by the bloodstream to plug another vessel (embolus). The clot may plug a blood vessel in the lungs (pulmonary embolism), brain (stroke), gastrointestinal tract, kidneys, or leg.
Thrombolytic	Having the property of destroying or breaking up dangerous clots in blood vessels to improve blood flow and prevent damage to tissues and organs.
Tolerance	Diminution of a response to a stimulus (to a drug in the context of this book) after prolonged or repeated exposure.
Ulcerative colitis	Ulcerative colitis is a form of inflammatory bowel disease (IBD). It causes swelling, ulcerations, and loss of function of the large intestine.
Uremic	The presence of excessive amounts of urea and other nitrogenous waste products in the blood, as occurs in moderate to severe renal function impairment.
Uterine fibroids	A benign neoplasm of the smooth muscle of the uterus, also called Leiomyomas. Tumors of this kind develop in the myometrium and generally occur in women between 30 and 50 years of age.

APPENDIX C

Ionization and the pH Partition Hypothesis

Most drugs are weak acids or weak bases. In solution, they exist as an equilibrium between un-ionized and ionized forms. When two aqueous phases of different pH are separated by a lipophilic membrane, there is a tendency for the compounds to concentrate on the side with greater ionization. To explain this phenomenon, the pH partition hypothesis assumes that movement across a membrane is transcellular and passive, and that only the un-ionized form is assumed to be sufficiently lipophilic to traverse membranes. If it is not, theory predicts that there is no transfer, regardless of pH. The ratio of ionized and un-ionized forms is controlled by both the pH and the pK_a of the drug according to the Henderson–Hasselbalch equation. Thus, for acids,

$$pH = pK_a + \log_{10}\left(\frac{\text{Ionized concentration}}{\text{Un-ionized concentration}}\right) \quad \text{Eq. C-1}$$

and for bases,

$$pH = pK_a + \log_{10}\left(\frac{\text{Un-ionized concentration}}{\text{Ionized concentration}}\right) \quad \text{Eq. C-2}$$

As $\log_{10}(1) = 0$, the pK_a of a compound is the pH at which the un-ionized and ionized concentrations are equal. The pK_a is a characteristic of the drug (Fig. C-1). Consider, for example, the anticoagulant warfarin. Warfarin is an acid with pK_a 4.8; that is, equimolar concentrations of un-ionized and ionized drug exist in solution at pH 4.8. Stated differently, 50% of the drug is un-ionized at this pH. At one pH unit higher (5.8), the ratio is 10 to 1 in favor of the ionized drug; that is, 10 of 11 total parts or 91% of the drug now exists in the ionized form, and only 9% is un-ionized. At 1 pH unit lower than the pK_a (3.8), the percentages in the ionized and un-ionized forms are 9 and 91, the converse of those at pH 5.8.

Fig. C-2 shows changes in the percent ionized with pH for acids and bases of different pK_a values. The pH range 1.0–8.0 encompasses values seen in the gastrointestinal tract and the renal tubule. Several considerations are in order and are exemplified by movement across the gastrointestinal barrier. First, very weak acids, such as phenytoin and many barbiturates, whose pK_a values are greater than 7.5, are essentially un-ionized at all pH values. For these acids, drug transfer across the membrane should be rapid and independent of pH, provided the un-ionized form is permeable and in solution. Second, the fraction un-ionized changes dramatically only for acids with pK_a values between 3.0 and 7.5. For these compounds, a change in rate of transfer with pH is expected and has been observed. Third, although transfer across the membrane of still stronger acids—those with pK_a values less than 2.5—should theoretically also depend on pH, in practice, the fraction un-ionized is so low that movement of compound across the gut membranes may be slow even under the most acidic conditions.

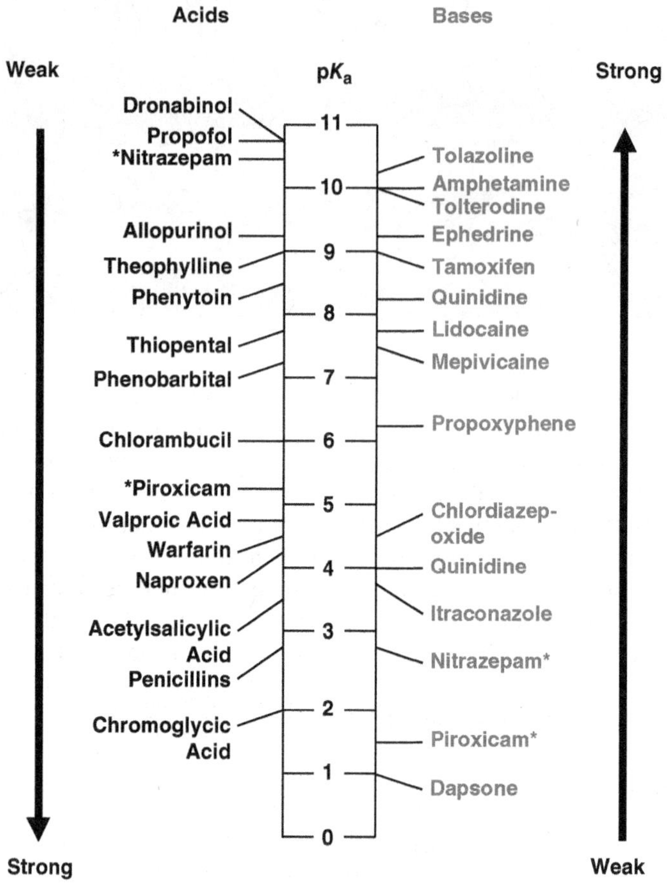

FIGURE C-1 The pK_a values of acidic and basic drugs vary widely. Drugs marked with an asterisk are amphoteric; they have both acidic and basic functional groups.

As originally proposed, the pH partition hypothesis relates to events at equilibrium, with the assumption that this condition is reached when the un-ionized concentrations on both sides of the membrane are equal. Yet it has been applied most widely to predict the influence of pH on the *rates* of absorption and distribution. The likely influence of pH on a rate process depends, however, on where the rate limitation lies. Only if the limitation is in permeability is an effect of pH on rate expected. If the limitation is in perfusion, the problem is not one of movement of drug through membranes and, therefore, any variation in pH is unlikely to have much effect on the rate process. Where the equilibrium lies, however, is independent of what process rate-limits the approach toward equilibrium. Accordingly, the distribution of an ionizable drug across a membrane at equilibrium, when the membrane is permeable only to un-ionized drug, tends to be affected by differences in pH across the membrane.

STUDY PROBLEMS

1. What pH does the Henderson–Hasselbalch predict for a weak acid with a pK_a of 8, when the ratio of the nonionized to ionized species is 1:100?

A. 4 **B.** 6 **C.** 8
D. 9 **E.** 10

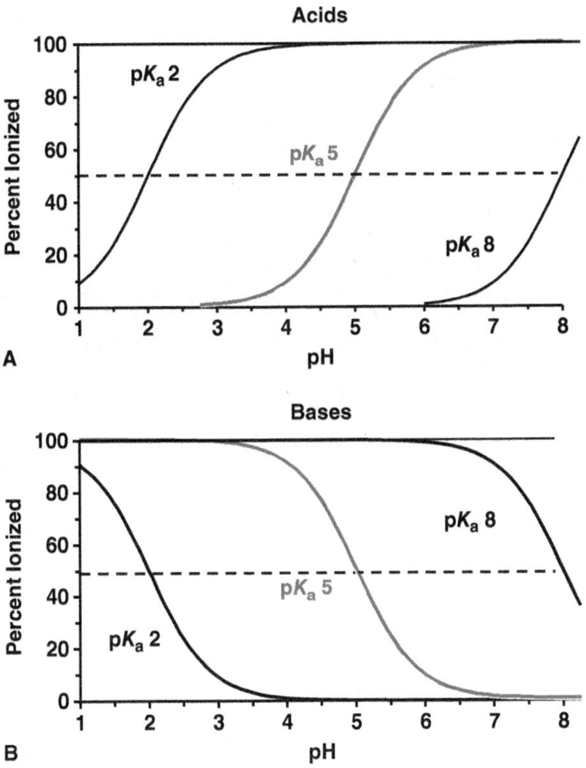

FIGURE C-2 **A.** Weak acids with pK_a values greater than 8.0 are predominantly (*above dashed line*) un-ionized at all pH values between 1.0 and 8.0. Profound changes in the fraction ionized occur with pH for an acid whose pK_a value lies within the range of 3.0–8.0. Although the fraction ionized of even stronger acids may increase with pH, the absolute value remains high at most pH values shown. **B.** For weak bases, the trends are the converse of those for weak acids. Ionization decreases toward higher pH values.

2. Ninety one percent of a weak base is ionized at a pH of 9. Approximately, what is its pK_a?

A. 7 **B.** 8 **C.** 9

D. 10 **E.** 11

3. a. Phenobarbital, a weak acid, has a pK_a of 7.2.
Calculate the percent ionized: (1) in blood (pH 7.4) and (2) in urine at (pH 6.4).
The percent ionized is:

$$\frac{\text{Ionized concentration} \times 100}{\text{Ionized concentration} + \text{Un-ionized concentration}} \qquad \text{Eq. C-3}$$

or

$$\left(\frac{\dfrac{\text{Ionized concentration}}{\text{Un-ionized concentration}}}{\dfrac{\text{Ionized concentration}}{\text{Un-ionized concentration}} + 1}\right) \times 100 \qquad \text{Eq. C-4}$$

b. Itraconazole, a weak base, has a pK_a of 3.8. Calculate the percent ionized:
(1) In the stomach when the pH there is 1.
(2) In the blood (pH 7.4).

APPENDIX D

Assessment of AUC

Several methods exist for measuring the area under the concentration–time curve (AUC). One method, discussed here, is the simple numeric estimation of area by the *trapezoidal rule*. The advantage of this method is that it requires only a simple extension of a table of experimental data. Other methods involve either greater numeric complexity or fitting of an equation to the observations and then calculating the area by integrating the fitted equation.

Consider the concentration–time data, in the first two columns of Table D-1, obtained following oral administration of 50 mg of a drug. What is the total AUC?

Fig. D-1 is a plot of the concentration against time after extravascular drug administration. If a perpendicular line is drawn from the concentration at 1 hour (7 mg/L) down to the time-axis, then the area bounded between zero time and 1 hour is a trapezoid with an area given by the product of average concentration and time interval. The average concentration is obtained by adding the concentrations at the beginning

TABLE D-1 | Calculation of Total AUC Using the Trapezoidal Rule

Time (hr)	Concentration (mg/L)	Time Interval (hr)	Average Concentration (mg/L)	Area (mg-hr/L)
0	0	–	–	–
1	7	1	3.5	3.5
2	10	1	8.5	8.6
3	5	1	7.5	7.5
4	2.5	1	3.75	3.75
5	1.25	1	1.88	1.88
6	0.61	1	0.93	0.92
8	0.15	2	0.38	0.76
			Area (0–8 hr)	26.91
			Area remaining after last measurement (C_{last}/k)	0.22
			Total area	27.13

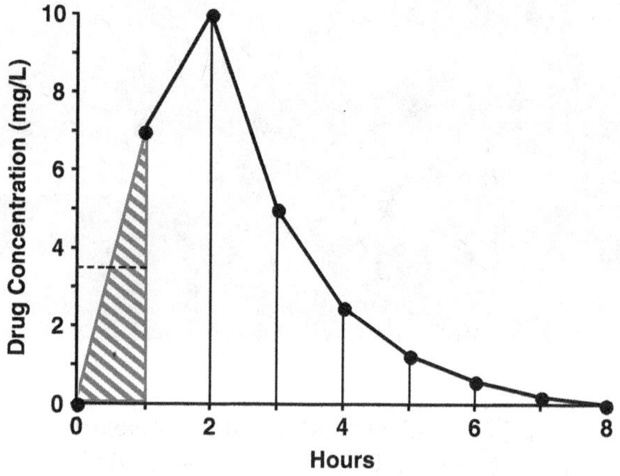

FIGURE D-1 Plot of concentration-time data from Table D-1. The dotted line is the average concentration in the first interval.

and end of the time interval and dividing by 2. Since, in the first interval, the respective concentrations are 0 and 7 mg/L and the time interval is 1 hour, it follows that:

$$\underset{\text{Area of trapezoid within the first time interval}}{AUC_1} = \underset{\text{Average concentration over the first interval}}{\frac{(0+7)}{2}\text{mg/L}} \times \underset{\text{First time interval}}{1\text{ hr}} \quad \text{Eq. D-1}$$

or

$$AUC_1 = 3.5 \text{ mg-hr/L} \quad \text{Eq. D-2}$$

In this example, the concentration at zero time is 0. Had the drug been given as an intravenous (IV) bolus, the concentration at zero time might have been the extrapolated value, $C(0)$.

The area during each time interval can be obtained in an analogous manner to that outlined above. The total AUC over all times is then simply given by

$$\text{Total AUC} = \text{Sum of the individual areas} \quad \text{Eq. D-3}$$

Usually, *total* AUC means the area under the curve from zero time to infinity. In practice, infinite time is taken as the time beyond which the area is insignificant.

The area remaining under the curve after the last time point can be estimated from

$$\text{Area Remaining} = \frac{C_{last}}{k} \quad \text{Eq. D-4}$$

This relationship comes from integration of the concentration with time after the last measured concentration, that is,

$$\text{Area Remaining} = \int_0^{\infty} C_{last} \cdot e^{-kt} \cdot dt = \frac{C_{last}}{k} \quad \text{Eq. D-5}$$

The calculations used to obtain the AUC, displayed in Fig. D-1, are shown in Table D-1. In this example, the AUC to 8 hours from the trapezoidal rule is 26.91 mg-hr/L. The area remaining under the curve, obtained from C_{last} (0.15 mg/L) divided by k (0.693/hr), obtained from the terminal decline of a semilogarithmic plot (not shown) of the data in Table D-1, is 0.22 mg-hr/L. The total area (AUC) is therefore 27.13 mg-hr/L.

TABLE D-2 | Plasma Concentrations of Zileuton (Zyflo) Following a 600-mg Oral Dose

Time (hr)	0	0.5	1	1.5	2	3
Concentration (mg/L)	0	2.14	2.95	3.25	3.27	2.68
Time (hr)	4	6	8	10	12	14
Concentration (mg/L)	2.15	1.12	0.631	0.341	0.185	0.101

STUDY PROBLEM

1. Table D-2 lists the plasma concentrations of zileuton (Zyflo), a drug used in the treatment of asthma, following a 600-mg oral dose. (Adapted from Wong SL, Awni WM, Cavanangh JH, et al. The pharmacokinetics of single oral doses of zileuton 200 to 800 mg, its enantiomers, and its metabolites, in normal healthy volunteers. *Clin Pharmacokinet* 1995;29(Suppl 2):9–21.)

   Using the trapezoidal rule, determine the AUC from 0 to 14 hours after the single 600-mg oral dose. Remember that the area of each trapezoid formed by the successive concentrations is the product of the average concentration $[(C(t) + C(t-1))/2]$ and the time interval between them $[(t) - (t-1)]$.

$$\text{Area of each trapezoid} = \frac{[C(t) + C(t-1)]}{2}[(t) - (t-1)]$$

   Recall that the total area is the sum of the areas of each of the successive trapezoids up to 14 hours plus the area remaining after the last measurement. The elimination rate constant (from a semilogarithmic plot of the data, not shown) is 0.3058/hr.

APPENDIX E

Amount of Drug in the Body on Accumulation to Plateau

DRUG ACCUMULATION

Accumulation of drug in the body is addressed here for multiple intravenous doses of fixed size and dosing interval. Consider the situation in which a dose of drug is given as an IV bolus every dosing interval, τ. Recall that after each dose the fraction remaining in the body at time t is e^{-kt}. The fraction of drug remaining at the end of a dosing interval τ, therefore, is $e^{-k\tau}$. When time is equal to 2τ, the fraction remaining is $e^{-2k\tau}$. The amount of drug in the body after multiple doses is simply the sum of amounts remaining from each of the previous doses. The amount in the body just after the next dose is shown in Table E-1 for four successive equal doses given every τ.

It is apparent from the table that the maximum amount of drug in the body just after the fourth dose, $A_{max,4}$, is the fourth dose plus the sum of the amounts remaining from each of three previous doses (sum of terms in row 4 of Table E-1). That is, letting $r = e^{-k\tau}$,

$$A_{max,4} = \text{Dose}\ (1 + r + r^2 + r^3) \qquad \text{Eq. E-1}$$

Just after the Nth dose, the amount in the body is

$$A_{max,N} = \text{Dose}\ (1 + r + r^2 + r^3 \cdots + r^{N-2} + r^{N-1}) \qquad \text{Eq. E-2}$$

Multiplying by r,

$$A_{max,N} \bullet r = \text{Dose}\ (r + r^2 + r^3 + r^4 \cdots + r^{N-1} + r^N) \qquad \text{Eq. E-3}$$

Subtracting Equation E-3 from Equation E-2, yields

$$A_{max,N} \bullet (1 - r) = \text{Dose}\ (1 - r^N) \qquad \text{Eq. E-4}$$

Therefore,

$$A_{max,N} = \text{Dose}\frac{(1-r^N)}{(1-r)} \qquad \text{Eq. E-5}$$

TABLE E-1 | Drug Remaining in the Body Just After Each of Four Successive Doses

Time	First Dose	Second Dose	Third Dose	Fourth Dose
0	Dose			
τ	Dose·$e^{-k\tau}$	Dose		
2τ	Dose·$e^{-2k\tau}$	Dose·$e^{-k\tau}$	Dose	
3τ	Dose·$e^{-3k\tau}$	Dose·$e^{-2k\tau}$	Dose·$e^{-k\tau}$	Dose

As r equals $e^{-k\tau}$ and $N \cdot \tau$ is the time elapsed, the value of r^N is e^{-kNt}. Hence,

$$A_{max,N} = \text{Dose}\frac{\left(1-e^{-k \cdot N \cdot \tau}\right)}{\left(1-e^{-k \cdot \tau}\right)} \qquad \text{Eq. E-6}$$

At the end of the dosing interval, it follows that the minimum amount in the body after the Nth dose, $A_{min,N}$, is

$$A_{min,N} = A_{max,N} \cdot r = \text{Dose}\frac{\left(1-r^N\right) \cdot r}{(1-r)} \qquad \text{Eq. E-7}$$

or

$$A_{min,N} = A_{max,N} \cdot e^{-k \cdot \tau} = \text{Dose}\frac{\left(1-e^{-k \cdot N \cdot \tau}\right) \cdot e^{-k \cdot \tau}}{\left(1-e^{-k \cdot \tau}\right)} \qquad \text{Eq. E-8}$$

STEADY STATE

As the number of doses, N, increases, the value of r^N ($e^{-k \cdot N \cdot \tau}$) approaches zero, since r is always a value less than 1. The maximum and minimum amounts of drug in the body during an interval approach upper limits. Then, the amount lost in each interval equals the amount gained, the dose. For this reason, drug in the body is then said to be at *steady state* or *at plateau*. Here, the maximum, $A_{max,ss}$, and the minimum, $A_{min,ss}$, are readily obtained by letting $r^N = 0$ in Equations E-5 and E-6 and in Equations E-7 and E-8, respectively, to give

$$A_{max,ss} = \frac{\text{Dose}}{1-r} = \frac{\text{Dose}}{1-e^{-k \cdot \tau}} \qquad \text{Eq. E-9}$$

$$A_{min,ss} = \frac{\text{Dose} \cdot r}{1-r} = \frac{\text{Dose} \cdot e^{-k \cdot \tau}}{1-e^{-k \cdot \tau}} = A_{max,ss} - \text{Dose} \qquad \text{Eq. E-10}$$

STUDY PROBLEM

1. The amount of diazepam remaining in the body (A) with time after a single intravenous dose in an individual subject is summarized by the equation

$$A(\text{mg}) = 10 \cdot e^{-0.5t}$$

where t is in days.

a. Complete the second column (first dose) of Table E-2, which has the same format as Table E-1, by calculating the amount of diazepam remaining in the body from the first dose at 1, 2, and 3 days, respectively.

b. A second 10-mg dose is given at $\tau = 1$ day. The amount remaining at 2τ and 3τ are therefore equal to Dose $\cdot$ $e^{-k\tau}$ and Dose $\cdot$ $e^{-2k\tau}$, respectively. Calculate these values and also place them in Table E-2. Also, calculate the amount remaining at time τ after the third dose.

c. Calculate the maximum ($A_{ss,max}$) and minimum ($A_{ss,min}$) amounts of diazepam in the body at steady state.

TABLE E-2 | Amount of Diazepam in the Body Just After Each of Four Successive Daily 10-mg Doses

Time[a]	First Dose	Second Dose	Third Dose	Fourth Dose
0	10 mg	—	—	—
τ		10 mg	—	—
2τ			10 mg	—
3τ				10 mg

[a] $\tau = 1$ day.

d. How closely does the sum of the amounts remaining after the 4 doses in Table E-2 approach $A_{ss,max}$ calculated in part c? Is you answer what you might have expected and explain the basis of your expectation.

APPENDIX F

Answers to Study Problems

CHAPTER 2

1. G. All three of the reasons listed explain why plasma has become the common site of measurement.
2. A. Relatively, the drug concentration will be much higher in *blood cells* than in plasma in Statement I and, therefore, the concentration in whole blood will be higher than that in plasma. In Statements II and III, drug is restricted to plasma, and blood cells act as a diluent, rendering the whole blood concentration lower than in plasma.
3. A. Protein-bound drugs are too large to pass readily across cells membranes and interact with enzymes and receptors; only unbound drug is small enough to do so. Nonetheless, as long as the ratio of unbound to bound drug in plasma remains constant, total drug concentration in plasma may be used as an alternative to unbound drug concentration to track, and interpret, events in the body. This condition is violated when disease, such as renal and hepatic disease, alters this concentration ratio, or when another drug displaces the bound drug from its binding site in plasma. The fact that a drug is highly bound generally does not automatically violate the condition, especially if, as is often the case, the plasma concentration at therapeutic levels is well below the capacity (total sites available for binding) of the binding protein. Then the fraction unbound remains essentially unchanged over the therapeutic plasma concentration range.
4. F. Most sites of action reside in tissues, and while response may be monitored, one is unable to measure drug concentration there without invasive procedures. Drug is conveyed to tissues and removed from them via the blood stream, so it does reflect drug entering and leaving the body. Once drug at the target site is in equilibrium with drug in plasma, drug in plasma may be used to reflect drug there. However, distribution to tissues takes time, and during this period, events in plasma may poorly reflect events at the site of action, and sometimes can be quite misleading.
5. c. **The primary route of drug elimination is formation of its metabolite.** The primary route of metabolite elimination is fecal excretion. The other three statements are essentially correct.
6. a. **The measured value (shown in Fig. F-1 by the line with the black-filled circles) is the sum of the concentrations of the drug and its major metabolite.**
   b. **The drug disappears much more quickly than the measured value (sum of drug and metabolite).** As activity resides with the drug only, activity would not track the measured concentration. Drug effect would quickly wear off, whereas

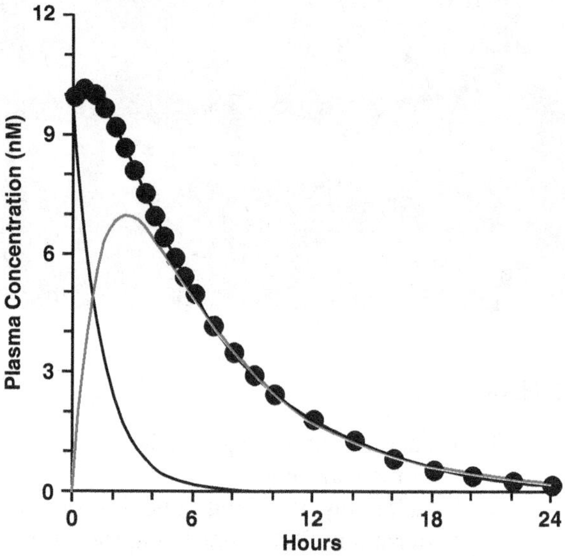

FIGURE F-1

the measured concentration would continue to be present. Totally wrong estimates would be obtained for the kinetic parameters of the drug itself. Also, the initial small rise in the measured plasma concentration after an intravenous bolus would be hard to explain.

7. a. **Correct.** At the maximum, the rate of change of amount of drug in the body is zero.
   b. **Correct.** The rate of absorption is now zero. Thereafter, the only reason for the decline of drug in the body is elimination. Under these conditions, the rate of change of drug in the body is the rate of elimination.
   c. **Incorrect.** The rate of change of drug in the body is zero at the peak time. Here, the rates of absorption and elimination are equal.
   d. **Incorrect.** The rate of absorption equals the rate of change of amount of drug in the body plus the rate of elimination.
8. a. **First-pass effect refers to loss of administered drug during its systemic input.** It generally applies to the metabolism of drugs in the gut wall and liver following oral administration. As a consequence, for a given oral dose of drug, less reaches the systemic circulation than when the same dose is administered intravenously.
   b. **Yes.** Drug can be metabolized in the local tissue before reaching the systemic circulation following intramuscular, subcutaneous, or sublingual administration. First-pass loss is often considerable for large molecular weight protein drugs when given intramuscularly or subcutaneously because of a long residence in the interstitial fluids and passage through the lymphatic system where proteolytic enzymes reside (see Chapter 8).
9. **Yes.** They are forms of administering drugs by a route "outside" the enteric tract, but the term *parenteral* generally is restricted to injection by intradermal, intramuscular, intravenous, and subcutaneous routes.
10. **Absorption or disposition, or both, can be different for the *R*- and *S*-isomers.** Measurement of the sum of the two isomers can therefore give erroneous information following administration of a racemic mixture. The overall kinetic profile

is then not that of either isomer. The difference in the kinetics becomes particularly important in therapy when the isomers have different therapeutic or adverse activities.

CHAPTER 3

1. C. An objective measure is one in which quantitative information is available. Subjective measures, on the other hand, refer to measures that are more of a "feeling" or "sense" of what is observed. Answer I is incorrect because it describes a biomarker. Answer II is incorrect because a safety marker is a response related to the safety (e.g., an adverse effect) of a drug.
2. C. To remove kinetics as an issue, the pharmacodynamic comparison of potency should be based on the exposure under steady-state conditions at the active site. Being unable to measure drug there, the unbound concentration in plasma is the best alternative. Dose (Statement I) and C_{max} (Statement II) are less useful because no further information is provided on how well or how quickly each of the drugs is absorbed or how quickly each is distributed and eliminated.
3. d. **The statement is accurate.** Statements a, b, and c are not correct. Statement e is generally correct, but over time the baseline may change. The drug effect may remain the same, but the measured response would then change.
4. G. **All three statements are correct.** One can go from no effect to maximum effect in the plot mentioned only if each individual has the same or very similar C_{50} and large γ values. Answer II is the definition of C_{50}. Answer III is also correct as the unbound concentration is the key measure of potency. However, the total concentration can be used in the current case as it differs by the same factor for both drugs.
5. **Drugs that act on receptors are said to be *agonists* or *antagonists*, depending on whether they increase (agonist) or diminish (antagonist) the functional response of the receptor.**
6. a. **A placebo effect is the response observed with time after the administration of a placebo, corrected for baseline.** If there has been no independent assessment of the baseline, then the response observed with the placebo reflects a composite of the baseline and the placebo effect. In some instances, the baseline is known to change very little with time over the period of interest, in which case an accurate assessment of the placebo effect is gained by correcting the measured response after giving placebo by the baseline observed before the placebo has been administered. In other instances, the baseline varies with time, and needs to be assessed independently in order to determine the placebo effect. A placebo treatment phase is needed to allow correction of the response observed after drug treatment for the response resulting from the patient's expectation—consciously or subconsciously induced perhaps by the prescriber, clinician, friends, or news media—and thereby to gain a measure of the true effect of the drug. One common approach mentioned in the chapter is the double-blind crossover study, in which neither patient nor clinician knows whether drug or placebo has been administered, and the code is broken only at the end of the study.

   b. **The results demonstrate that zidovudine has a beneficial effect, increasing the blood CD4 cell count above the baseline, but that the maximum benefit is not seen until the patient has been approximately 5 weeks on treatment.** Had there been no baseline measurement, one might have concluded that the benefit associated with zidovudine gently diminishes over the subsequent 90 weeks of this 4-year study, whereas, taking into account the progressive baseline decline of the CD4 count with time, the effect of zidovudine (difference between the two curves) is relatively constant throughout the 100-week study.

7. a. **The response is graded.** This is apparent because the plot is of the magnitude of response against the alprazolam concentration. Had it been a quantal response, the plot would have been one of the cumulative probability of the event against concentration.

   b. E_{max} **= 16%.** Notice that as the results are expressed as a percentage of the baseline, response has no units.

   c. C_{50} **= 7 μg/L.** It is the concentration corresponding to a E that is 50% of E_{max}.

   d. **The slope or steepness factor (γ) is much greater than 1.** Had $\gamma = 1$, then, by appropriate substitution into Equation 3-2 of this chapter, the concentrations corresponding to 20% and 80% of the maximal response (3.2% and 12.8% in the figure) are 0.25 and 4 times C_{50}, that is 2 and 32 μg/L, respectively, a 16-fold range. Note that examination of the plot shows that the corresponding concentrations are approximately 4 and 14 μg/L, a much narrower (3.5-fold) range. A more detailed analysis of the plot shows that γ is approximately 3.

8. a. **The response is quantal.** Although serum alanine aminotransferase (ALT) is a continuous measure such that changes in ALT may vary with drug exposure in a graded manner, this measure has been made quantal by defining hepatic toxicity as occurring when the ALT value is threefold or more than the normal value. The likelihood or incidence of this occurring is then examined as a function of drug exposure.

   b. **Many adverse outcomes take time to develop and require reasonably prolonged exposure to the drug.** This appears to be the case in this example. Under these circumstances, the incidence of the harmful effect depends not so much on the drug concentration at any particular time but on the overall exposure to the drug, which is best reflected by AUC.

9.

Measured, Drug, and Placebo Responses to Spiriva® 6 Hours after Its Inhalation*			
Measure	Measured Response	Drug Response	Placebo Response
FEV_1 (L)	1.27	0.19	0.03
FEV_1 (% of baseline)**	121	18	3

*Your answers may differ slightly from those provided in this table. This arises due to differences in reading off values by eye from Fig. 3-12.

**The baseline is 1.05 on the assumption that the response 1 hour before any treatment (drug or placebo) is a good measure of it and that it does not change with time.

10. C_{20} **= 50 μg/L,** C_{50} **= 200 μg/L.** The values were calculated by substituting values for E/E_{max}, C_{50}, and γ in the following equation and solving for C_{20} and C_{80}.

$$\frac{E}{E_{max}} = \frac{C^{\gamma}}{C_{50}^{\gamma} + C^{\gamma}}$$

$$\frac{E}{E_{max}} = \frac{C_{20}^{2}}{C_{50}^{2} + C_{20}^{2}} = 0.2$$

$$\frac{E}{E_{max}} = \frac{C_{80}^{2}}{C_{50}^{2} + C_{80}^{2}} = 0.8$$

CHAPTER 4

1. C. **Statement III is correct.** The rate of passive diffusion is directly proportional to the concentration difference; the larger the difference, the higher is the rate. Statement I is wrong; cell membranes comprise a lipid interior and polar exterior. Statement II is wrong; while hepatic membrane may rate-limit movement of many drugs across them, for small highly permeable molecules, the rate of movement across this cell membrane is often limited by blood flow, a perfusion limitation.
2. E. **Active transport requires energy (Statement III) and is concentration dependent (Statement I) with saturation of the transport at high concentrations.** However, Statement II is wrong; the energy involved in an active transport system maintains a concentration gradient at equilibrium.
3. **a > d > c > b:** Cerebral capillaries have the highest resistance to drug permeation (the blood–brain barrier). Next is the intestinal epithelial cell, across which even small hydrophilic compounds have difficulty in permeating, and rely on either paracellular absorption or on an active transporter. The fenestrations in muscle capillaries allow even moderately large molecules (up to 5000 g/mol) to freely permeate, while the large fenestrations of the glomerulus tend to allow even larger compounds up to about 30,000 g/mol to pass through.
4. H. **None of the statements is correct.** P-glycoprotein is found in the cell membrane, not in the interior of the cell. It is an efflux transporter and a concentrating transporter (ATP dependent).
5. B. **Statement II is correct.** Lipophilic acids generally cross intestinal membranes *more slowly* at higher than at lower pH values (Statement I is incorrect). A lipophilic weak base is expected to cross a membrane *more slowly* at a pH below than at one above its pK_a (Statement III is incorrect).
6. C. **Statement III is correct.** Generally, the thinner the membrane, the higher is its permeability to drugs. Statements I and II are both false. Permeability and surface area are two different measures. The net rate of penetration across a membrane depends on permeability (velocity of the permeating compound through the membrane), surface area, and the difference in concentration of the permeating species across the membrane. By lowering the concentration of unbound compound protein binding decreases the rate of permeation for a given total concentration, but does not change the permeability of the permeating species, unbound drug.
7. c. **Systemically absorbed leflunomide acid metabolite can be removed by orally or nasogastrically administered charcoal, but to be effective, the charcoal treatment needs to be repeated frequently at high doses for many days to ensure that a sink for the drug exists along most of the gastrointestinal tract for a sufficient length of time.** Notice that it takes days for this compound to be removed even in the presence of prolonged oral dosing with charcoal (see Table 4-3). A single dose of charcoal as proposed in Statements b and e would reside in the intestine for too short a time and in a limited portion of the intestinal tract to be effective. It is inappropriate to give even a low dose of charcoal intravenously (Statement a), as there is no ready and rapid mechanism for its removal from the body. Statement d is incorrect because the procedure can be useful for this drug.
8. **Hydrophilic—A water (hydro)–loving (philic) property.** Generally, a hydrophilic substance is readily soluble in water.

Hydrophobic—A water (hydro)–hating or fearing (phobic) property. Substances with this property are poorly soluble in water, but readily dissolve in many organic solvents.

Lipophilic—A fat (lipo)–loving (philic) property. A substance with this property is generally highly soluble in organic solvents and relatively insoluble in water.

Lipophobic—A fat (lipo)–hating or fearing (phobic) property. A substance with this property is relatively insoluble in lipid solvents, but dissolves in water.

9. **Both influx and efflux transporters are involved in drug absorption in the gastrointestinal tract.** Influx transporters aid in the absorption of some compounds (e.g., the antibiotic amoxicillin, B vitamins, and vitamin C), whereas efflux transporters tend to reduce the absorption of others (e.g., the immunosuppressive agent cyclosporine, used to prevent organ transportation, and digoxin, used in the treatment of atrial fibrillation). **Transporters are important in drug distribution, particularly in the central nervous system.** Efflux transporters, such as P-glycoprotein, reduce brain exposure to some substances such as the newer antihistamines, thereby reducing the sedative properties of these agents, as well as the reasonably hydrophilic β-adrenergic blocking agent, atenolol, used in the treatment of hypertension. **Transporters are also extensively involved in drug elimination in the kidneys** (secretion, e.g., *p*-aminohippuric acid, and active reabsorption, e.g., vitamin C and glucose) **and in the liver** (biliary excretion, e.g., pravastatin).

10. a. **Not true.** Equilibrium is reached when the net flux of compound across a membrane is zero. This condition can be achieved with both equilibrating and concentrating transporters. The difference between equilibrating and concentrating transporters, which are both facilitative transporters, is that the concentrating transporters are capable of producing a much higher concentration of the diffusible form of the drug on one side than the other of the membrane, at equilibrium. Equilibrating transporters facilitate the rate of achievement of equilibrium, but do not change the concentration of the diffusible form of the drug on both sides of the membrane at equilibrium.

    b. **True.** Had the initial rate of movement into a tissue increased in direct proportion to tissue blood flow rate, reflecting the ease with which the compound distributes into the tissues, then distribution would have been limited by blood flow, a perfusion rate limitation. The failure to do so indicates that distribution is limited by the barrier property of the tissue, a permeability rate limitation.

    c. **True.** Molecular size and lipophilicity (and permeability) of the drug, and blood flow in the intestine are assumed to be the same, as "all other factors are the same." At pH 6.4, the weak acid (pK_a 10) is almost completely un-ionized, whereas the weak base (pK_a 10) is extensively ionized, thereby slowing its absorption.

CHAPTER 5

1. H. **None is correct.** As Drug A in Statement I has a clearance that is twice that of Drug B, but they both have the same volume of distribution, the half-life of Drug A would be one-half that of Drug B. In Statement II, the two drugs would have very different clearances, and therefore the AUC values for the same dose would not be the same. In Statement III, it is possible for both drugs to have the same *V* values, and therefore the same initial concentration, if the ratio of *CL*/half-life is the same for both of them.

2. G. **All three of the statements are correct.**
3. **d is the only correct one.** It is correct because it takes 2 half-lives to eliminate 37.5 mg of a 50-mg dose; it takes 1 half-life to eliminate half of a 100-mg dose. The other statements (a–c) are incorrect because:

Statement a. The elimination rate constant is

$$k = \frac{0.693}{10 \text{ hr}} = 0.0693 \text{ hr}^{-1}$$

Statement b. 40 hours corresponds to 4 half-lives. In one $t_{½}$ (10 hours), 50% of the drug has been eliminated; by 2 $t_{½}$ (20 hours), 75% has been eliminated; by 3 $t_{½}$ (30 hours), 87.5% has been eliminated; and by 4 half-lives (40 hours), 93.75% of the dose has been eliminated. The same result is obtained from any one of the following equations.

$$100 \cdot \left(1 - e^{-k \cdot t}\right) = 100 \cdot \left(1 - e^{-0.693 \times 4}\right) = 100 \cdot \left(1 - (1/2)^4\right)$$

Statement c. The fraction of the dose remaining at 30 hours is that at 3 half-lives. One-half remains at 1 half-life (10 hours); 0.25 at 2 half-lives (20 hours); and 0.125 at 3 half-lives (30 hours). It could also have been calculated from

$$e^{-k \cdot t} = e^{-0.0693 \times 20} = (1/2)^3 = 0.125$$

4. b. **12.5%.** As the half-life is 2 days, 6 days is 3 half-lives. At this time, 12.5% of the absorbed dose should remain in the body.
5. **The time courses of the two drugs are shown in Fig. F-2.**
6. a. $V = 80$ **L**

$$V = \frac{\text{Dose}}{C(0)} = \frac{2000 \text{ µg}}{25 \text{ µg/L}} = 80 \text{ L}$$

b. **Half-life = 13.86 hours**

$$\text{Half-life} = \frac{\ln(2)}{k} = \frac{0.693}{0.05 \text{ hr}^{-1}} = 13.86 \text{ hr}$$

c. $CL = 4.0$ **L/hr**

$$CL = k \cdot V = 0.05 \text{ hr}^{-1} \times 80 \text{ L} = 4.0 \text{ L/hr}$$

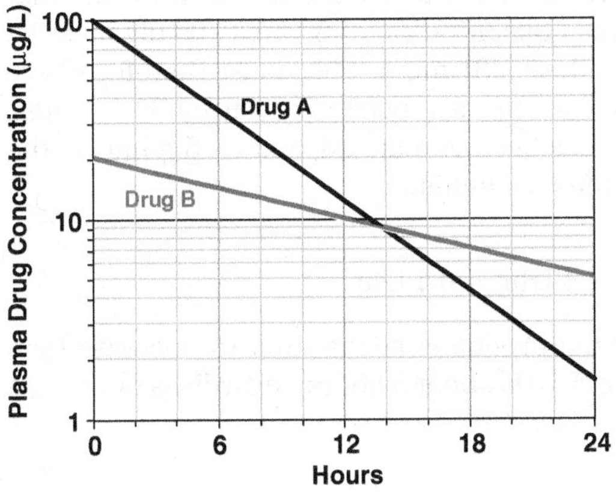

FIGURE F-2

d. **$C(24) = 15\ \mu g/L$**

$$C = C(0)\ e^{-0.05t} = 50\ \mu g/L \cdot e^{-0.05 \times 24\ hr} = 15\ \mu g/L$$

Note: $C(0)$ for a 4-mg dose is 50 μg/L, as the value for a 2-mg dose is 25 μg/L.

7. a. **Rate of elimination = 15 mg/hr**

$$\text{Rate of elimination} = CL \cdot C = 0.5\ L/hr \times 30\ mg/L = 15\ mg/hr$$

b. **Half-life = 12.5 hours**

$$\text{Half-life} = \frac{0.693 \cdot V}{CL} = \frac{0.693 \times 9\ L}{0.5\ L/hr} = 12.5\ hr$$

c. **Amount in body = 540 mg**

$$\text{Amount in body} = V \cdot C = 9\ L \times 60\ mg/L = 540\ mg$$

d. **Plasma concentration (12 hours) = 40 mg/L**

$$\text{Plasma concentration} = \frac{\text{Dose}}{V} e^{-k \cdot t} = \frac{700\ mg}{9\ L} e^{\frac{-0.693 \times 12\ hr}{12.5\ hr}} = 40\ mg/L$$

8. a. **Clearance is 4 L/hr; theophylline has a low hepatic extraction ratio.**

$$CL = \frac{\text{Dose}}{\text{AUC}} = \frac{500\ mg}{125\ mg\text{-}L/hr} = 4\ L/hr$$

b. **Yes, the initial rapidly declining phase is the distribution phase.** This conclusion is based on area considerations. The fraction of the dose eliminated within the first 30 minutes is given by

$$\frac{\text{Fraction eliminated in first 30 min}}{\text{Fraction totally eliminated}} = \frac{CL \cdot \text{AUC}(0, 30\ \text{min})}{CL \cdot \text{AUC}(0, \infty)} = \frac{\text{AUC}(0, 30\ \text{min})}{\text{AUC}(0, \infty)}$$

$$= \frac{13.1\ mg\text{-}L/hr}{125\ mg\text{-}L/hr} = 0.105$$

Thus, with only 10.5% of the area in the first 30 minutes, it is reasonable to describe the first phase as the distribution phase of this drug.

c. **Eighty percent of the dose has left the plasma by 5 minutes. The most likely tissues involved include the lungs, liver, kidneys, and brain because these are the most highly perfused tissues and hence receive most of the drug in the early moments after its administration.** Knowing that the plasma volume is 3 L, at a plasma concentration of 33 mg/L, 99 mg must be there. The remainder of the 500-mg dose, 401 mg or 80%, must therefore have left the plasma and distributed out into tissues, because even by 30 minutes, only 10.5% of the theophylline dose has been eliminated, and by 5 minutes, the fraction of theophylline eliminated must be minimal.

d. **Renal clearance = 0.4 L/hr**

$$CL_R = fe \cdot CL = 0.1 \times 4\ L/hr = 0.4\ L/hr$$

e. **Half-life = 5 hours.** The time for the plasma concentration to decrease by a factor of 2 in the terminal part of Fig. 5-10 is about 5 hours, regardless of the two concentrations chosen (with $C_1 = 2 \times C_2$).

f. **Volume of distribution is 29 L**

$$V = \frac{CL}{k} = \frac{\frac{\text{Dose}}{\text{AUC}}}{\frac{0.693}{\text{Half-life}}} = \frac{\frac{500 \text{ mg}}{125 \text{ mg-hr/L}}}{\frac{0.693}{5 \text{ hr}}} = 28.9 \text{ L}$$

g. **Amount remaining in body at 8 hours = 168 mg. From Fig. 5-10 at 8 hr $C = 5.8$ mg/L**

$$A = V \cdot C = 29 \text{ L} \times 5.8 \text{ mg/L} = 168.2 \text{ mg}$$

The value could also be calculated as follows. As the amount eliminated up to time $t = CL \cdot \text{AUC}(0 - t)$ and $\text{AUC}(0 - t)$ is the difference between the total area and the area remaining under the curve after time t (125 – 83 mg-hr/L), the amount remaining in the body is $CL \cdot \text{AUC}(t - \infty) = [\text{Dose}/\text{AUC}(0 - \infty)] \cdot \text{AUC}(t - \infty) = [500 \text{ mg}/125 \text{ mg-hr/L}] \times 42 \text{ mg-hr/L} = 168$ mg.

9. a. **The plasma concentration–time profiles of diazepam, nortriptyline, and warfarin following a 10-mg intravenous dose are displayed in the semilogarithmic plot in Fig. F-3 below.**
   b. The plasma concentration–time profile for each drug following a 10-mg intravenous bolus dose, displayed in Fig. F-3, is calculated from

$$C = \frac{\text{Dose}}{V} \cdot e^{-\frac{CL}{V} \cdot t}$$

Notice that despite the similarity in half-lives, for the same dose, the plasma concentration–time profiles for the three drugs are very different. They differ in the absolute concentrations and hence in the values of AUC. Clearly, clearance and volume of distribution control half-life, and not the converse.

10. a. **See Fig. F-4 on next page.**
   b. **Half-life = 0.7 hour**
   c. **Using the relationship AUC = $C(0)/k$, AUC = 0.200 mg–hr/L.**
   d. **Clearance = 147 L/hr.** CL = Dose/AUC = 33 mg × (304 g/mol/340 g/mol)/0.200 mg-hr/L.
   e. **Volume of distribution = 1.96 L/kg.** $V = CL/k$ = 147 L/hr/1/hr = 147 L/75 kg.

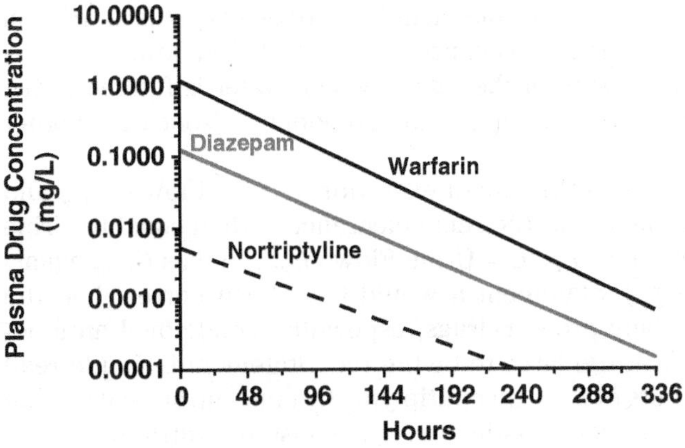

FIGURE F-3

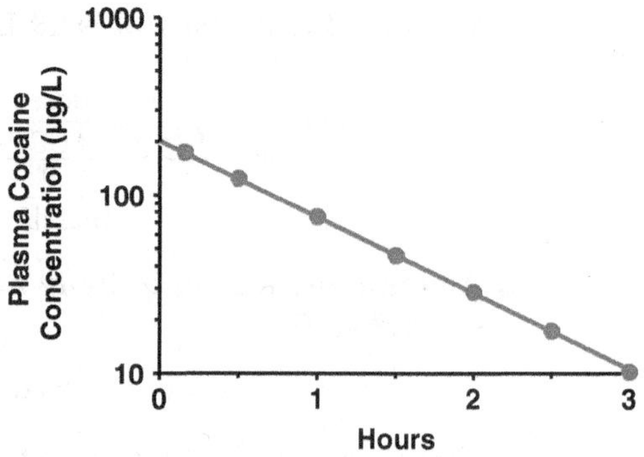

FIGURE F-4

CHAPTER 6

1. H. **All the statements are incorrect.** Statement I is wrong because, for a given plasma concentration and blood perfusion rate, the higher the affinity of a tissue for a drug (K_p), the longer (not shorter) it takes to deliver to the tissue the amount of drug at equilibrium. Statement II is wrong because the ranking of the time for tissues to reach distribution equilibrium depends not only on the perfusion rate but also on the tissue to plasma equilibrium distribution ratio (K_p), which can differ from one tissue to another. Statement III is also wrong because the lower the binding within tissues (higher fu_T), the smaller (not larger) is the volume of distribution.
2. B. **Statement II is true.** For the volume of distribution to be 850 L, the average value of K_p must be >10, with values likely to be much higher than 10 in some tissues and lower in others. Statement I is too restrictive. While a drug with a volume of distribution of 15 L and $fu = 0.1$ may distribute intracellularly, it might not. It could be restricted to the extracellular water (15 L) and bind within the interstitial space with $fu_T = 0.1$. A telling point would be the lipophilicity of the compound. If it is reasonably high, intracellular distribution would be expected. Statement III is wrong; for such a drug, its expected volume of distribution is 15 L (not 42 L) in a 70-kg patient.
3. C. **Statement III is true.** When the hepatic extraction ratio is high, clearance is perfusion rate–limited, and relatively insensitive to changes in either plasma protein binding or intrinsic clearance. Statement I is the unbound clearance ($CL_b \cdot C_b = CL_u \cdot Cu$ *and* $fu_b = Cu/C_b$). Statement II is wrong; when the extraction ratio is low, clearance is insensitive to changes in hepatic blood flow.
4. c. Creatinine clearance is a measure of the rate at which water is filtered in the glomerulus, the glomerular filtration rate, from both kidneys. None of the other statements is correct.
5. c. **Statement c is correct.** When the rate of excretion = Urine Flow · C_{urine} and the urine concentration equals Cu, the renal clearance is then equal to Urine Flow · fu (Rate of excretion = $CL_R \cdot C$ = Urine Flow · C_{urine} and as C_{urine} equals Cu, CL_R = Urine Flow · fu). Statement a would have been correct had the answer been GFR · fu. Many protein drugs, especially monoclonal antibodies, have a much higher MW, too large to be filtered. Statement b should read Urine Flow · fu; CL has units of flow, so multiplying by concentration gives the wrong units. Similarly, Statement d is incorrect because the filtration rate is GFR · Cu.

6.

Hepatic Extraction Ratio	Hepatic Blood Flow	Unbound Fraction in Blood	Intrinsic Clearance	Total (Plasma) Clearance
1. High	↑	↔	↔	↑
2. Low	↔	↓	↔	↓
3. High	↔	↔	↑	↔
4. Low	↔	↑	↔	↑
5. High	↔	↓	↔	↔
6. **Low**	↓	↔	↔	↔

↑, increase; ↔, little or no change; ↓, decrease.

7. G **All three statements are reasonable generalizations.**

8. a. **A low extraction ratio drug.** Even based on a plasma clearance of 4.2 L/hr, the conclusion would be that tacrolimus has a low hepatic extraction ratio. Furthermore, with a plasma-to-blood ratio of 0.05, resulting in a very low blood clearance of only 0.21 L/hr, there can be no doubt as to the low extraction ratio status of this drug.

   b. **Extensive uptake into blood cells.** With such extensive binding to plasma proteins (fraction bound 0.99), one would have anticipated that most of the drug in the blood should be located in plasma, whereas the plasma-to-blood concentration ratio of only 0.03 indicates that the majority of tacrolimus in blood resides in blood cells. This can occur only if the affinity of blood cells (in particular, erythrocytes) for tacrolimus is very much greater than that of plasma proteins, or because transporters concentrate drug in the cells.

   c. **Clearance would increase, and half-life shorten, with induction.** With tacrolimus being a drug of very low extraction ratio, induction of CYP3A4 (by increasing hepatocellular metabolic activity) is expected to increase clearance. And, because induction is not expected to cause any change in drug distribution, and hence in V, it follows that half-life should decrease, since $t_{1/2} = 0.693 \cdot V/CL$.

9. a.

Organ	K_p	Q/V_{tissue}	Time to 50% of Equilibrium (min)[a]
Lungs	1	10	**0.07**
Heart	3	0.6	**3.5**
Kidneys	40	4	**7**
Liver	15	0.8	**13**
Skin	12	0.024	**347**

[a]It takes 1 half-life to reach 50% of the equilibrium tissue concentration, and $t_{1/2} = \frac{0.693 \cdot K_p}{Q/V_{tissue}}$. The organs are ranked by the time to reach 50% of the equilibrium value.

Note the large differences in the time for equilibration. It ranges from being extremely rapid for lungs that receive the entire cardiac output to the very slow equilibration in skin owing to a combination of very low perfusion and high affinity for the drug. Note also that drug in the heart equilibrates faster than drug in the kidneys, even though the kidneys are more highly perfused. This is the result of a higher affinity of the drug for renal tissue.

   b. **If distribution into heart tissue was permeability rate–limited, then the time to reach distribution equilibrium would be longer than that had distribution been perfusion rate–limited.** However, at equilibrium, the heart concentration is the same wherever the rate limitation lies; it depends only on the affinity that this organ has for the drug.

10. a. **Theophylline is a low extraction ratio drug.** CL is 4 L/hr, and even in the extreme case that the plasma/blood concentration ratio is 2, implying none entering blood cells, CL_b cannot exceed 8 L/hr, which is considerably less than either hepatic or renal blood flow.

b. **Yes, there is definitely net reabsorption.** $CL_R = 0.4$ L/hr $(fe \cdot CL)$, which is less than filtration clearance $(fu \cdot \text{GFR} = 0.6 \times 7.5 \text{ L/hr} = 4.5 \text{ L/hr})$.

c. (1) a. **The fraction of theophylline in the body unbound is 0.87.**

$$\text{Fraction unbound} = \frac{\text{Amount in body unbound}}{\text{Total amount in body}} = \frac{Cu \times 42 \text{ L}}{C \times V} = \frac{fu \times 42 \text{ L}}{V}$$

$$= \frac{0.6 \times 42 \text{ L}}{29 \text{ L}} = 0.87$$

Hence, 87% of theophylline in the body is unbound at equilibrium.

b. **Unbound concentration = 10.4 mg/L.**

$$Cu = \frac{\text{fraction unbound in body} \times \text{Dose}}{42 \text{ L}} = \frac{0.87 \times 500\text{mg}}{42 \text{ L}} = 10.4 \text{ mg/L}$$

(2) a. **Volume of distribution is 16 L, when *fu* = 0.3.**

$$V = Vp + \frac{fu \bullet V_T}{fu_T}$$

With only fu changing, it is possible to predict the volume of distribution for a given value of fu. The approach is as follows. Upon rearrangement, one obtains

$$\frac{V_T}{fu_T} = \frac{V - Vp}{fu}$$

where V_T is the aqueous volume outside of plasma into which drug distributes at equilibrium. As theophylline distributes into all body water spaces, volume 42 L, and the plasma volume $Vp = 3$ L, it follows that $V_T = 39$ L. Therefore, as $V = 29$ L when $fu = 0.6$, it follows that

$$\frac{V_T}{fu_T} = \frac{29 \text{ L} - 3 \text{ L}}{0.6} = 43.3 \text{ L}$$

Substituting this ratio back into the equation for V, for $fu = 0.3$,

$$V = Vp + \frac{fu \bullet V_T}{fu_T} = 3 \text{ L} + 0.3 \times 43.3 = 16 \text{ L}$$

b. **Unbound concentration = 9.4 mg/L. The unbound concentration of theophylline is relatively insensitive to changes in the fraction unbound in plasma.**

$$\text{Fraction unbound} = \frac{\text{Amount in body unbound}}{\text{Total amount in body}} = \frac{fu \times 42 \text{ L}}{V} = \frac{0.3 \times 42 \text{ L}}{16 \text{ L}} = 0.79$$

Hence,

$$Cu = \frac{\text{fraction unbound in body} \times \text{Dose}}{42 \text{ L}} = \frac{0.79 \times 500 \text{ mg}}{42 \text{ L}} = 9.4 \text{ mg/L}$$

Thus, for a twofold decrease in *fu*, despite the expected similar fold decrease in *V* (from 29 to 16 L), the fraction of theophylline in the body unbound decreases by only about 9%. In practical terms, this means that for 500 mg in the body, the unbound concentration would decrease only from 10.3 mg/L (0.87 × 500 mg/42 L) to 9.4 mg/L (0.79 × 500 mg/42 L), a small drop, and of little clinical value. This example stresses the importance of focusing attention in drug therapy on the pharmacologically active unbound drug, especially when, as here, there are significant changes in the fraction of drug unbound in plasma. Basing conclusions on the total plasma concentration under these circumstances can be highly misleading. *Note:* Although the conclusion that *Cu* will minimally change with a change in *fu* could have been readily answered knowing that 87% of drug in the body is unbound when *fu* = 0. 6, in making quantitative decisions it is important to go through the formal analysis, as the magnitude of change is not always so apparent.

CHAPTER 7

1. H. **All the statements are incorrect.** Statement I is incorrect because there was no significant change in AUC. Statement II is incorrect because the absorption was slower, not faster, when lying down. Statement III is incorrect because the drug was absorbed more slowly when taken with food.
2. b. **Conclusion b is valid.** Conclusion a is invalid as one cannot declare bioequivalence for Product B. Conclusion c is invalid because tightening the confidence interval with a larger number of subjects is not likely to keep the interval within the acceptable range of 0.8–1.25. Conclusions d and e are invalid as only for Product A can bioequivalence be declared.
3. a. **Statement a is correct.** Statement b is incorrect because the absorption half-life is 1 hour (0.693/0.693/hr), so at 2 hours, 25% should remain at the injection site. Statement c is incorrect as the half-life is 1 hour. Statement d is incorrect because 87.5% should be absorbed at 3 hours. Statement e is incorrect because there is no information on the elimination half-life of the drug.
4. A. **Only Relationship I is a first-order kind of an equation.** Relationships II and III are typical of zero-order absorption.
5.

Formulation	k_a	F
Immediate-release	Increased	No change
Modified-release	Decreased	Probably no change, but it is not possible to assess the total AUC.
Poor formulation	No change. The peak time appears to be unchanged.	Decreased

6. **See Fig. F-5.** The dashed black line shows the effect of reducing the extent of absorption. The solid colored line shows the effect of slowing absorption to the point that the terminal decline is now determined by k_a, instead of k.
7. a. **Statement incorrect.** The slower the absorption process, the lower is the peak plasma concentration, and the later its occurrence after a single dose. The lower peak concentration occurs because, with slower absorption, more drug remains at the absorption site, when the rate of elimination matches the rate of absorption. The peak occurs later because it takes longer for the plasma concentration to rise to a value at which the rate of elimination matches the rate of absorption.

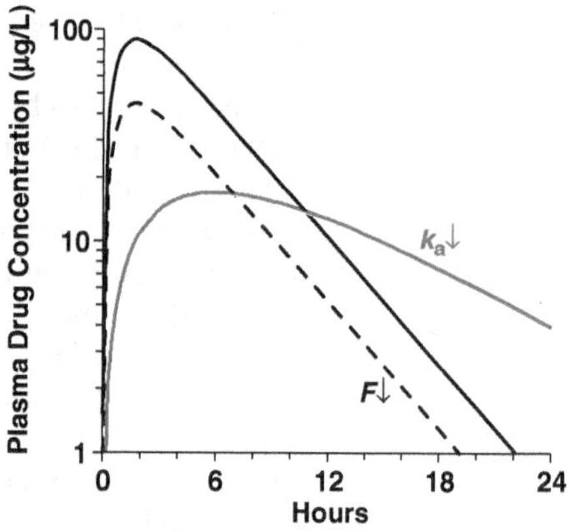

FIGURE F-5

b. **Correct.** For a given oral dose, AUC is a measure of the total amount eliminated for a given value of clearance. Moreover, total amount eliminated equals the total amount absorbed systemically. Hence, because clearance tends to remain relatively constant in a subject, AUC is a measure of the amount of drug absorbed systemically.
c. **Correct.** When absorption is the rate-limiting step in the overall elimination of drug from the body, elimination cannot proceed any faster than absorption. The terminal half-life of decline of the plasma concentration then reflects absorption, rather than elimination, of the compound.
d. **Needs qualification.** In some situations, there may be an increase in bioavailability (extent) and a shortening of the peak time (due to $k_a \uparrow$), but they do not necessarily go together. For example, the bioavailability may be increased in hepatic disease for a drug normally metabolized extensively during the first pass through the liver. However, the absorption rate constant for drug reaching the liver may not be affected.
e. **Correct.** The rate of absorption is constant and independent of the amount remaining to be absorbed as long as some drug remains to be absorbed.

8. a. **F_{rel}(oral/SC) = 0.14; F_{rel}(rectal/SC) = 0.19; F_{rel}(nasal/SC) = 0.16**
Relative bioavailability

$$\frac{F(\text{oral})}{F(\text{SC})} = \left(\frac{\frac{52.2}{25}}{\frac{90.3}{6}}\right) = 0.14 \quad \frac{F(\text{rectal})}{F(\text{SC})} = \left(\frac{\frac{71.6}{25}}{\frac{90.3}{6}}\right) = 0.19 \quad \frac{F(\text{nasal})}{F(\text{SC})} = \left(\frac{\frac{47.8}{20}}{\frac{90.3}{6}}\right) = 0.16$$

b.

Observation	Subcutaneous Solution	Oral Tablet	Rectal Suppository	Nasal Spray
C_{max} (μg/L)[a]	289	52.2	71.6	59.8
C_{max}/AUC (hr^{-1})[b]	0.77	0.32	0.32	0.27

[a]Per 25 mg of sumatriptan.
[b]C_{max}/AUC has been used as a measure of relative speed of drug input when comparing across formulations and routes of administration for the same drug. Its value should be independent of the dose administered.

Note that absorption is fastest after subcutaneous administration. The t_{max} is also the shortest by this route.

c. One explanation is a much more rapid systemic absorption after the subcutaneous dose.

9. a. **A delayed esophageal transit profoundly affects the rapidity, but not the extent, of absorption of acetaminophen.** The peak concentration is much lower (delayed transit group, 3.9 mg/L; normal transit group, 6.3 mg/L) and delayed (90 vs. 40 minutes), but the AUC values (697 mg-min/L and 773 mg-min/L) are reasonably comparable.
   b. **Drug disposition is the rate-limiting step.** Displayed semilogarithmically, the declines in the plasma concentration for the two groups are parallel. The slopes would probably be different if absorption had been the rate-limiting step.
   c. **To ensure rapid absorption, acetaminophen should be taken while upright with plenty of water.**

CHAPTER 8

1. d. **Dissolution is key.** A tablet can disintegrate, but the drug must dissolve to be absorbed; solid particles do not pass across the intestinal wall. Under fasting conditions, the time of day a tablet is taken and the pH of the colon probably have very little influence on the speed of the absorption process for most drugs.
2. d. **Statement d is correct.** Statement a is incorrect because large pellets are held in the stomach for a longer, not a shorter, period of time when taken with a fatty meal. Statement b is incorrect because the transit times of large and small pellets are about the same in the small intestine, independent of whether the product is taken fasted or with a fatty meal. Statement c is incorrect as there is very little, if any, effect of pellet size on their gastric retention when taken on a fasted stomach. Statement e is incorrect as the small intestine transit times are more like 3–4 hours than 6 hours.
3. G. **All three statements are correct.**
4. G. **All three statements are correct.**
5. **Five examples of reasons for low oral bioavailability from the following list or any other reasonable example.**
   - Lack of complete release of drug from the dosage form where the intestine is sufficiently permeable to allow absorption to occur.
   - Instability of drug in stomach (low pH).
   - Drug is too water-soluble to be absorbed across lipophilic gastrointestinal membranes and too large to readily permeate paracellularly.
   - Metabolism of drug in gut wall or lumen.
   - Efflux of drug from the gut wall.
   - Extensive extraction of drug during first pass through the liver.
   - Decomposition of drug by microflora in the large intestine.
   - Formation of a virtually insoluble complex with materials within the gastrointestinal lumen.
   - Effect of food, other drugs, gastrointestinal disease, and abnormalities.

   Drug examples of each scenario are listed in Tables 8-3 and 8-7.
6. For all situations, eating a meal (especially one with a high fat content) slows gastric emptying compared with that occurring on a fasted stomach.
   a. Being water-soluble and given as an immediate-release tablet, the drug would be expected to dissolve rapidly in the stomach, effectively becoming a solution. A slowed gastric emptying rate would then slow the rate of delivery of drug to the small intestine, where absorption occurs with an **expected lower C_{max} and later t_{max}. The extent of absorption (as measured by AUC) would not be affected** because food has no material effect on small intestinal transit time, and being highly permeable, the drug is likely to be absorbed along much of the intestinal tract. However, when immediate response is desired, the product should

be taken on a fasted stomach. Acetaminophen, taken to relieve a headache, is an example of a drug in this category.

b. For a sparingly soluble lipophilic compound, normally, dissolution may not only rate-limit absorption but also affect oral bioavailability, if dissolution is not complete by the time a compound has entered the large intestine; continued water absorption in the large intestine compacts the solid materials there and may hinder further dissolution. This is the case with the drug in question; its bioavailability is only 26%. By slowing gastric emptying and facilitating gastric mixing, food helps dissolution of compound within the stomach to occur for longer before drug reaches the small intestine, where absorption is favoured. Additionally, a high-fat meal may facilitate dissolution by providing a sink for the dissolved lipophilic drug. **The overall expected effect is a higher C_{max}, longer t_{max}, and higher AUC.** The antifungal drug, itraconazole, is an example in this category. To improve bioavailability, it is recommended to be taken with a (preferably high-fat) meal.

c. Large (>7 mm), single nondisintegrating entities tend to be retained in the stomach as long as food is there. Only on a fasted stomach is a large entity ejected from the stomach relatively quickly, by the action of housekeeping waves. **Therefore, delivery of a single enteric-coated product into the small intestine, where removal of the enteric coating and absorption occurs, is significantly delayed. The time of leaving the stomach is highly variable.** Once the enteric coating is removed, however, subsequent release and absorption of the compound should be the same, regardless of food. If, however, the release of drug is delayed after reaching the small intestine, the extent may be reduced as well. Delayed-release capsules of erythromycin, an anti-infective agent, or didanosine, a drug used to treat HIV, are examples. For these products, the enteric coating is on small pellets contained in the capsule. This allows the pellets to enter the small intestine after the capsule disintegrates, so that there is no great delay in drug absorption. If taken with food, the drug is slowed somewhat, as seen with small pellets in Fig. 8-12.

The slowdown is not as extensive as that observed with aspirin contained in enteric-coated tablets; the enteric coating around the entire tablet is to prevent gastric irritation rather than decomposition. Here, the time drug absorption starts is greatly delayed and highly variable.

7. a. **Elimination.** The terminal half-life of the drug appears to be the same for both routes of administration.

b. $\boldsymbol{F = 0.128}$.

$$AUC_{p.o.} = 0.566 \ \mu\text{g-hr/L}$$

$$AUC_{iv} = 4.44 \ \mu\text{g-hr/L}$$

$$F = \frac{0.566}{4.44} = 0.128 \quad \text{(same dose given by both routes)}$$

$\boldsymbol{CL = 31.5}$ **L/hr.**

$$CL = \frac{\text{Dose}_{iv}}{AUC_{iv}} = \frac{2 \ \mu\text{g/kg} \times 70 \ \text{kg}}{4.44 \ \mu\text{g-hr/L}} = 31.5 \ \text{L/hr}$$

c. $\boldsymbol{F_H = 0.69}$.

$$F_F = F_G = 1$$

$$F_H = 1 - E_H = 1 - \frac{CL_{H,b}}{Q_H} = 1 - \frac{CL_b(1 - fe)}{Q_H}$$

Since $CL_b = CL \bullet \frac{C}{C_b}$; $Q_H = 60 \times 1.35$ L/min $= 81$ L/hr; and $fe = < 0.01$,

$$F_H = 1 - \frac{CL(1 - fe)}{Q_H} \bullet \frac{C}{C_b} = 1 - \frac{31.5 \times 0.8}{81 \text{ L/hr}} = 0.69$$

d. **No, the value of F in 7b (0.128) is much lower.** There must be one or more additional explanations for the low F. Possible reasons are provided among the answers to Problem 5. Given the use of the compound in primarily intensive-care settings and the need for rapid and reliable response, the compound was developed clinically as an intravenous infusion. The low (and variable) oral bioavailability and time to achieve therapeutic concentrations limited the use of the oral route for the current indication.

8. There are several factors that influence the speed and extent of systemic absorption of protein drugs following i.m. and s.c. administration. For example:
   - **Molecular size of the drug molecule.** Larger proteins, especially those greater than 20,000 g/mol, are primarily absorbed systemically via the lymphatic system, because of a marked decrease with molecular size in the permeability of blood capillaries.
   - **Degradation**. Degradation within the interstitial fluid and the lymphatic system often results in reduced bioavailability.
   - **Site of injection is important.** Both rate and extent of absorption can be affected by the location of the injection, even by the same route, e.g., subcutaneous. The number of lymph nodes and the length of lymphatic vessels traversed before returning to the systemic blood circulation are important for large proteins.
   - **Exercise and rubbing**. Exercise and rubbing influence the speed of systemic absorption, as does the volume of fluid injected.

9. a. **Clearance = 0.80 L/hr; Volume of distribution = 7.7 L**

$$CL = \left[\frac{\text{Dose}}{\text{AUC}}\right]_{iv} = \frac{\frac{40 \text{ units}}{\text{kg}} \times 60 \text{ kg}}{3010 \text{ unit-hr/L}} = 0.80 \text{ L/hr}$$

$$V = \frac{CL}{k} = \frac{0.80 \text{ L/hr}}{0.693/6.7 \text{ hr}} = 7.7 \text{ L}$$

b. Bioavailability = 0.46

$$F = \frac{(\text{AUC/Dose})_{sc}}{(\text{AUC/Dose})_{iv}} = \frac{1372}{3010}$$

The molecular size of erythropoietin (34,000 g/mol) is such that the majority of a dose probably enters the systemic circulation via the lymphatic, rather than the vascular, system. For loss to occur during the absorption process, the drug must be metabolized (degraded) in the interstitial fluid near the injection site or within the lymphatic system.

c. **Reduced bioavailability, absorption rate-limiting elimination after subcutaneous administration.** In part, this is due to the lower bioavailability from the subcutaneous route, but with a bioavailability of 0.46, this alone cannot explain the C_{max} following subcutaneous administration being 10-fold lower than that after intravenous dosing. The other reason is the slow absorption from the subcutaneous site such that much drug still remains at the absorption site when C_{max} is reached, a characteristic of "flip-flop" kinetics, that is, when elimination is rate-limited by absorption.

CHAPTER 9

1. D. **Statements I and II are correct.** Statement III is incorrect because there must be a pharmacodynamic explanation for the response lasting so long, that is, long after the drug has been eliminated.
2. c. **Statement c is the most accurate.** Statement a is incorrect because a counterclockwise hysteresis loop is expected. Statement b is incorrect because hastening of the loss of the key constituent would have the opposite effect—a decrease in its concentration and, therefore, a decrease in the response to the drug. Statement d is incorrect, because the duration should increase by a half-life for every doubling of the dose.
3. A. **Statement I is correct because the concentration does not rise; it starts high and declines.** There cannot be two responses at the same concentration. Statement II is incorrect as one expects an essentially linear decline in response with time during this range of responses. Statement III is incorrect as the duration of response is expected to increase linearly with the logarithm of the dose.
4. G. **All three are good explanations.** The linear decline in the blood pressure lowering suggests that the data are obtained in Region II of the concentration–response curve (Fig. 9-6), where the response varies with the logarithm of the concentration. As the drug response lasts much longer than drug persists in the body, the possibility of a metabolite being the active form of the drug (Statement I) is a logical explanation of the observations. The decline of the concentration of an active metabolite with a considerably longer half-life would then govern the decline of the response. This is the most likely explanation for the observed results and is, indeed, the actual one. A pharmacodynamically rate–limited explanation (Statement II) may also explain the observations. The drug may affect a body constituent that has very slow kinetics. Statement III is also expected to be correct as there appears to be little change in response in this time frame. What is not clear from the limited data available is the appropriate regimen for this prodrug.
5. a. **E_{max} = 30 mm Hg; C_{50} = 4 µg/L; $\gamma = 2$.**

From the graph, E_{max} appears to be about 30 mm Hg. The value of C_{50} is the concentration at which the response is 50% of the maximum. From the graph this is about 4 µg/L. The value of γ can be obtained from any two points on the graph. For example,

$E = 25$ mm Hg when $C = 9$ µg/L
$E = 5$ mm Hg when $C = 1.8$ µg/L
Thus,

$$\frac{E}{E_{max}} = \frac{C^{\gamma}}{C_{50}{}^{\gamma} + C^{\gamma}} = \frac{25}{30} = \frac{9^{\gamma}}{4^{\gamma} + 9^{\gamma}} = 0.833$$

$$= \frac{5}{30} = \frac{1.8^{\gamma}}{4^{\gamma} + 1.8^{\gamma}} = 0.167$$

Rearranging,

$$0.833 \times 4^{\gamma} = 9^{\gamma} \times (1 - 0.833) \text{ and}$$

$$0.167 \times 4^{\gamma} = 1.8^{\gamma} \times (1 - 0.167)$$

On taking the ratio of the last two equations,

$$5 = \frac{5^{\gamma}}{5} \qquad \text{Thus, } \gamma = 2$$

b. **13.9 hours.** The concentration drops from 9 to 1.8 μg/L in 6 hours. Therefore,

$$\ln C = \ln C(0) - k \cdot t$$

$$\ln 1.8\ \mu g/L = \ln 9\ \mu g/L - \frac{0.693}{6\ hr} \cdot t$$

$$t = 13.9\ hr$$

c. **Approximately linearly.** Response varies with the logarithm of the concentration in this concentration range:

$$\text{Response} = m \cdot \ln C - b$$

The logarithm of the plasma concentration declines linearly with time:

$$\ln C = \ln C(80\%) - k \cdot t$$

where $C(80\%)$ is the concentration on entering Region II (80% E_{max}) of the concentration-response relationship. On substituting the second equation into the first, it is evident that the response should decline linearly in this region. The decline depends on both the slope of the response versus ln C and on the half-life (k).

$$\text{Response} = \text{Constant} - m \cdot k \cdot t$$

where the constant is $m \cdot \ln C(80\%) - b$.

6. a. **See Fig. F-6** for how your plot of reduction in systolic blood pressure against plasma concentration should look. Counterclockwise hysteresis is observed.

b. Possible explanations include:

- Formation of an active metabolite.
- Delay in equilibration of drug at active site with drug in plasma.
- Occurrence of sequential time-delaying events between binding to receptor and the elicitiation of the response.

7. a. Examples in which changes in response with time are rate-limited by the kinetics of the drug are the **decrease in exercise tachycardia produced by propranolol,** the relief of pain with naproxen, and **muscle paralysis produced by neuromuscular blocking agents.** Examples in which changes in response with

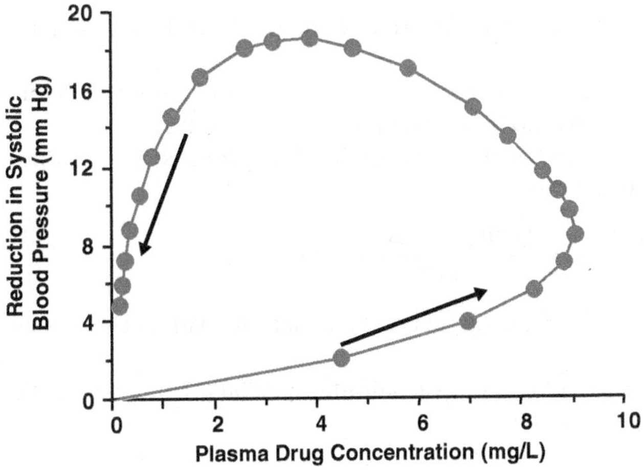

FIGURE F-6

time are rate-limited by the dynamics of the affected system are the **lowering of body temperature with antipyretics,** such as ibuprofen, and the **lowering of the plasma prothrombin complex by warfarin.**

b. **The change in the blood leukocyte count following administration of paclitaxel is an example of a response that is rate-limited by the dynamics of the measured system.** Notice that paclitaxel is almost completely eliminated within 2 days; yet the effect on blood leukocyte count extends over 3 weeks. Leukocytes in blood, like many components in the body, reflect a balance between production and destruction. The direct effect of paclitaxel is inhibition of leukocyte production, which occurs in the bone marrow. The inhibition of leukocyte production is then manifested later in time with a fall in the blood leukocyte count. The exact sequence of events is not fully understood, but it appears that part of the delay in the fall and subsequent return of the blood leukocyte count occurs because only certain phases in the development of the leukocyte, in particular the mitotic phase, are sensitive to paclitaxel. Once paclitaxel has been eliminated, time is needed to produce more leukocytes to restore the blood pool back to normal.

8. a. **The slope is $-m \cdot k$.** A linear decline of response with time is expected when response lies within the region of 80%–20% of the maximum response. Recall, in this region, intensity of response is proportional to the logarithm of plasma concentration, C, with slope m. That is, *response* = $m \cdot \ln C$ + constant. However, as concentration declines exponentially with time, it follows that $\ln C = \ln C(80\%) - k \cdot t$, from which it is seen that response = $m(\ln C(80\%))$ + constant $- m \cdot k \cdot t$. That is, the decline in response with time = $m \cdot k \cdot t$; the slope is $-m \cdot k$.

b. **The apparent half-life of propranolol is 2.3 hours.** The slope of intensity of effect versus time ($-m \cdot k$) = –3.5%/hr. Given that m = +11.5%, it follows that k, the apparent elimination rate constant of propranolol, must be equal to 0.3/hr. Hence, the corresponding half-life (0.693/k) is 2.3 hours. The elimination rate constant and half-life are apparent in that only propranolol is assumed to be active, thus ignoring the possibility that a metabolite may contribute to the observed response.

c. **The minimum amount of propranolol needed in the body is 6 mg.** After a 20-mg dose, the effect remains above 15% for 4 hours (see Fig. 9-18). Hence:

$$A_{min} = \text{Dose} \cdot e^{-k \cdot t_D} = 20\ \text{mg} \times e^{-0.3\ \text{hr}^{-1} \times 4\ \text{hr}} = 6\ \text{mg}$$

d. **6.3 and 8.2 hours.** After a 20-mg dose, the effect remains above 15% for 4 hours (see Fig. 9-18).

(1) After a 40-mg dose, a doubling of the dose, the duration of effect is expected **to increase by 1 half-life,** 2.3 hours (for a total of 6.3 hours).

(2) The duration is expected to **increase an extra 4.2 hours,** since the duration of effect following 70 mg is:

$$t_D = \frac{\ln(\text{Dose}/A_{min})}{k} = \frac{\ln(70\ \text{mg}/6\ \text{mg})}{0.3\ \text{hr}^{-1}} = 8.2\ \text{hr}$$

9. a. **t_D = 11.4 hours** [A_{min} ($C_{min} \cdot V$) = 32 mg] using the equation given in the answer in 8d(2).

b. **t_D after 200 mg = 18.3 hours** (11.4 hours + half-life (= 0.693/0.1/hr = 6.93 hr)).

c. **(1) 22.8 hours, and (2) 8.9 hours.**

d. **Doubling the dose increases the duration of effect by one half-life, 6.9 hours.** The effect of doubling the half-life depends on the mechanism of the change. A decreased clearance leads to a doubling of the duration of effect, whereas in this example, duration is decreased when the cause of the increased half-life is a doubling of the volume of distribution.

CHAPTER 10

1. G. **All three statements are correct.**
2. c. **One can have a wide therapeutic window for a small therapeutic index drug.** The example given was warfarin. The dose at which the anticoagulant effect is too large is not much greater than that at which therapy is satisfactorily achieved within each individual, but across the patient population, as therapeutic window is typically defined, the window of concentrations associated with therapy is quite wide (1-4 mg/L). Statements a, b, and d are all essentially correct.
3. c. **Statement c is correct.** The major limitation of the process is how to weigh the beneficial against the adverse responses. Statement a is incorrect because measuring plasma concentration to guide therapy is *uncommon* in clinical practice, and only for a few drugs are there good direct and simple correlations of therapeutic and adverse responses with systemic exposure. Statement b is incorrect as the adjectives are reversed–narrow or wide therapeutic window and small or large (also low or high) therapeutic index. d is incorrect because there are many examples of drug therapy consisting of a single dose. A few examples were given in this chapter, and more will be accounted for later in the book.
4. **Response is often better correlated with drug exposure than dose for several reasons.** First, although changes in response can be correlated with plasma concentration over time after a single dose of drug, these cannot be correlated with a single value, dose. Second, even after chronic dosing, response is often better correlated with plasma concentration at plateau than dose. This is because bioavailability and clearance often vary widely in the patient population, thereby resulting in a wide variation in drug (and active metabolite) exposure for the same maintenance dose. However, as discussed in the text, there are exceptions.
5. **The existence of a steep adverse effect–exposure relationship does not, in itself, make a drug one with a narrow therapeutic window.** The primary consideration is the degree of overlap in the relationships of efficacy and adverse effects with increasing exposure. Both relationships may be steep, but if there is minimal overlap between the two, such that essentially all responsive patients can be adequately treated at a range of exposures that have minimal probability of producing an adverse effect, then the therapeutic window of the drug is wide. Only when the two relationships overlap, such that there is a low probability of achieving efficacy without harm, is the therapeutic window narrow. Obviously, a steep adverse effect–exposure relationship means that on approaching the region of drug exposure where adverse effects become likely, a small increase in exposure markedly increases the probability of adverse effects being experienced within the patient population.
6. **One potential benefit of drug combinations to treat a specific disease is that because the dose of each drug in the combination needed to produce a given therapeutic effect is often lower than that needed for any individual**

drug if used alone, and adverse effect profiles tend to be drug specific, the therapeutic window of the combination tends to be wider than that of any of the drugs within the combination. Also, combining drugs that attack the disease or condition by different mechanisms can enhance efficacy beyond that which can be achieved with only one drug. An example of the former is the use of a combination of low doses of a thiazide diuretic, an angiotensin-converting enzyme inhibitor or angiotensin receptor inhibitor, and a β-adrenergic blocking drug to treat hypertension. The use of drug combinations to treat human immunodeficiency virus infections, AIDS, and tuberculosis is an example of the latter.

7. Examples given in Chapter 9 of situations in which complexity exists when attempting to correlate response with drug exposure include: **the development of tolerance to a drug; when metabolites contribute significantly to drug response; when single-dose therapy is totally effective; and when response is a function of both dose and duration of treatment.**

CHAPTER 11

1. b. **The time to reach 75% of plateau is 2 half-lives.** The greater the infusion rate, the higher is the plateau concentration, but the time to reach 75% of the plateau should remain the same. All of the other statements are correct.
2. H. **None of the three statements is correct.**
   I. The plateau concentration expected is 0.5 mg/L when infused at 5 mg/hr.

$$C_{ss} = \frac{R_{inf}}{CL} = \frac{5 \text{ mg/hr}}{10 \text{ L/hr}} = 0.5 \text{ mg/L}$$

   II. The time to reach 50% of the plateau is one half-life, 5 hours, not half of a half-life (2.5 hours).
   III. The calculated initial concentration is 0.55 mg/L.

$$C(0) = \frac{\text{Dose}}{V} = \frac{\text{Dose}}{CL/k} = \frac{\text{Dose} \cdot 0.693}{CL \cdot t_{1/2}} = \frac{40 \text{ mg} \times 0.693}{10 \text{ L/hr} \times 5 \text{ hr}} = 0.55 \text{ mg/L}$$

3. d. **Only d is expected to be *not* true.** The greater the affinity of the drug for fat, the more drug there will be in the body when distribution equilibrium is achieved. This should lead to a longer time to remove drug from the body and a longer recovery time. Propofol is an example of a drug with these characteristics.
4. a. **No.** A given concentration is reached more quickly the higher the infusion rate, and the steady-state concentration is increased when the infusion rate is increased. However, one expects the time to reach a given fraction of the new steady state to remain the same, regardless of the infusion rate.
   b. **No.** A decrease in clearance will increase both the plateau concentration and the half-life of the drug, resulting in an increase in the time to achieve plateau.
   c. **No.** The drugs would reach steady state at the same time if their half-lives are the same. For this to be so, in addition to having the same clearance, the drugs must also have the same volume of distribution, which is very unlikely.
   d. **Yes.**The amounts of the drugs at plateau can be the same if the ratio *CL/V* is constant, that is, when the drugs have the same half-life, but this is uncommon.
   e. **Yes.** The time to go from one steady state to another, whether higher or lower, depends only on the half-life of a drug.

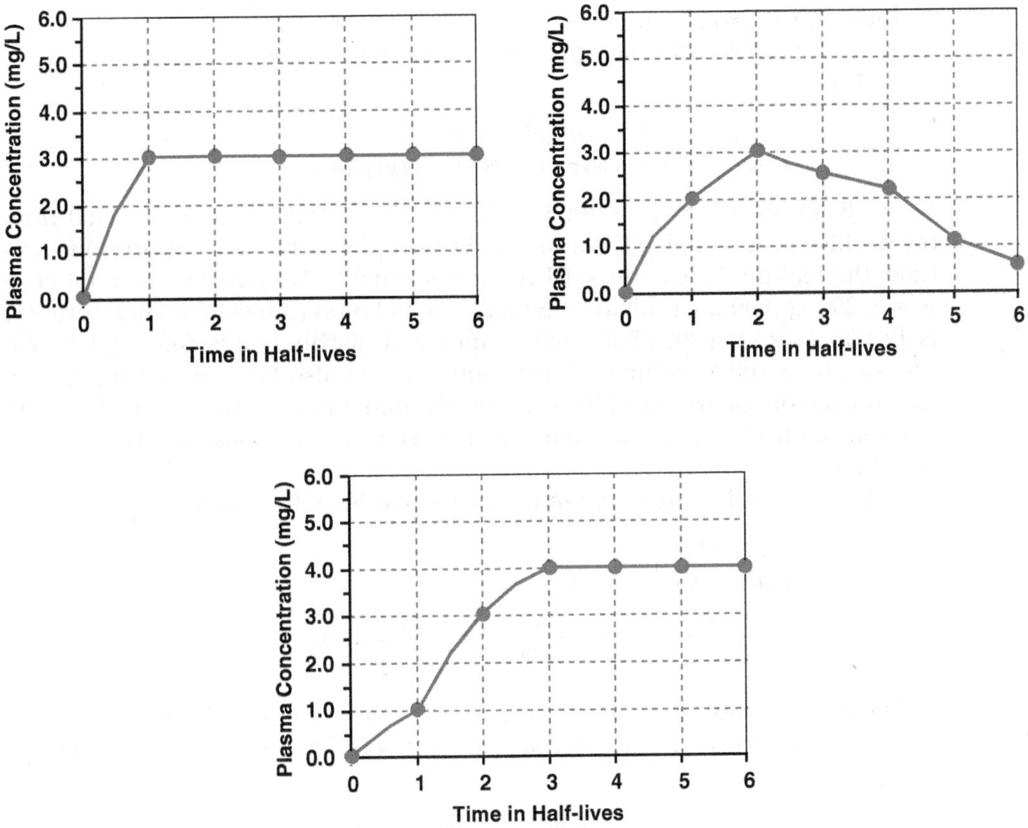

FIGURE F-7

5. **See Fig. F-7.**

6. a. **Time should be in hours rather than days, because the half-life is 1 hour.** From the decline in the plasma concentration after discontinuing drug administration, the half-life in the graph appears to be about 1 day, a value totally inconsistent with the value, 1 hour, from the literature, as calculated from:

$$t_{1/2} = \frac{0.693 \times V}{CL} = \frac{0.693 \times 28.8 \text{ L}}{20 \text{ L/hr}} = 1 \text{ hr}$$

The authors had not caught their mistake before it was published.

b. **First infusion rate = 1.6 mg/hr.**

C(μg/L)	Time(hr)	
40	$1\ t_{1/2}$	$C_{ss} = 2 \times C$ at 1 half-life (40μg/L) = 80 μg/L, had the infusion rate been maintained.
60	$2\ t_{1/2}$	$C_{ss} = \frac{4}{3} \times C$ at 2 half-lives (60μg/L) = 80 μg/L

$$R_{inf} = CL \cdot C_{ss} = 20 \text{ L/hr} \times 80 \text{ μg/L} = 1600 \text{ μg/hr or } 1.6 \text{ mg/hr}$$

Second infusion rate = 1.0 mg/hr.

C (μg/L)	Time (elapsed, hr)	C (μg/L)	Time (elapsed, hr)
60	0	52.5	$2\ t_{1/2}$
55	1 half-life	51.25	$3\ t_{1/2}$

Therefore, $C_{ss} = 50\ \mu g/L$.
$R_{inf} = CL \cdot C_{ss} = 20\ L/hr \times 50\ \mu g/L = 1000\ \mu g/hr$ or 1.0 mg/hr.

c. **1.44 mg.**

$$C(0) = 50\ \mu g/L \qquad V = 28.8\ L$$
$$\text{Dose} = C(0) \cdot V = 50\ \mu g/L \times 28.8\ L = 1440\ \mu g = 1.44\ mg$$

7. **$t_{1/2}$ = 5.8 hours, *CL* = 12 L/hr, V = 100 L.** The half-life is best obtained from the decline after stopping the infusion. From a plot of ln (concentration) versus time, the half-life is 5.8 hours. Clearance is equal to Dose/AUC. The total dose was 2420 mg [500 mg (bolus) + 120 mg/hr × 16 hours (infusion)]. Therefore, *CL* is 12 L/hr (2420 mg/202.28 mg-hr/L). Volume of distribution is CL/k ($1.443 \cdot CL \cdot t_{1/2}$) or about 100 L. Volume of distribution could also have been crudely estimated from the bolus dose (500 mg) and the initial concentration. The 5-minute concentration was 5.0 mg/L when 500 mg was given as a bolus. $V = \text{Dose}/C(0) = 500\ mg/5\ mg/L = 100\ L$.

8. a. **Rate of input into the systemic circulation is 19.6 μg/min**

$$C_{ss} = 40\ \mu g/L$$
$$\text{Rate of input} = CL \times C_{ss}$$
$$= \frac{7\ ml/min}{kg} \times 70\ kg \times \frac{1\ L}{1000\ ml} \times \frac{40\ \mu g}{L} = 19.6\ \mu g/min$$

b. **The total amount delivered systemically over 24 hours is 28.2 mg.** Assuming that the product releases for an additional 4 to 6 hours, the amount input per day is:

$$19.6 \frac{\mu g}{min} \times \frac{1440\ min}{day} \times \frac{1\ mg}{1000\ \mu g} = \frac{28.2\ mg}{day}$$

c. **Yes, the oral bioavailability (*F* = 0.47) is essentially the same as for the immediate-release capsule (*F* = 0.5).** The estimated bioavailability is:

$$F = \frac{28.2\ mg/day}{60\ mg/day} = 0.47$$

d. Under fasting conditions, the modified-release system should transit the stomach in about 1 hour, and the small intestine in an additional 3 hours. Thus, most of the release (20/24) occurs in the large intestine. Furthermore, the constant plasma concentration after 6 hours indicates that the constantly released drug is absorbed at the same rate, regardless of where it is in the large bowel. The absorption of the drug must therefore not be permeability rate–limited there. Also supporting these conclusions is the similarity of the oral bioavailabilities of the two dosage forms, one in which drug is released very quickly and absorbed in the small intestine, and the other in which release is prolonged over 24 hours and mostly absorbed in the large intestine. Thus, systemic absorption of nifedipine must be independent of location of release along the gastrointestinal tract.

9. a. **Clearance = 100 mL/min (or 6 L/hr or 0.075 L/hr/kg).**

$$C_{ss} = 2400\ ng/mL = 2.4\ \mu g/mL$$
$$CL = \frac{R_{inf}}{C_{ss}} = \frac{3\ \mu g/kg\ \text{per min} \times 80\ kg}{2.4\ \mu g/mL} = 100\ mL/min$$
$$\text{or } 6\ L/hr \text{ or } 0.075\ L/hr \text{ per kg}$$

b. **$V = 19$ L.**

$$k = \frac{0.693}{2.2\ \text{hr}} = 0.315\ \text{hr}^{-1} = 0.00535\ \text{min}^{-1}$$

$$V = \frac{CL}{k} = \frac{100\ \text{mL/min}}{0.00535\ \text{min}^{-1}} = 19{,}048\ \text{mL}\ \text{or}\ 19\ \text{L}$$

or 0.24 L/kg

c. **1200 µg/L.** It should be one-half of the 2400 µg/L observed at the 3 µg/kg/min infusion rate.

d. **The dip occurs because distribution to the tissues is not instantaneous.** Drug from the bolus quickly distributes to the tissues, while drug from the infusion more slowly rises toward steady state as the tissues are filled. The dip may also be explained in terms of the two-compartment model. The bolus dose is placed into the central compartment and, having a small volume, a large initial concentration is produced. With time, drug rapidly distributes into the peripheral compartment until steady state (rate of elimination = rate of input) is achieved.

10. a. **Half-life = 1.8 hours.** There is no evidence of a rapid distribution phase after stopping the intravenous infusion or after pulling out the rectal device at 24 hours, suggesting that a one-compartment model is a good representation of the drug's kinetic behavior.

From the plot of the post-infusion data in Fig. 11-16B, the half-life is about 1.83 hours.

$$k = \frac{0.693}{1.83\ \text{hr}} = 0.378\ \text{hr}^{-1}$$

b. **AUC(IV infusion) = 68.57 mg-hr/L; AUC(rectal device) = 36.58 mg-hr/L**

Calculation of Total AUC of Droperidol After an Intravenous Infusion and the Use of a Rectal Device Using the Trapezoidal Approximation

Time (hr)	Concentration (mg/L)	Time Interval (hr)	Average Concentration (mg/L)	Area (mg-hr/L)
IV Infusion				
0	0	–	–	–
0.5	0.9	0.5	0.45	0.225
2	1.8	1.5	1.35	2.025
4	2.6	2	2.2	4.4
6	2.5	2	2.55	5.1
8	2.5	2	2.5	5.0
10	2.7	2	2.6	5.2
14	2.7	4	2.7	10.8
18	2.9	4	2.8	11.2
24	2.9	6	2.9	17.4
26	1.4	2	2.15	4.3
28	.61	2	1.005	2.01
30	.30	2	0.455	0.91
			AUC(0,30)	*68.57*
			Extrapolated Area[a]	1.2
			Total area	69.77

[a]The extrapolated area, given by $C(30)/k$, equals 1.2 (0.455/0.378) for the infusion, and 0.37 (0.14/0.378) for the rectal device.

(continued)

Time (hr)	Concentration (mg/L)	Time Interval (hr)	Average Concentration (mg/L)	Area (mg-hr/L)
Rectal Device				
0	0		–	–
0.5	0	0.5	0	0
2	0.49	1.5	0.245	0.3675
4	0.99	2	0.74	1.48
6	1.83	2	1.41	2.82
8	1.84	2	1.835	3.67
10	1.93	2	1.885	3.77
14	1.52	4	1.725	6.9
18	1.43	4	1.475	5.9
24	1.41	6	1.42	8.52
26	0.65	2	1.03	2.06
28	0.29	2	0.47	0.94
30	0.14	2	0.215	0.43
			AUC(0,30)	36.575
			Extrapolated Area[b]	0.57
			Total area	*37.14*

[b]extrapolated area 0.215/0.378 = 0.57, giving a total area of 37.14

c. ***CL* = 43.0 L/hr**

$$CL = \frac{\text{Dose}}{\text{AUC}} = \frac{125\ \mu\text{g/hr} \times 24\ \text{hr}}{69.77\ \mu\text{g-hr/L}} = 43.0\ \text{L/hr}$$

d. **V = 114 L**

$$V = \frac{CL}{k} = \frac{43.0\ \text{L/hr}}{0.378\ \text{hr}^{-1}} = 113.8\ \text{L}$$

e. ***F* = 0.53**

$$F = \frac{\left(\text{AUC}/\text{Dose}\right)_{\text{Rectal}}}{\left(\text{AUC}/\text{Dose}\right)_{\text{iv}}} = \frac{\left(37.14\ \mu\text{g-hr/L}/3\ \text{mg}\right)_{\text{Rectal}}}{\left(69.77\ \mu\text{g-hr/L}/3\ \text{mg}\right)_{\text{iv}}} = \frac{37.14\ \mu\text{g-hr/L}}{69.77\ \mu\text{g-hr/L}} = 0.53$$

Calculated Expected *F* is 0.47. With a plasma-to-blood concentration ratio of 1.0, the blood clearance is the same as plasma clearance. Assuming the liver is the only site of loss, the hepatic extraction ratio would be the ratio of hepatic blood clearance to hepatic blood flow ($E_H = CL_{b,H}/Q_H$ = 43.0L/hr/(1.35L/min × 60 min) = 0.53). The hepatic availability would then be 0.47 ($1 - E_H$). The expected value (0.47) is close to the observed value (0.53) suggesting that first pass hepatic extraction explains the observation. The slight difference between the two values could easily be accommodated by a slight adjustment of hepatic blood flow (Q). Calculation shows that it would need to be 1.55L/min, to bring prediction in line with observation, well within the physiological range.

f. **The rectal device worked reasonably well in terms of the systemic exposure profile.** A little larger rectal dose would have nearly superimposed the rectal and iv curves from 4 to 24 hours. Two issues are of further concern: First, as the drug is used for the prevention and treatment of nausea and vomiting, the slow absorption during the first few hours is a concern. Second, the curve shown is of mean data. There is no information given above on the variability in the delivery of drug from this device.

CHAPTER 12

1. H. **None of the statements is correct.** Statement I is incorrect because the amount eliminated in the first dosing interval is always *less* than the amount systemically absorbed from the first dose. Otherwise, accumulation would never occur. Statement II is incorrect because the accumulation index depends on both the dosing frequency and the half-life. Statement III is incorrect because the amount of drug lost within a dosing interval at plateau equals the amount of the oral maintenance dose absorbed ($F\cdot$Dose), which is not the administered dose when $F < 1$.
2. G. **All of the statements are correct.** The drug is given 100 mg IV every half-life (12 hours). The amount in the body just after the third dose, two half-lives, is 175 mg (100 + 50 mg remaining from the second dose + 25 mg remaining from the first dose). The maximum amount at plateau is 200 mg (100 mg/(1 – 0.5)); therefore, the minimum amount at steady state (one half-life later; the dosing interval) is 100 mg. 24 hours (2 half-lives) after the last dose, the amount in the body is 200 mg × ¼ = 50 mg.
3. d. **200 mg.** The dosing interval (1 day) is one-half of a half-life. The fraction remaining at the end of a dosing interval is $0.5^{0.5}$ or $e^{-0.693 \times 24/48 \text{ hrs}}$, that is, 0.707. Thus, the fraction lost within the dosing interval is 0.293, so that the 60-mg dose represents just 29.3% of the initial amount in the body at the beginning of the interval, which must have been 60/0.293 or 205 mg at steady state. The value also could have been calculated from $D_L = D_M/(1 - e^{-k\tau})$.
4. E. **Statements I and III are correct.** Statement II is incorrect because such a condition (pharmacodynamic rate limitation) would allow a much *longer* dosing interval to be used than what one would predict on the basis of pharmacokinetic principles alone.
5. a. **This statement is true.** Because some drug always remains in the body from previous doses, however, the accumulation is small when the drug is given infrequently relative to its half-life.

   b. **This statement is true.** Recall that the accumulation index at plateau is given by

$$\text{Accumulation index}\,(R_{ac}) = \frac{A_{max,ss}}{A_{max,1}} = \frac{A_{min,ss}}{A_{min,1}} = \frac{1}{(1 - e^{-k\cdot\tau})}$$

   from which it is seen that the index depends only on $k\cdot\tau$ (*or* $0.693\tau/t_{1/2}$) where $\tau/t_{1/2}$ is the dosing interval relative to the half-life of the drug. The index is therefore a function of the half-life relative to the dosing frequency ($1/\tau$). For a given half-life, the more frequent the administration (the smaller the value of τ), the greater is the extent of accumulation.

   c. **This statement is incorrect.** The time to reach plateau depends only on the half-life of the drug; the shorter the half-life, the sooner the plateau is reached. Dosing the drug more frequently increases the extent of accumulation, but has no effect on the time to reach plateau.

d. **This statement is incorrect.** The average plateau plasma concentration is independent of the volume of distribution, as can be seen from its absence from the relationship,

$$C_{av,ss} = \frac{F \cdot Dose}{CL \cdot \tau}$$

6. **The statement is very much conditioned on the pharmacodynamics of the drug.** For situations in which the therapeutic effect is dependent only on drug concentration regardless of time, then maintaining a constant level of exposure is desirable. Moreover, if tolerance develops to any of the adverse effects, then maintenance of constant exposure of drug is an added benefit. However, when tolerance develops to the therapeutic effect of the drug or constant exposure increases the risk and severity of adverse events, then, clearly, maintenance of a constant concentration is undesirable. These issues, with examples, are further discussed in this chapter and further in Chapter 14.

7. a. **Yes.** The drug has a half-life of 18 hours. Thus, 60 hours (3.33 half-lives) corresponds to the time to achieve 90% of plateau. Accordingly, on taking the dose at 0, 12, 24, 36, 48, and 60 hours, a plateau is practically reached following the 6th dose.

b. (1) **25.4 mg calculated using Eq. 12-1.**

Dose Number	1	2	3	4	5	6
Fraction remaining at 60 hours	0.10	0.16	0.25	0.40	0.63	1
Amount remaining at 60 hours (mg)	1.0	1.6	2.5	4.0	6.3	10

(2) **27 mg**

$$A_{max,ss} = \frac{Dose}{(1 - e^{-k \cdot \tau})} = \frac{Dose}{\left(1 - e^{-\frac{0.693 \times 12\ hr}{18\ hr}}\right)} = 27\ mg$$

c. **17 mg**

$$A_{min,ss} = A_{max,ss} - Dose = 17\ mg$$

It could also have been calculated from $A_{min,ss} = A_{max,ss} \cdot e^{-k \cdot 12}$.

8. a. **Average steady-state concentrations: acetaminophen = 7.14 mg/L; ibuprofen = 13.3 mg/L; naproxen = 72.0 mg/L.**

	Equation	Acetaminophen	Ibuprofen	Naproxen
$C_{av,ss}$ (mg/L)	$\frac{F \cdot Dose}{CL \cdot \tau}$	$\frac{0.9 \times 1000 mg}{21 L/hr \times 6 hr} = 7.14$	$\frac{0.7 \times 400 mg}{3.5 L/hr \times 6 hr} = 13.3$	$\frac{0.95 \times 500 mg}{0.55 L/hr \times 12 hr} = 72$

Note that despite the longer dosing interval and the relatively modest maintenance dose, because of its much lower clearance, the $C_{av,ss}$ of naproxen is much higher than that of the other two drugs.

b. **Ibuprofen reaches the plateau soonest.** The time to reach a plateau depends only on the half-life; the shorter the half-life, the sooner the plateau is reached. The half-lives of the three drugs are:

	Equation	Acetaminophen	Ibuprofen	Naproxen
$t_{1/2}$ (hr)	$\frac{0.693 \cdot V}{CL}$	$\frac{0.693 \times 67 L}{21 L/hr} = 2.21$	$\frac{0.693 \times 10 L}{3.5 L/hr} = 1.98$	$\frac{0.693 \times 11 L}{0.55 L/hr} = 14$

Note that in practice, the difference in the half-lives of acetaminophen and ibuprofen is inconsequential. For both drugs, the plateau is effectively achieved by the time the second dose is given, 6 hours after the first one. With naproxen, there is a case for giving a loading dose if the full therapeutic effect is needed as soon as possible; otherwise, it would take about 2 days to reach plateau.

c. **Naproxen accumulates the most extensively, even though the frequency of its administration is the least.** The degree of accumulation, given by the accumulation index, is

	Equation	Acetaminophen	Ibuprofen	Naproxen
Accumulation index	$\frac{1}{(1-e^{-k\cdot\tau})}$	$\frac{1}{\left(1-e^{-\frac{21\text{L/hr}\times6\text{hr}}{67\text{L}}}\right)}$ = 1.18	$\frac{1}{\left(1-e^{-\frac{3.5\text{L/hr}\times6\text{hr}}{10\text{L}}}\right)}$ = 1.14	$\frac{1}{\left(1-e^{-\frac{0.55\text{L/hr}\times12\text{hr}}{11\text{L}}}\right)}$ = 2.22

Notice that the greatest degree of accumulation occurs with naproxen, because it is given more frequently relative to its half-life than the other two drugs.

d. **The maximum concentrations at plateau are: ibuprofen = 31.9 mg/L; naproxen = 95.7 mg/L.**

	Equation	Ibuprofen	Naproxen
$C_{max,ss}$ (mg/L)	$\frac{F\cdot\text{Dose}}{V\cdot(1-e^{-k\cdot\tau})}$	$\frac{0.7\times400\text{mg}}{10\times\left(1-e^{-\frac{3.5\text{L/hr}\times6\text{hr}}{10}}\right)}=31.9$	$\frac{0.95\times500\text{mg}}{11\times\left(1-e^{-\frac{3.5\text{L/hr}\times12\text{hr}}{11}}\right)}=95.7$

e. **The minimum concentrations at plateau are: ibuprofen = 3.91 mg/L, naproxen = 52.5 mg/L.**

	Equation	Ibuprofen	Naproxen
$C_{min,ss}$ (mg/L)	$C_{max,ss}\,e^{-k\cdot\tau}$	$31.9\times e^{-\frac{3.5\text{L/hr}\times6\text{hr}}{10}}=3.91$	$95.7\times e^{-\frac{0.55\text{L/hr}\times12\text{hr}}{11}}=52.5$

f. **Relative fluctuation: ibuprofen = 2.1; naproxen = 0.6.**

	Equation	Ibuprofen	Naproxen
Relative fluctuation	$\frac{C_{max,ss}-C_{min,ss}}{C_{av,ss}}$	$\frac{31.9-3.91}{13.3}=2.1$	$\frac{95.7-52.5}{72}=0.60$

Note: The fluctuation of naproxen concentration is much less than that of ibuprofen, even though it is given every 12 hours compared with every 6 hours. This is primarily a function of the disproportionately longer half-life of naproxen.

9. a. **The relative fluctuations of albuterol in the extended-release and immediate-release dosage forms are comparable or may even be higher for the latter as noted in the table below, despite the lower frequency of administration of the former.** This is seen by noting the similarities in the maximum and minimum concentrations and also noting that the average concentrations are also similar.

	Equation	IR Product	ER Product
Relative fluctuation	$\frac{C_{max,ss}-C_{min,ss}}{C_{av,ss}}$	$\frac{13.5-9.5}{11.2}=0.36$	$\frac{13.0-9.8}{11.0}=0.29$

b. **Yes.** The oral bioavailabilities of albuterol for the two formulations are equal. This follows from the observation that the AUCs within a 12-hour interval for the same dose are equal.

c. **Yes.** Recall from Chapter 7 that the slower the kinetics of absorption, the later is the time of the peak concentration.

d. **No.** Other factors besides half-life also need to be considered. One factor is whether the time course of the clinical response is rate-limited by the dynamics of the affected system or by the kinetics of the drug. If it is the latter, the case for an extended-release product exists. Another factor is whether metabolites contribute significantly to response; if so, their pharmacokinetics and relative activities should be considered. Still other factors include: whether the exposure–response relationship is stable with time (that is, for example, no tolerance development); the width of the therapeutic window of the drug; and the impact of the kinetics of release on local adverse effects.

10. **The time course for the development of full clinical response is determined primarily by the dynamics of the affected system.** The effect of the venlafaxine may be viewed as the difference in the HAM-A scores between the treatment and placebo phases (Fig. F-8, *colored triangle*). This difference is seen to increase progressively until about 8 weeks. Thereafter, the difference remains relatively stable. Based on the pharmacokinetics of both venlafaxine and its active metabolite, with half-lives of 5 and 11 hours, respectively, steady state of these compounds is anticipated to be reached by the third day of dosing. Yet, clearly, the clinical effect takes much longer to be fully manifested. This strongly suggests that the time course of the development of the full clinical response is determined primarily by how the body responds to drug exposure, rather than being controlled by the pharmacokinetics of the drug, or its metabolite. Notice also the strong placebo effect with a temporal pattern similar to that seen with patients on venlafaxine treatment, suggesting that some of the determinants controlling the temporal profile of the HAM-A score, which has a strong subjective element, are also operative with the placebo.

The preparation evaluated is a once-a-day modified-release dosage form that releases venlafaxine more slowly than the twice-daily immediate-release (IR) product. One might argue that there is a questionable need for a slow-release dosage form of this drug because the sluggish clinical response clearly must be responding to the average exposure of drug and metabolite and because once-daily administration of the IR product should be adequate. However, drug therapy is a balance between the beneficial and adverse effects. Giving the same daily dose of venlafaxine in the IR

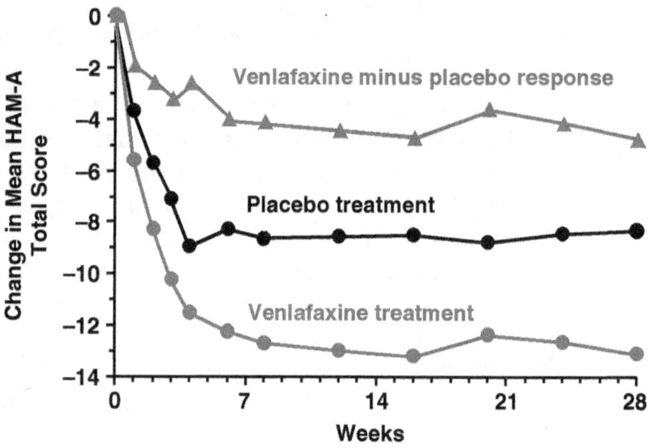

FIGURE F-8

product produces much higher concentrations of drug in the gastrointestinal tract and systemically, thereby decreasing the tolerability of the drug by increasing the likely risk and severity of adverse effects, such as nausea. In addition, the convenience of once-daily administration tends to improve adherence by patients to prescribed regimens, although, more generally, how much benefit is derived depends on both the drug and the condition being treated, as discussed more fully in Chapter 14.

11. a. **No. But relative to elimination, yes.**

The plasma concentrations of the enantiomers after a single dose peak at 18 and 30 hours, indicating that absorption continues for some time. However, relative to the respective half-lives of 128 and 409 hours, the peak concentrations are indeed rapidly achieved with minimal elimination of the enantiomers occurring by the times of their respective t_{max} values.

b. **Both *V* and *CL* increase for (+) - MQ relative to those of (−)-MQ.**

The following discussion applies to the single-dose data. A difference in C_{max} (0.36 mg/L for (−)-MQ versus 0.12 mg/L for (+)-MQ) reflects a difference in *V/F*. If *F* is not changed, then *V* is greater for (+)-MQ.

The difference in AUC(0 – ∞), 20 mg-hr/L for (+)-MQ and 190 mg-hr/L for (−)-MQ), reflects a difference in *CL/F* (Dose/AUC). If *F* is unchanged, then *CL* is almost 10-fold greater for (+)-MQ.

c. $\boldsymbol{C_{max,ss}}$ **= 1.45 mg/L.**

$$C_{max,ss} = \frac{C_{1,max}}{1 - e^{-k \cdot \tau}} = \frac{0.36}{1 - e^{-\frac{0.693}{409} \cdot 168}} = 1.45 \text{ mg/L}$$

$$k = \frac{0.693}{409 \text{ hr}} \qquad \tau = 24 \text{hr/day} \times 7 \text{ days} = 168 \text{ hours}$$

The observation was 1.42 mg/L, an almost identical value.

d. **Yes, but not for individuals with half-lives greater than about 650 hours.**
The (−)-MQ isomer has an average half-life of 430 hours on multiple dosing, seen on stopping administration. Thirteen weeks is 2184 hours (168 hr/week × 13) or about 5.1 half-lives (2184/439 hours). However, its standard deviation is 255 hours. Therefore, some individuals may have much longer half-lives. If 2184 hours is 3.32 half-lives, the corresponding half-life is 657 hours. For those individuals with half-lives of this value or higher, steady state is not yet achieved.

e. $\boldsymbol{R_{ac}}$ **= 4.0**

$$R_{ac} = \frac{1}{1 - e^{-k\tau}} = \frac{1}{1 - e^{-\frac{0.693 \times 168}{409}}} = 4.0$$

f. **Relative fluctuation at steady state: (+)-MQ = 0.83; (−)-MQ = 0.35.**

$$\text{Relative fluctuation} = \frac{C_{ss,max} - C_{ss,min}}{C_{ss,av}}$$

For (+)-MQ,

$$\text{Relative fluctuation} = \frac{0.26 - 0.11}{0.18} = 0.83$$

For (−)-MQ,

$$\text{Relative fluctuation} = \frac{1.42 - 1.01}{1.17} = 0.35$$

The difference in the values is explained by (+)-MQ having a much shorter half-life (~ 173 hours) than (−)-MQ (~ 430 hours), therefore showing greater fluctuation on the once-weekly regimen.

g. **Yes, for both treatment and prevention.** The accumulation index for once-weekly dosing was 4.0 (Part e above). Thus, a loading dose of 4 or 5 tablets seems reasonable to rapidly achieve the steady-state level normally achieved on once-a-week dosing. The half-life is so long that the single dose comprises the dosage regimen. Indeed, if a patient does not respond to the drug in 48–72 hours, an alternative therapy must be considered.

The requirement of 2–3 doses before going to an endemic area allows some accumulation to occur before being exposed to the parasite. Three weeks is 504 hours (3 × 168 hours). This is well over one average half-life. Thus, the plasma concentration is now more than 50% of the steady-state value.

CHAPTER 13

1. C. **Rifampin is a strong inducer of the CYP3A4 enzyme that cause a decrease in the bioavailability of this high first-pass drug and raise its clearance as well, resulting in a decreased response to midazolam.** Itraconazole and clarithromycin, on the other hand, are inhibitors of CYP3A4 that metabolize midazolam (see Fig. 13-9). They are expected to cause an increase in exposure and hence in the response to midazolam.
2. D. **Statements I and II are correct.** A rough rule is that clearance, whether by the liver or the kidneys, decreases by about 1%/year in adults, that is, after age 20. In children (>2 years of age), the rule of the clearance increasing in proportion to body surface area is usually a good first approximation for children with near normal weight and height for age. It follows from Statements I and II that Statement III is incorrect.
3. D. **Statements I and II are correct.** Statement III is partially incorrect. Certain rare adverse effects are said to be idiosyncratic in nature, not because the cause of them is unknown, but because they are peculiar to the individual and are therefore genetic in origin.
4. d. **Statement d is definitely incorrect because enzyme induction should produce a *decrease*, not an *increase*, in systemic exposure to the affected drug. All the remaining statements are correct.**
5. **Six major sources of variability in drug response are genetics, age, body weight, disease, concurrent drugs, and nonadherence to a regimen.** The relative importance of each depends on the drug, the response, and the patient population being treated. Genetics is often the most important but least understood of these sources of variability, and only recently has knowledge and technology become available that promises to help predict likely outcomes from genomic information. In addition, there is sometimes a significant degree of covariance among these sources. For example, during childhood, much of the influence of age on pharmacokinetic parameters can be explained by body size. Of all the major sources of variability, the one that is probably the most important across the spectrum of pharmacotherapy is nonadherence.
6. **Understanding variability, particularly quantifying it, in drug response is very important in the optimization of drug administration for the individual patient.** There is a view that one dose fits all. However, as our understanding of variability in drug response and the relative contributions of pharmacokinetics

and pharmacodynamics as well as important factors influencing such variability improves, it is clear that often, there is a need to adjust the dosage regimens of many drugs to the individual. One important distinction to be made is between *inter*individual and *intra*individual variability. **Large interindividual variability in pharmacokinetics and pharmacodynamics is often reflected in a range of dose strengths being made available for a drug. Large intraindividual variability would make stabilization of drug therapy for an individual patient difficult unless the therapeutic index of the drug is very wide.** Fortunately, in most cases, intraindividual variability is much smaller than interindividual variability.

7. a. **Yes.** It would be prudent to consider reducing the dosing rate in the patient with a renal function of 20% of that in the typical patient. This drug ($fe = 0.96$) is almost exclusively dependent on renal function for its elimination. All the activity resides with the drug and, on repetitive dosing, drug would accumulate more extensively than it normally would, unless the dosing rate is reduced.
   b. **No.** Because only 2% of the dose is normally excreted unchanged, the pharmacokinetics of the drug would not be expected to change much in a patient with poor renal function. The metabolite might accumulate, but it is inactive.
   c. **Yes.** With all the (inactive) drug converted to the active metabolite, which depends exclusively on renal excretion for its elimination, the dosing rate of drug should be reduced to avoid excessive accumulation of the active metabolite.
   d. **No.** Because all the activity resides with the primary metabolite, which is then further metabolized to inactive metabolites, there would be no need to adjust the dosing rate of the drug in the patient with poor renal function.
   Note: Another consideration is the therapeutic index of the drug and metabolites. If the index is wide, making no adjustment in the dosage regimen of the drug may still not result in an adverse clinical outcome. Still, it is generally prudent to reduce the dosage when there is impaired removal of drug or of significant active metabolites.

8. **Pharmacodynamic sources of variability can be distinguished from pharmacokinetic sources in drug response by concurrently measuring drug (and metabolite, if important) exposure (usually in plasma) and response in the patient population receiving the drug.** Preferably, concentration and response should be determined in the same patient, but this is not always possible or appropriate. For example, the taking of a blood sample, with its associated trauma, may influence the response itself. If those in whom pharmacokinetic measurements are different from those in whom response outcomes are assessed, then the resulting analysis may not allow a relationship to be established, such as between exposure and the severity of an adverse effect. Also, preferably, any pharmacodynamic relationship should be based on unbound drug concentration, particularly in situations in which plasma protein binding is known to vary appreciably within the patient population.

   Examples of inherited variability in pharmacokinetics include **clearance of metoprolol due to polymorphism of CYP2D6; clearance of S-warfarin due to polymorphism of CYP2C9; and clearance of azathioprine due to polymorphism of thiopurine *S*-methyltransferase.** In each of these cases, the drug can be any substrate for which its elimination is predominantly mediated by the respective enzyme.

   Examples of inherited variability in pharmacodynamics include: **response to trastuzumab (Herceptin) in the treatment of primary breast cancer due to polymorphism of the HER2 proto-oncogene; FEV_1 (forced expiratory volume in 1 second) to β-adrenergic agonists such as albuterol due to**

polymorphism of the receptor; development of cough in some patients on angiotensin-converting enzyme (ACE) inhibitors due to polymorphism in the bradykinin B_2 receptor. Other examples are provided in the chapter.

9. a. Answers are provided in the table below.

Subject	1	2	3	4	5
Cu_{ss} (mg/L)	0.25	0.24	**0.27**	**0.24**	0.28
CL (L/hr)	**8.0**	12.5	6.7	13.3	**8.7**
V (L)	**16.1**	34.3	**16.4**	57.7	35.1

b. **Volume of distribution is the most variable and Cu_{SS} the least variable because these have the largest and smallest coefficients of variation, respectively.** Given that fu varies within the group by a factor of 1.6 (0.16/0.1), while V varies by a factor of 3.58 (57.7/16.1), it follows that distribution within the tissues appears to be the major source of variability in V.

c. **Therapeutically, unbound concentration is more important than total plasma concentration.** As such, given that the unbound concentration is very similar among the subjects, they can all receive the same rate of infusion (assuming that the interindividual variability in pharmacodynamics is small). The time to approach plateau does vary considerably across the sampled population, as seen by the variability in half-life. If the decision is to give a loading dose to achieve the same unbound concentration, here, too, the dose needed is quite variable among subjects, which can be seen by calculating Dose, from the relationship Dose $= V \cdot C = V \cdot Cu/fu$, as the value of V/fu is also quite variable (161, 229, 182, 360, and 292 L) among the subjects. Clearly, a very different conclusion for maintenance dosing rate would have been reached had the erroneous decision been made to calculate the rate using the pharmacokinetic parameters based on the total plasma concentration.

10. a.

Age Group	Mean Age and Weight (kg)	Recommended Daily Dose (mg)	Predicted Daily Dose (mg)[a]
Adult (18 y of age and older)	22 y; 66 kg	10	**10**
Child (6–14 y of age)	10 y; 32 kg	5	**5.8**
Child (2–5 y of age)	8 y; 15.5 kg	4	**3.4**
Child (12–24 mo of age)	18 mo, 11 kg	4	**2.6**

[a]Calculated using the formula given.

Note: If the pediatric dose had been calculated on body weight, it would have been too low, particularly for a 1- to 2-year-old child (11 kg/70 kg × 10 mg = 1.6 mg). The predictions and the recommendations are close except for the youngest group.

b. **No.** Asthma is primarily a childhood disease. Allergic rhinitis can occur at any age, but a 60-year-old adult undoubtedly does not represent a "typical aged" patient on this drug.

c. There are two major assumptions: **First, oral bioavailability is the same as in adults.** The formula used to calculate child dosage only corrects for anticipated change in clearance. However, let's assume that parity in absorption is reasonable in children >2 years old, as their physiological function is similar to that in adults. In the specific case of montelukast, there is a chewable tablet and a granule dosage form for facilitating administration in children. **Second, pharmacodynamics is unchanged, that is, the exposure–response relationship is the same in children as in adults.** As pointed out in the chapter, this may not always be the case, but in the absence of any specific data, it is a reasonable starting point.

d. **Shortening the dosing interval should generally be a consideration.** With clearance varying with body surface area, and volume of distribution with body weight, the expectation is that the half-life of a drug will be shorter in young children than in adults. So a shorter dosing interval to avoid excessive fluctuation in systemic exposure is a worthwhile consideration. Specifically, the half-life of montelukast in adults is 2.7–5.5 hours, and it is recommended to be taken once daily in the evening, suggesting a pharmacodynamic rate limitation in the response to the drug or that the drug is only needed at nighttime. This condition appears to apply to children as well, as once daily dosing is recommended for them too.

11. a. **Distribution kinetics.** Distribution to the tissues takes time. It appears to be essentially complete in an hour or so. A rapid distribution phase is not apparent for the oral doses because absorption is probably slower than (rate-limits) distribution.

b. **High hepatic extraction ratio.** One can quickly draw this conclusion from the high plasma clearance, 1.33 L/min after an IV dose, and knowledge that only 3.5% of an intravenous dose is excreted unchanged in the urine. More specifically, the blood clearance is:

$$CL_b = CL \cdot \frac{C}{C_b} = 1.33\ (\text{L/min}) \times .85 = 1.13\ \text{L/min}$$

The hepatic blood clearance, assuming nonrenal clearance occurs hepatically, is:

$$CL_{b,H} = (1 - fe) \cdot CL_b = (1 - 0.035) \times 1.13 = 1.09\ \text{L/min}$$

The hepatic extraction ratio is then:

$$E_H = \frac{CL_{H,b}}{Q_H} = \frac{1.09\text{L/min}}{1.35\text{L/min}} = 0.81$$

c. **Because of an increase in the bioavailability in the cirrhotic patients.** Recall that

$$F = \frac{\left(\frac{\text{Dose}}{\text{AUC}}\right)_{\text{oral}}}{\left(\frac{\text{Dose}}{\text{AUC}}\right)_{\text{i.v.}}}$$

Therefore,

$$\frac{\left(\frac{\text{AUC}}{\text{Dose}}\right)_{\text{oral}}}{\left(\frac{\text{AUC}}{\text{Dose}}\right)_{\text{i.v.}}} = \frac{1}{F}$$

The value of F in cirrhotics is 0.55, but only 0.22 in healthy subjects.

d. **The tissue binding must be increased (fu_T decreased); in the cirrhotic patients; fu was not changed.**
This conclusion is based on the relationship:

$$V = V_P + V_T \cdot \frac{fu}{fu_T}$$

CHAPTER 14

1. E. **Statements I and III are correct.** The elimination rate constant can be calculated by substituting the peak (7.2 mg/L) and trough (1.8 mg/L) concentrations and the interval between these observations (7.0 hours) into the following equation.

$$1.8 \text{ mg/L} = 7.2 \text{ mg/L} \times e^{-k \times 7.0 \text{ hr}}$$

which, on rearrangement, gives

$$k = \ln(7.2/1.8)/7.0 = 0.2 \text{ hr}^{-1}$$

And, therefore, $t_{1/2} = 3.5$ hr.

Statement II is incorrect as the volume of distribution can be estimated from the peak and trough concentrations. There should be little of the infused drug (one half-hour infusion) lost during the first hour, and the drug is now essentially at steady state. The volume of distribution is then crudely:

$$V = \frac{\text{Dose}}{C_{\text{peak}} - C_{\text{trough}}} = \frac{100 \text{ mg}}{7.2 \text{ mg/L} - 1.8 \text{ mg/L}} = 18.5 \text{ L}$$

With a dosing interval of 8 hours, at the end of the third infusion (24 hours, approximately 6 half-lives), steady state has been reached.

2. B. **Statement II is incorrect.** Monitoring of plasma concentrations may be useful when a drug has a low therapeutic index, and *pharmacokinetics* accounts for much of the interpatient variability in the dose–response relationship.

3. A. **Statement I is correct.** A drug with a high accumulation index accumulates extensively on repeated administration. This is a pharmacokinetic reason why a loading dose may be needed. Practically, it may not be prudent to give a loading dose for a number of reasons as presented in this chapter.

4. c. **Statement c is correct.** Statement a is incorrect because one is *less*, not more, likely to show greater peak toxicity when the drug is taken frequently than when it is taken infrequently, relative to the drug's half-life because on frequent dosing drug accumulates extensively, so that each dose adds relatively little to what is already in the body. Statement b is incorrect because tolerance to its adverse hypotensive effect to terazosin develops with time, allowing greater doses to be given. Statement d is incorrect because plasma concentration monitoring can be useful when variability in dose–response lies mostly in its *pharmacokinetics*, not in its pharmacodynamics, as is the case for phenytoin.

5. **See values in table below and the two curves drawn in Fig. F-9 (next page).**

$$e^{-k\tau} = e^{-\frac{0.693}{20 \text{ hr}} \times 24} = 0.435 \quad F \cdot \text{Dose} = 0.9 \times 7.5 \text{ mg} = 6.75 \text{ mg}$$

a. **7.5 mg daily**

Time (hr)	A_{max} (mg)	Time (hr)	A_{min} (mg)
0+	6.75	24	2.94
24	9.69	48	4.21
48	10.96	72	4.77
72	11.52	96	5.01
96	11.78	120	5.12
120	11.87	144	5.16
144	11.91		

b. Third and fourth doses missing on days 2 and 3

Time (hr)	A_{max} (mg)	Time (hr)	A_{min} (mg)
0+	6.75	24	2.94
24	9.69	48	4.21
48	4.21	72	1.83
72	1.83	96	0.80
96	7.55	120	3.28
120	10.03	144	4.36
144	11.11		

Notice that the missed doses result in the almost complete loss of meloxicam from the body, which may deprive a patient of benefit with this drug. The reason for the large loss of drug is that, in effect, only one dose is given during a three-day period (72 hours), which is long relative to the 20-hour half-life of this drug. Clearly, good adherence to the dosage regimen is important for such a drug, if adequate exposure is needed to be maintained to ensure efficacy. The problem of the missed doses may be less acute if the half-life of the drug had been very much longer, or if pharmacodynamics rate-limits the response.

c. $C_{av,ss}$, = 0.80 mg/L.

$$C_{av,ss} = \frac{F \bullet \text{Dose}}{\tau \bullet CL} = \frac{0.9 \times 7.5 \text{ mg}}{24 \text{ hr} \times 0.35 \text{ L/hr}} = 0.80 \text{ mg/L}$$

$$CL = k \bullet V = \frac{0.693 \times 10 \text{ L}}{20 \text{ hr}} = 0.35 \text{L/hr}$$

d. Extensively reabsorbed.
The renal clearance (CL_R) is 0.002 × 350 mL/hr = 0.70 mL/hr or 0.012 mL/min. If filtered only, $CL_R = fu \cdot \text{GFR} = 0.006 \times 100$ mL/min = 0.6 mL/min or 36 mL/hr As CL_R is much less than $fu \cdot$ GFR, the drug must be extensively reabsorbed in the renal tubule.

e. Fraction unbound unchanged. The highest concentration is about 1.2 mg/L ($C = A/V$ = 12 mg/10 L) after a regimen of 7.5 mg daily. This corresponds to a

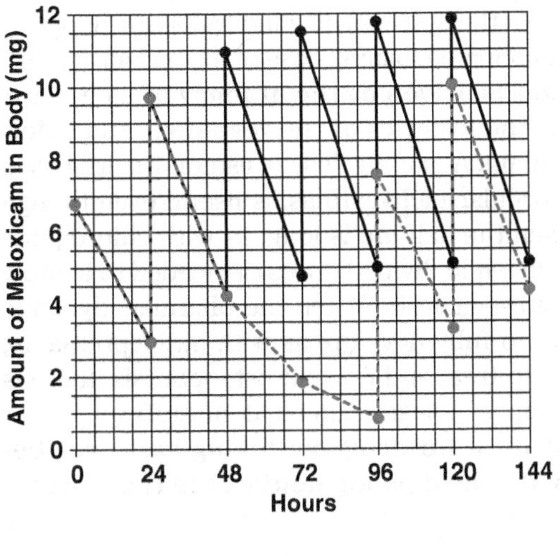

FIGURE F-9 Amount of meloxicam in the body following: 7.5 mg once daily (*black*) and the same regimen but the third and fourth doses were not taken (*color*).

concentration of 2.4 mg/351.4 mg/mmol or 0.0068 mM after a regimen of 15 mg daily. This value is small compared with the molar concentration (0.6 mM) of albumin, the protein to which it primarily binds. Therefore, the fraction unbound in plasma, which depends on the sites available for binding, is expected to be constant over the therapeutic range.

6. a. **In one strategy, the initial dosage regimen for a patient is calculated on the basis of the population pharmacokinetic and pharmacodynamic information, together with the patient-specific data, such as age, body weight, renal function, and other characteristics, such as genotypic information, which are known to explain some of the interindividual variability in the dose–response relationship.** Drug therapy is subsequently managed by monitoring the effects observed; that is, the dose is increased when the desired response is inadequate, or decreased when an adverse response is excessive. Digoxin and ganciclovir are examples of drugs administered using this strategy.

   The second strategy is one in which an individual's requirements are determined by starting with a low dose and slowly raising the dosage, if needed, until the optimal therapeutic response, without undue adverse effects, is achieved. How quickly the dose is adjusted depends on the kinetics of the drug and its responses. Flecainide, antiepileptics, and many antidepressants are examples of drugs administered using this second strategy.

   b. **Stratifying dosage for infants, children, and frail elderly patients is clearly needed.** Stratification before starting therapy may also be prudent when the patient has compromised renal function, hepatic disease, or a genetically related condition in which drug metabolism or drug response is known to be affected. Further adjustment of dosage may also be required if concurrently administered drugs interact with the introduced drug. Taking such patient-specific information into account can reduce the occurrence and intensity of harmful events and help to more rapidly establish an individual's optimal dosage requirements.

7. a. **Giving a loading dose in several sequential doses allows development of the full beneficial effect of a drug while minimizing the risk of undue adverse events.** The use of sequential doses of chloroquine for treating chloroquine-sensitive malaria is an example given in the chapter.

   Another example (discussed in Chapter 12) of this situation is the loading of digoxin (a drug with a half-life of 1.5–2 days) in the treatment of congestive cardiac failure. Here, the purpose of sequential (often 6-hourly) doses is to titrate the patient to the response desired. The procedure is largely historical in origin. It was established when only crude plant products were available and the active ingredient and its dose were essentially unknown. Nonetheless, evidence indicates that adopting this approach is safer than giving an anticipated loading dose of digoxin all at once.

   b. **The administration of loading doses is driven by the urgency of a need for response, the kinetics of the drug, the kinetics of the response, and tolerance to the adverse effects of the drug.** A loading dose of esmolol, a drug used in treating life-threatening supraventricular tachycardias, is useful even though the drug has a 9-minute half-life. When the half-life is long, as with chloroquine (half-life of 40 days), a loading dose (given in divided doses) is needed to acutely treat patients with chloroquine-sensitive malaria. When the pharmacodynamic effect takes weeks, months, or years to fully develop, as with antidepressants, antihyperlipidemic agents, and drugs to treat and prevent osteoporosis, there is no need for a loading dose; a maintenance dosage regimen alone suffices.

   c. **Loading doses are sometimes not used for drugs with long half-lives because the time delay associated with the development of the therapeutic**

response is longer than the time required to accumulate the drug. Another reason is that adverse effects associated with rapid loading are not tolerable, as is the case with flecainide acetate, valproic acid, and terazosin.

8. **Plasma drug–concentration monitoring is useful when, for a low therapeutic index drug, much of the interpatient variability in response (beneficial or adverse) is accounted for by variability in pharmacokinetics.** This is the case with the antiepileptic drug, phenytoin, and the immunosuppressive drug, cyclosporine. The concept of a therapeutic concentration window has its greatest usefulness here. The response to the drug is then reasonably well predicted from the measured concentration. The usefulness of plasma drug concentration monitoring is further enhanced in situations in which the drug is given prophylactically because the desired effect is then the absence of an undesired outcome, such as an epileptic fit or organ transplant rejection. Clearly, plasma concentration monitoring has little to no value when most of the variability in the dose–response relationship is of pharmacodynamic origin. Recall also that low *intra*patient variability in both pharmacokinetics and pharmacodynamics is required for a low therapeutic index drug; otherwise, a patient could not be well controlled on the drug.
9. **Nitroglycerin—development of tolerance to therapeutic effect; terazosin—tolerance to adverse effect.** These were the two examples given in the text. Tolerance to narcotic analgesics (not in text) develops to both therapeutic (analgesic) and adverse (respiratory depression) effects, such that the patient needs and can tolerate more of these drugs when given chronically.
10. **β-blockers, corticosteroids.** These two examples of drugs requiring a slow reduction of dosage to reduce adverse effects are given within the text of the chapter. Other examples are those of withdrawing from nicotine abuse (heavy smoking) and withdrawing from narcotic analgesics for those who are highly addicted.

APPENDIX C

1. E. **pH = 10.** At this pH, the weak acid will be mostly ionized.

$$pH = pK_a + \log\left(\frac{A^-}{HA}\right) = 8 + \log\left(\frac{100}{1}\right) = 10$$

2. D. **pK_a 10**

$$pH = pK_a + \log\left(\frac{B}{BH^+}\right) = pK_a + \log\left(\frac{0.09}{0.91}\right) = 9$$

3. a.

(1) **61.4%.** Taking the antilog of Equation C-1,

$$\frac{\text{Ionized Concentration}}{\text{Un-ionized Concentration}} = 10^{pH-pK_a} = 10^{7.4-7.2}$$

Substituting into Equation C-4, the percent ionized in blood is

$$\frac{1.58 \times 100}{1.58 + 1} = 61.4\%$$

(2) **9.09%.** Similarly, for the urine

$$\frac{\text{Ionized Concentration}}{\text{Un-ionized Concentration}} = 10^{pH-pK_a} = 10^{6.4-7.2}$$

Substituting into Equation C-4, percent ionized in urine at pH 6.2 is

$$\frac{0.158 \times 100}{0.158 + 1} = 10.03\%$$

b.

(1) **99.8%.** Taking the antilog of Equation C-2 and rearranging,

$$\frac{\text{Ionized Concentration}}{\text{Un-ionized Concentration}} = 10^{pK_a - \text{pH}} = 10^{3.8-1.0} = 631$$

Substituting into Equation C-4 the percent ionized in a pH 1.8 stomach is

$$\frac{631 \times 100}{631 + 1} = 99.8\%$$

(2) **0.025%.** Similarly, for the blood

$$\frac{\text{Ionized Concentration}}{\text{Un-ionized Concentration}} = 10^{pK_a - \text{pH}} = 10^{3.8-7.4} = 10^{-3.6} = 2.5 \times 10^{-4}$$

Substituting into Equation C-4, the percent ionized in blood is

$$\frac{2.5 \times 10^{-4} \times 100}{2.5 \times 10^{-4} + 1} = 0.025\%$$

APPENDIX D

1. **Total area under the curve = 17.512 mg-hr/L.**

Time (hr)	Plasma Concentration (mg/L)	Time Interval (hr)	Average Concentration[a] (mg/L)	Area[b] (mg-hr/L)
0	0	–	–	–
0.5	2.14	0.5	1.070	0.535
1	2.95	0.5	2.545	1.273
1.5	3.25	0.5	3.100	1.550
2	3.27	0.5	3.260	1.630
3	2.68	1	2.975	2.975
4	2.15	1	2.415	2.415
6	1.12	2	1.635	3.270
8	0.631	2	0.875	1.750
10	0.341	2	0.486	0.972
12	0.185	2	0.263	0.526
14	0.101	2	0.143	0.286
			AUC(0–14):	17.182
			Area remaining: (C_{last}/k)	0.330
			Total area (AUC)	*17.512*

[a]Average concentration within a sampling interval $C_{av} = \frac{[C(t) + C(t-1)]}{2}$.

[b]Average concentration times time interval.

APPENDIX E

1. a and b **See Table below.** Note that the sum of the amounts remaining from the first 3 doses plus the last dose, last row, is identical to the sum of the values in column 2. Thus, the accumulation expected after multiple doses can be readily predicted from data following a single dose.

Amount of Diazepam (mg) in the Body Just After Each of four Successive Daily Doses				
Time	First Dose	Second Dose	Third Dose	Fourth Dose
0	10			
τ[a]	**6.07**	10		
2τ	**3.68**	**6.07**	10	
3τ	**2.23**	**3.68**	**6.07**	10

[a]$\tau = 1$ day.

c. **$A_{max,ss}$ = 25.4 mg, $A_{min,ss}$ = 15.4 mg**

$$A_{max,ss} = \frac{\text{Dose}}{\left(1-e^{-k\tau}\right)} = \frac{\text{Dose}}{\left(1-e^{-0.5/\text{day}\times 1\text{ day}}\right)} = 25.4 \text{ mg}$$

$$A_{min,ss} = A_{max,ss} - \text{Dose} = 15.4 \text{ mg}$$

or

$$A_{min,ss} = A_{max,ss} \cdot e^{-0.5\text{ day}^{-1}\times 1\text{ day}} = 15.4 \text{ mg}$$

d. **The sum of the amounts remaining from each of the 4 doses (sum of numbers in row 3τ, or column "First Dose") is 21.98 mg.** The maximum amount at steady state is 25.4 mg. The approach of the peak amounts to steady state start at time = $-\tau$ (not in Chapter). As we are now 4 days into the regimen, the amount in the body should be $(1 - e^{-k\tau})$ of the steady-state value., i.e., $A_{max,ss} = A_{max,4}/(1 - e^{-k\tau})$ With $k = 0.5$/day and $t = 4$ days, the steady-state amount is 24.5 mg, the same value as that obtained from the table.

INDEX

Note: Page numbers followed by *f* denote figures; those followed by *t* denote tables